Treating Contemporary Families

Treating Contemporary Families

Toward a More Inclusive Clinical Practice

Edited by
Scott Browning &
Brad van Eeden-Moorefield

 AMERICAN PSYCHOLOGICAL ASSOCIATION

Published by
American Psychological Association
750 First Street, NE
Washington, DC 20002
https://www.apa.org

Order Department
https://www.apa.org/pubs/books
order@apa.org

In the U.K., Europe, Africa, and the Middle East, copies may be ordered from Eurospan
https://www.eurospanbookstore.com/apa
info@eurospangroup.com

Typeset in Charter and Interstate by Circle Graphics, Inc., Reisterstown, MD

Printer: Gasch Printing, Odenton, MD
Cover Designer: Gwen Grafft, Minneapolis, MN

Library of Congress Cataloging-in-Publication Data

Names: Browning, Scott, editor. | Van Eeden-Moorefield, Brad, editor.
Title: Treating contemporary families : toward a more inclusive clinical practice /
  edited by Scott Browning and Brad van Eeden-Moorefield.
Description: Washington, DC : American Psychological Association, [2022] |
  Includes bibliographical references and index.
Identifiers: LCCN 2021032207 (print) | LCCN 2021032208 (ebook) |
  ISBN 9781433836657 (paperback) | ISBN 9781433839177 (ebook)
Subjects: LCSH: Family psychotherapy.
Classification: LCC RC488.5 .T715 2022 (print) | LCC RC488.5 (ebook) |
  DDC 616.89/156—dc23
LC record available at https://lccn.loc.gov/2021032207
LC ebook record available at https://lccn.loc.gov/2021032208

https://doi.org/10.1037/0000280-000

Printed in the United States of America

10 9 8 7 6 5 4 3 2 1

Contents*

---

*For the clinical sections in Chapters 3 through 10, the first author listed is considered the lead author of the section, while authors listed after that are considered equal secondary coauthors of the section. Secondary coauthors are listed in the same order as their work appears in the section.

Contributors

Allie Abraham, PsyD, private practice, King of Prussia, PA, United States

Francesca Adler-Baeder, PhD, Auburn University, Auburn, AL, United States

Tamara D. Afifi, PhD, University of California–Santa Barbara, Santa Barbara, CA, United States

Maya Autret, MA, PhD candidate, Montclair State University, Montclair, NJ, United States

Jacquelyn J. Benson, PhD, Washington University School of Medicine, St. Louis, MO, United States

Kristen Benson, PhD, LMFT, Marriage and Family Program, Appalachian State University, Boone, NC, United States

Autumn M. Bermea, PhD, Ohio State University, Columbus, OH, United States

Tashel C. Bordere, PhD, University of Missouri–Columbia, Columbia, MO, United States

Matthew Bowen, PhD, Department of Military Science, James Madison University, Harrisonburg, VA; private practice, Charlottesville, VA, United States

Scott Browning, PhD, ABPP, Chestnut Hill College, Philadelphia, PA, United States

Kyle Burke, PsyD, Northeast Treatment Centers, Philadelphia, PA, United States

Marianne Celano, PhD, ABPP, Emory University, Atlanta, GA, United States

Marilyn Coleman, EdD, University of Missouri–Columbia, Columbia, MO, United States

Angus Craig, PhD, private practice, Auckland, New Zealand

Salvatore D'Amore, PhD, Université Libre de Bruxelles, Brussels, Belgium

Lindsey Sank Davis, PhD, William James College, Newton, MA; Harvard University, Cambridge, MA; private practice, Brookline, MA, United States

Dena DiNardo, PsyD, private practice, Philadelphia, PA, United States

Charles Fishman, PhD, University of Hawaii at Manoa, Manoa, HI, United States

Peter Fraenkel, PhD, The City College of the City University of New York, New York, NY, United States

Lawrence Ganong, PhD, University of Missouri–Columbia, Columbia, MO, United States

Claudia García-Leeds, PhD, Chestnut Hill College, Philadelphia, PA, United States

Erika Grafsky, PhD, Virginia Polytechnic Institute and State University, Blacksburg, VA, United States

Kim D. Gregson, PhD, LMFT, Gregson Consulting, LLC, Auburn, AL, United States

Cadmona A. Hall, PhD, LMFT, FT, Adler University, Chicago, IL, United States

Rachel Hull, PsyD, Chestnut Hill College, Philadelphia, PA, United States

C. Wayne Jones, PhD, Center for Family Based Training, Bala Cynwyd, PA; University of Pennsylvania, Philadelphia, PA, United States

Kelley Kenney, EdD, Kutztown University, Kutztown, PA, United States

Mark Kenney, MEd, NCC, LPC, Chestnut Hill College, Philadelphia, PA; DeSales University, Center Valley, PA, United States

Christine Kodman-Jones, PhD, Center for Family Based Treatment and Bala Child and Family Associates, Philadelphia, PA, United States

Miguel Lewis, PsyD, CGP, ABPP, West Palm Beach VA Medical Center, West Palm Beach, FL, United States

Alison Mazur, MA, PhD candidate, University of California–Santa Barbara, Santa Barbara, CA, United States

Susan McGroarty, PhD, New Jersey Psychological Association, Livingston, NJ; Behavioral Medicine Inspira Medical Center, Mullica, NJ, United States

Bindu Methikalam, PhD, Chestnut Hill College, Philadelphia, PA, United States

Chris Otmar, MA, PhD candidate, University of California–Santa Barbara, Santa Barbara, CA, United States

Patricia L. Papernow, PhD, Institute for Stepfamily Education, Hudson, MA, United States

Bryan M. Peightal, PsyD, Cabrini University, Radnor Township, PA; Autism Spectrum Diagnostics and Consulting, Doylestown, PA, United States

Abigail J. Rolbiecki, PhD, MPH, MSW, University of Missouri–Columbia, Columbia, MO, United States

Cheryll Rothery, PsyD, Chestnut Hill College, Philadelphia, PA, United States

Christopher Royer, PsyD, private practice, Mechanicsburg, PA, United States

Allison Rozovsky, MS, PsyD candidate, Chestnut Hill College, Philadelphia, PA, United States

Michelle Sherman, PhD, ABPP, University of Minnesota, Minneapolis, MN, United States

Catherine Solheim, PhD, University of Minnesota, Minneapolis, MN, United States

Camille St. James, PsyD, Chestnut Hill College, Philadelphia, PA, United States

Ileana Ungureanu, MD, PhD, LMFT, CFTP, Governors State University, University Park, IL, United States

Brad van Eeden-Moorefield, MSW, PhD, CFLE, Montclair State University, Montclair, NJ, United States

Amy C. Wagner, PhD, LMFT, ABPP, private practice, Evanston, IL, United States

Anne Williams-Wengerd, MA, PhD candidate, University of Minnesota, Minneapolis, MN, United States

Yiqing Youngman, PsyD, The Center, LLC, King of Prussia, PA; La Salle University, Philadelphia, PA, United States

Acknowledgments

We wish to acknowledge the gift of working with Susan Reynolds of American Psychological Association (APA) Books. Having Susan embrace this idea for a book was a great boost to the project, and as always, Susan offered support and effective criticism. We also wish to thank two women who were instrumental in editing, reviewing, and organizing this manuscript: Maya Autret and Allie Rozovsky. And, of course, we wish to acknowledge the remarkable team of research and clinical scholars who worked together to create a text that merges research and clinical practice in a manner that is original, inclusive, and highly effective.

Scott wishes to thank Joanne Ahearn and Owen Ahearn-Browning. To have a loving and supportive family is a critical component of completing such a project. In addition, Scott is grateful to Josh Fetterman for his consultation on the validity and reliability testing for the Genogram Based Interactional Measure. Finally, Scott wants to thank Brad van Eeden-Moorefield; he is an exceptional scholar, writer, and coeditor, and this project would have never been possible without his many talents, patience, and friendship.

Brad wishes to thank the many students he has worked with over his career who always push him to teach to "real life" (i.e., make the link among research, practice, and supporting families explicit). He also thanks Scott Browning for being such an amazing colleague, friend, and scholar. It is a privilege when you are able to work with people who are as talented, gracious, and humble as Scott.

Treating Contemporary Families

1

OUR APPROACH TO INCLUSIVE EVIDENCE-BASED PRACTICE WITH CONTEMPORARY FAMILIES

SCOTT BROWNING AND BRAD VAN EEDEN-MOOREFIELD

We are excited to introduce you to this book! Our core aim is to provide readers, most of whom we believe will be students in clinical graduate programs, as well as those currently licensed to practice, insight into how research findings can be used to inform clinical practice (i.e., evidence-based practice) and how this *bridge*, as some refer to it, between research and practice can be used to promote inclusiveness. We also believe the broader process works in reverse, with clinical practice able to inform research (e.g., areas in need of study, interpretation of contemporary findings) in important ways (Grzywacz & Allen, 2017). Building this bridge is quite elusive, though. Specifically, it is a challenge to find shared goals and languages across researchers and clinicians. To complicate the process further, the process of bridging research and practice often fails to explicitly include the voices of those who the bridge actually is supposed to serve—individuals and families in our communities. In fact, the people whom we, as research and clinical scholars, want to help often are left out of the process altogether except as "data points" in a research study or "recipients" of therapy. Certainly, this is changing (e.g., participatory action research models, strengths-based practices), and we encourage

https://doi.org/10.1037/0000280-001
Treating Contemporary Families: Toward a More Inclusive Clinical Practice, S. Browning and B. van Eeden-Moorefield (Editors)

more widespread inclusion of those for whom our work is supposed to support.

Although this book also does not directly include the voices of those individuals and families we seek to support and help because it is beyond the scope of this text, we do focus on building a more inclusive research–clinical bridge and advocate bringing those we serve into these discussions. That said, we do not quite see this connection as a bridge. In fact, the bridge metaphor seems to maintain this siloed idea of living in different lands such that we might use the bridge to visit each other from time to time, or maybe even stay over for a weekend. We see merit in the idea of a feedback loop as suggested by others (e.g., Grzywacz & Allen, 2017), especially for its emphasis on a continuous process. However, a feedback loop, although circular and closed, still feels pretty linear. We see the process as much more dynamic, fluid and iterative, and relational. In many ways it is a more constructivist take on things. Accordingly, maybe it is more productive to think of researchers and clinicians attending a wild 1970s painting disco party (a bunch of 4-year-olds having a party with finger paints works as a great alternative metaphor as well) with researchers bringing various shades of yellow paint and clinicians bringing shades of blue. As we mix and mingle (and share our paints), we begin to create new colors (shades of green) that continuously evolve and change the more we mix and mingle. We do this through the integration of our respective strengths (research knowledge and methods; clinical judgment and expertise). In the outside world, this does not happen easily or without intention. What is important to the process is having someone who can bring the canvas and help promote the mixing of paints. As editors, we are attempting to serve in this capacity and hereby invite you to our painting disco party!

Over our careers, we both traversed the roles of researcher and clinician, albeit to varying degrees. Because we have experienced both yellows and blues, we also have experienced a lot of green and many variations of green. We have come to speak both yellow and blue somewhat fluently, translating into green—a space that we believe most people actually inhabit. Frankly, we live in the green. Stated another way, we have committed our careers to facilitating dialogue and the exchange of disciplinary strengths and knowledge across research and clinical worlds. Our initial work together centered on this shared commitment and served as the beginning of our collaborative efforts, and friendship, to this day. Over our years working together, we have learned a great deal from each other about how to facilitate dialogue and build stronger collaborations between research and clinical scholars (Browning & van Eeden-Moorefield, 2017). We continue to grow ourselves, trying out new styles of collaboration along the way.

This book represents some new styles in terms of building collaborations and developing evidence-based practices, but, perhaps more important, we are trying out a new style of attending to diversity that we hope is a bit more inclusive of the people and families we study and serve. Given the paucity of research of diverse populations and culturally responsive clinical practices, despite mounting evidence that demonstrates strong health disparities among many diverse groups (e.g., Fleary et al., 2018; Kaestle, 2019), we believe the goals of this book had to center inclusion and promote the use of evidence-based practice. In what follows, we offer contextual information and briefly explain a few foundational terms that are essential for readers to understand when engaging this text and developing skills in the development of evidence-based practices in psychology (i.e., EBPP) in their practice. We then articulate the purpose and organization of this text and the process of collaboration, including some of the common elements across chapters, used to develop the evidence-based practices presented.

FOUNDATIONAL TERMINOLOGY AND CONTEXTUAL INFORMATION

The term *contemporary families* is central to this text. Contemporary families represent the full variety of family configurations, ways of being a family, ways of experiencing family life, and the diversity of each family member's identities, all situated within the most current historical context (Berger & Carlson, 2020). The term also acknowledges the ability for people to choose who (or what; e.g., family pets) is part of their family. The term is meant to be inclusive and stands in contrast to notions of there being a "one" family. The *One Family* notion, at least in the United States, has been used to uphold the standard North American family (i.e., SNAF; Smith, 1993) as the ideal family to which everyone should ascribe. That is, the SNAF is often used as the benchmark family rather than articulating a notion of family pluralities. Those families not fitting the SNAF ideal often are deemed unstable, deficient, and dysfunctional. Historically, the SNAF has been most represented in research and clinical practice, and when more diverse families are included, their form and function are often compared with the ideal and viewed from a deficit lens (e.g., van Eeden-Moorefield, 2018). This means available research evidence that can be used to inform clinical practice is limited or contains SNAF-like biases. Accordingly, any inclusive approach must begin with an inclusive definition of family and family life, and it must also use a critical perspective that recognizes potential biases, including personal biases, and limitations of existing research evidence. Finally, contemporary families, and practice with them, are dynamic and fluid.

As a field, psychotherapy is also quite dynamic and fluid, having been going through some dramatic shifts since the 1980s both in terms of funding (e.g., passage of the Mental Health Systems Act of 1980 to almost its entire repeal via the Omnibus Budget Reconciliation Act of 1981; managed care) and theoretically oriented treatment approaches (e.g., from psychodynamic to cognitive behavioral). In many ways, these are significantly intertwined, with much effort focused on reducing costs through outside (e.g., insurance companies) determinations of the number of treatment sessions deemed sufficient, which diagnoses and treatment approaches will be reimbursed, and a significant emphasis on one individual being the primary patient (*diagnostic focused*) even when the identified "patient" should be the entire family and or household (*systemic focused*). In short, people's mental health and well-being became secondary to an increasing emphasis across much of the health care system on profit over health. These shifts are not entirely new (see Duncan & Reese, 2012, 2015); however, they did increase the push to better establish evidentiary support for effectiveness of treatment as well as the development of more short-term treatment approaches. This has been beneficial in many ways.

As the importance of practicing in a responsible and evaluated manner became clearer to the field, a growing confusion arose as to what exactly constituted a treatment based in evidence and what is considered evidence. In 2006, the American Psychological Association (APA) created a Presidential Task Force on Evidence-Based Practice in Psychology. This Task Force widened the sources of "research evidence" that could be used to justify labelling a treatment as evidence based. Although a strict criterion (single diagnosis, randomized controlled trials, and treatment manuals) remains for what constitutes evidence-supported treatments (EST; see Duncan & Reese, 2012), increasingly, evidence-based practice (EBP) has increased in scope and use. This book recognizes that EST remains the gold standard for narrowly focused clinical issues (e.g., panic disorder), but emphasizes the use of EBP for the vast complexity of treating those in contemporary families. As noted by Scott Fraser (2018), "the field is moving toward a broader definition of effective psychotherapy practice" (p. 16).

On the basis of the work of the Task Force, APA (2006) articulated the tripartite model of evidence-based practice in psychology that suggests EBPP is created from the "integration of the best available research, with clinical expertise in the context of patient characteristics, culture, and preferences" (p. 273). "Best available research" refers to findings from scientific studies.

These studies can focus on intervention techniques, basic research, and assessment, for example, and can be conducting using a variety of methodological approaches. "Clinical expertise" includes such components as assessment, treatment planning and implementation, clinical decision making, interpersonal relationship skills, self-reflection, use of research evidence, and more. The third element, "patient characteristics, culture, and preferences," refers to thorough information related to a particular patient (the person or persons being treated). This also is where it is critical for clinicians to demonstrate knowledge of, and a balance between, what generally is known about a particular treatment concern and group of people or family types and their unique experience. This navigation of the nomothetic and the idiographic is one particularly important component for developing an inclusive practice. Of note, we opted to present EBPP visually using a Venn diagram (see Figure 1.1). We thought this captured EBPP well by demonstrating the integration of all three elements that combine to produce EBPP but also demonstrates some areas of overlap between two elements

FIGURE 1.1. Tripartite Model of Evidenced-Based Practice in Psychology (EBPP)

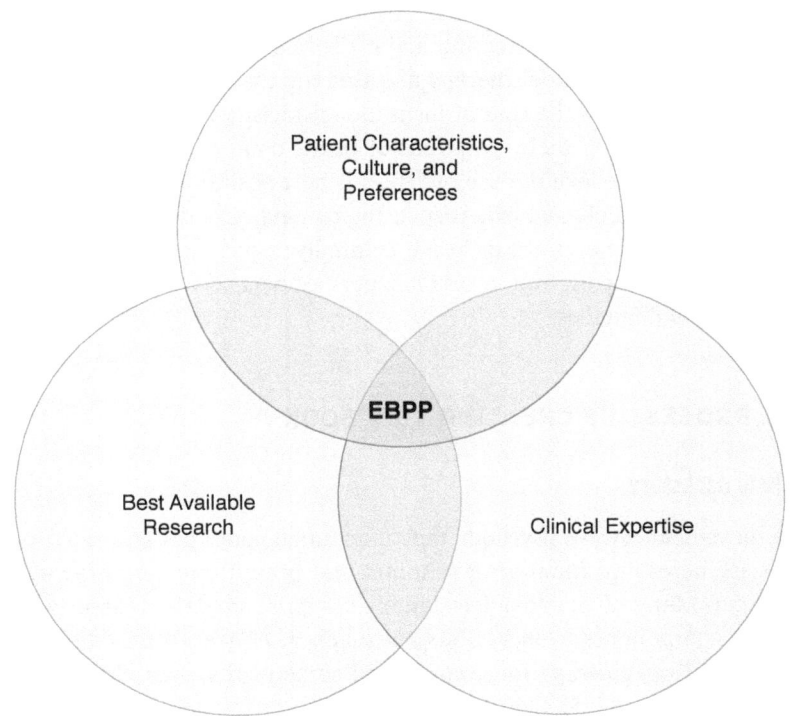

(e.g., the overlap of clinical expertise and patient characteristics, culture, and preferences). We believe those overlap areas demonstrate how EBPP is emergent as we collect more information relative to any one element. In fact, one of the final chapters in this text (Chapter 10 on medical changes related to vision and hearing loss experienced in families) represents this exact area because little research is available on family experiences with vision and hearing loss so clinicians must rely on two elements to develop best practice. This also is an example of how clinicians can share this with researchers to guide the development of new studies and areas of inquiry. Relatedly, APA (2021) recently published a set of 10 guidelines for EBPP in health care that further guide the process of EBPP. Although this document was not published until after this text was complete, we believe you will see a strong fit between the guidelines and the process engaged by the authors in this text.

Importantly, we want to reemphasize most of the U.S.-based models focus on treating White individuals and SNAF families with little attention paid to the presence and treatment of mental health disparities due to race, ethnicity, religion, socioeconomic status, sexual orientation, and many additional locations of diversity in spite of an increasingly diverse population in terms of individual and family identities (see Chapter 2, this volume). There is a big difference between treating major depressive disorder diagnostically using cognitive behavioral therapy and treating that person systemically in a way that considers the role of institutional racism, as an example, as an underlying source of their symptoms or in the context of an entire family. Accordingly, we believe the use of EBPPs is best positioned to use available research data and clinical expertise in the context of patient characteristics and lives to articulate a more inclusive, culturally responsive set of intervention strategies able to work from a systemic perspective and with the diversity of individuals and families.

THE PROCESS OF CREATING THIS BOOK

A Little Backstory

The movement toward psychotherapy integration continues at a rapid pace, with an increasing number of scholars and practitioners embracing the advances. Many of the advances largely comprise models created by integrating components from various approaches. APA even established the *Journal of Psychotherapy Integration*, and some of the most clarion voices in the field have stated clearly that psychotherapy integration is the future, and that future is now (Castonguay 2011; Fraser et al., 2012; Stricker & Gold, 1996; Wachtel, 1991). While established scholars each carve out their own integrative approach, the typical clinician goes to workshops and reads books that continue to introduce them to an approach that, although "new," seems strangely familiar. This pattern is largely due to the proliferation of integrative positions. One might say that nothing in psychotherapy is new, but instead has been repackaged and combined. Many of these new approaches are brilliantly constructed and have significant evidence to indicate their worth. Unfortunately, little practical guidance is provided on how to best integrate evidence-based practices in clinical settings in spite of this burgeoning part of the field.

This book is an outgrowth of the ongoing challenge to integrate research and practice, and it represents our continued commitment, as equal coeditors, to this endeavor. Early on, we reflected on our previous work together, advances in the field such as those outlined above, and our hopes for this newest iteration of our collaborations—our next 1970s painting disco party. Much of our early conversations focused on (a) the importance of helping researchers and clinicians create a shared starting point that also would help them create somewhat of a shared language, (b) the need to incorporate a more inclusive approach consistent with the diversity of contemporary families, and (c) the challenges and barriers we were likely to face along the way. We also wanted to try to do things a bit differently but also incorporate EBPP explicitly.

Purpose and Organization of the Book

The early discussions we had helped us articulate a purpose and organizational strategy for this text. As mentioned at the beginning of this chapter, the core aim of this book is to assist therapists, and students learning to be therapists, to conduct EBPP with a more diverse set of contemporary families experiencing a particular interactional problem (e.g., coparenting challenges). Accordingly, a second aim of this book is to provide a process so that clinicians working with contemporary families can more easily engage integrative psychotherapy. Rather than a diagnostic focus to the book, as mentioned earlier, most chapters examine a specific interactional challenge. Therefore, rather than concentrating on depression, as an example, this book is aimed at those practicing systemic treatment who are more concerned with interactional concerns (e.g., coparenting conflict). We started by identifying eight interactional problems (e.g., couple instability, loss and bereavement, boundary ambiguity) that typically come up frequently in clinical practice and that had supporting research. For each interactional problem, three or four contemporary family populations (e.g., stepfamilies, LGBTQ families, families with chronic mental illness) were selected. Consideration for inclusion of a specific family population was guided by (a) available research literature existed that could be drawn upon and (b) identification as a group either rarely included in clinical discussions despite engaging services or that are particularly vulnerable to the focal interactional problem, partly due to their social location.

In many ways, this text seeks to address key challenges to embedded systemic patterns. Various symptoms exist, and the full understanding and treatment of that condition are helpful. But, in addition, the system needs to adjust as well. Importantly, each interactional challenge also will be examined in light of specific family types—those families in which the identified concern is highlighted due to systemic pressures—such that we demonstrate how to adapt general integrative approaches for use with today's diverse families. For example, coparenting, although a general concern, is particularly problematic for couples who have a child on the autism spectrum as well as those coparenting across multiple households. Therefore, this book intends to identify specific interactional problems, highlight the extant research regarding the concern, and then identify specific clinical suggestions to assist therapists working with these diverse families.

As you have likely guessed by now, this chapter serves a more introductory role for the text. Chapter 2 provides an introductory discussion of inclusion and intersectionality in clinical practice, especially with regard to broad treatment approaches (cultural competency, cultural humility, cultural responsiveness) that aim to serve diverse populations. The core chapters of the text, Chapters 3 through 9, focus on specific interactional processes that are fairly common in clinical practice and for which there is good available research. Three to four family types are discussed in each chapter. The penultimate chapter is a clinical-only chapter intended to bring the book full circle, if you will. It focuses on an area (i.e., unplanned medical experiences) for which there is limited to no evidence to guide practice. In these instances, interventions are guided most by clinical decision-making, and we asked the authors to weigh in on some needed research areas that could confirm their clinical experiences or identify other ways to help these families (i.e., the use of clinical experience to inform future research agendas). We see this chapter as uniquely positioned to demonstrate how clinical experience, or views from the field, can be used to chart a needed research agenda to better serve families. We end the text with a chapter on outcome assessment.

Collaborative Process and Common Elements

To facilitate our goals for this work, several shared, common elements are used across the core chapters that were part of an explicit process used with the authors (the guidelines of our painting disco party), although some of the naming conventions evolved over time. Each of these elements was designed to align with the tripartite model of EBPP (APA, 2006) as well as to create a level of consistency across chapters. We call your attention to Table 1.1 to see the alignment. This table begins with a column listing each of the EBPP elements (e.g., clinical expertise; APA, 2006). Each core chapter has two main sections: a research section with a lead research author (some selected coauthors as well) and a clinical applications section with a lead clinical author as well as a group of equal second coauthors who served as experts for each specific family type. You will notice in the table which EBPP element can be found in which section of a given chapter. Across chapters, we used the same headings that further define which EBPP element is being articulated in which section of a chapter (see Column 3). Information included in a particular section is described in the final column. Our intent with this was to make sure that the connections among and between all elements of EBPP were always clear, thus making the process easier for readers to engage as they develop their own EBPPs. In fact, this would be a great class assignment for those still in school. We also believe some readers will read the entire book, whereas others might want to read sections pertaining only to a specific family type with whom they are currently working. The consistency of headings should aid both reading and use styles.

We also knew we needed something common and more substantive than a heading to add to each chapter that could also serve as a starting point for research and clinical scholars. Accordingly, we created a base table that would be used as the foundation of each chapter and that we hoped would facilitate a shared vision and communication style (we hoped the table would include yellows, blues, and produce shades of green, if you will). We provided full directions and an example table to the authors. We tasked them to first consider their respective research or clinical expertise to identify the key general focal factors that could exacerbate or ameliorate the interactional problem in their chapter. Focal factors were those factors that had clinical relevance. For example, helping ex-spouses establish a coparenting alliance can be influenced through intervention, whereas a demographic factor is less amenable to change, especially systemic change. We had them do the same for each of the included family types and then compare and discuss their lists to identify those few key factors to include in the chapter. This produced the final complete table you will see in each chapter (this was

TABLE 1.1. Alignment of Evidenced-Based Practice in Psychology (EBPP) and Chapters in This Text

EBPP elements[a]	Chapter section	Corresponding chapter headings	Description
Best Available Research	Research	Opening paragraphs (no heading used for the introduction)	The beginning of each research section introduces readers to the importance and scope of the interactional process covered in that chapter as well as a broad overview of what we know.
Best Available Research	Research	Research Evidence on (family type)	A unique research evidence section is provided for each family type covered within a chapter. It reviews what we know about the selected areas of clinical focus and indicates the quality of evidence.
Clinical Expertise	Clinical Applications	Clinical Expertise and Interpretation of Evidence: An Overview	The beginning of each clinical applications section provides the clinician's general overall perspective of the research presented, focusing on elements that stand out as particularly clinically relevant, informed by their clinical experiences and wisdom.
Clinical Expertise	Clinical Applications	Clinical Expertise and Interpretation of Evidence: (family type)	This section is unique to each family type and is where clinicians provide their understanding of key research information in conjunction with their experience working directly with a particular family type.
Clinical Expertise	Clinical Applications	Clinical Experience: Observations of Common Interactional Patterns	Clinicians used this section to share their clinical observations about typical, more nomothetic patterns specific to a family type.
Patient Characteristics, Culture, and Preferences	Clinical Applications	Case Context: Characteristics, Culture, and Preferences	This section provides an overview of the specific case used to illustrate EBPP including information garnered from the assessment process.
Evidence-Based Practice	Clinical Applications	Clinical Decisions: Intervention Implementation	This section describes the specific intervention(s) used with the case that brings together all of the EBPP elements. It also highlights some of the psychoeducational points shared with patients.

[a]From American Psychological Association (2006, 2021).

not always followed as closely as it should have been, mostly because of the challenges of the COVID-19 pandemic).

Thus, the content of each chapter (Chapters 3–9) identifies a small set of particular focal areas that research and clinical experience suggest are strong sites for intervention among families in general, either because they exacerbate or help ameliorate a presenting problem. Each chapter also identifies those general focal areas and unique focal areas that research and experience suggest are applicable to one or more of the selected four family types included in a given unit. This final set of focal factors included in the table also are bolded in text at their first substantive use in each main section. Again, our hope was to take out some of the guess work many of us do while reading and make things as clear and explicit as possible.

The research scholars wrote the research part of the unit and shared it with the editors and clinical authors for review and feedback, as well as so the clinical authors could then take the research evidence and use it to create their EBPP. Clinicians used the research evidence presented, along with their own expertise and judgment, to articulate specific psychoeducational and clinical interventions for a specific case. Clinical authors wrote their sections and shared them with the editors and research author for review and feedback. The process was largely iterative and produced the volume we share with you in the chapters that follow. To be clear, each chapter focuses on one specific interactional challenge (e.g., coparenting challenges) and how to address that across multiple types of families. This is in contrast to texts that often are entirely population specific (e.g., how to work only with Black families) or in which each chapter is devoted to one specific population (e.g., one chapter focuses on working with LGBTQ+ and another on Black families). Each type of text is important and serves a purpose.

We also recognize that books do not exist that focus on many of the intersectional locations of those we serve. Accordingly, we thought it would be more inclusive to embed multiple family locations within each chapter such that over the course of the book, readers would learn a variety of intervention techniques that could be used with certain diverse families or across multiple types of diverse families to treat several common family challenges. It also is a shift in focus from organizational schemes based on family structures to one based on family processes. Essentially, we see this text as providing numerous intervention strategies that can be used to better serve today's families—it enhances our toolbox and clinical decision making related to with whom and under what context to use a particular intervention. This also allows for a more integrated approach.

The Not So Aha Moment

Having engaged with this book, you may feel a desire to see more collaboration between researchers and practitioners and better understand how powerful it can be when these multiple perspectives are put into dialogue with one another. Certainly, as coeditors, we end this book with the satisfying recognition that collaboration, between research scholars and clinical scholars, is possible and can be deepened. We believed that going into this project, and we believe it as we complete it. A prescriptive procedure that compels true conversation between the two disciplines can create a product that is mutually beneficial. We expected this to be the case, and it was. We actually believe this could have been even more prescriptive but value having enough openness in the process that people can put themselves as fully and authentically into their work as possible. It is important for researchers to find aspects of their work that produce reliable findings and are useful to the practitioner. Likewise, therapy practitioners are able to relay specifically to researchers what direction their research might follow to have direct application. This might particularly be the case for enhancing research on and understanding of diversity when little or no research exists. Ultimately, when we collaborate, it is those we help who benefit most, and that is a shared goal among most of us.

We also recognize that the fields of research and practice need accessible forums to move toward a nexus. For too long the collaboration of research and practice has been aspirational. Clinicians and researchers need to demand that journals, books, and conferences create platforms in which inclusive efforts are encouraged and utilized. The best work takes the most intentional of efforts, efforts that often are undervalued by many of today's systems (they are not billable, as they say). We encourage readers to create synergistic relationships with one another and between research and clinical scholars. This is hard to do at the community level, especially if a university is not close by or does not have a relevant department with capacity for applied outreach and scholarship. It does seem—and this is from our observations—that the next generation of research and clinical scholars view collaboration (and painting disco parties) as highly valuable. This should enhance the current progress being made toward inclusive, integrative, and evidence-based practices and that excites us. We hope that you find this work as insightful and useful as we believe it is and that you are able to explore more intentionally some new shades of green.

REFERENCES

American Psychological Association. (2021). *APA guidelines on evidence-based psychological practice in health care.* https://www.apa.org/about/policy/psychological-practice-health-care.pdf

APA Presidential Task Force on Evidence-Based Practice. (2006). Evidence-based practice in psychology. *American Psychologist, 61*(4), 271–285. https://doi.org/10.1037/0003-066X.61.4.271

Berger, L. M., & Carlson, M. J. (2020). Family policy and complex contemporary families: A decade in review and implications for the next decade of research and policy practice. *Journal of Marriage and the Family, 82*(1), 478–507. https://doi.org/10.1111/jomf.12650

Browning, S., & van Eeden-Moorefield, B. (Eds.). (2017). *Contemporary families at the nexus of research and practice.* Routledge. https://doi.org/10.4324/9781315668598

Castonguay, L. G. (2011). Psychotherapy, psychopathology, research and practice: Pathways of connections and integration. *Psychotherapy Research, 21*(2), 125–140. https://doi.org/10.1080/10503307.2011.563250

Duncan, B. L., & Reese, R. J. (2012). Empirically supported treatments, evidence-based treatments, and evidence-based practice. In G. Stricker, T. A. Widiger, & I. B. Weiner (Eds.), *Handbook of psychology: Clinical psychology* (2nd ed., pp. 489–513). John Wiley & Sons. https://doi.org/10.1002/9781118133880.hop208021

Duncan, B. L., & Reese, R. J. (2015). The Partners for Change Outcome Management System (PCOMS) revisiting the client's frame of reference. *Psychotherapy: Theory, Research, & Practice, 52*(4), 391–401. https://doi.org/10.1037/pst0000026

Fleary, S. A., Nigg, C. R., & Freund, K. M. (2018). An examination of changes in social disparities in health behaviors in the US, 2003–2015. *American Journal of Health Behavior, 42*(1), 119–134. https://doi.org/10.5993/AJHB.42.1.12

Fraser, J. S. (2018). *Unifying effective psychotherapies: Tracing the process of change.* American Psychological Association. https://doi.org/10.1037/0000078-000

Fraser, J. S., Solovey, A. D., Grove, D., Lee, M. Y., & Greene, G. J. (2012). Integrative families and systems treatment: A middle path toward integrating common and specific factors in evidence-based family therapy. *Journal of Marital and Family Therapy, 38*(3), 515–528. https://doi.org/10.1111/j.1752-0606.2011.00228.x

Grzywacz, J. G., & Allen, J. W. (2017). Adapting the ideas of translational science for translational family science. *Family Relations, 66*(4), 568–583. https://doi.org/10.1111/fare.12284

Kaestle, C. E. (2019). Sexual orientation trajectories based on sexual attractions, partners, and identity: A longitudinal investigation from adolescence through young adulthood using a U.S. representative sample. *Journal of Sex Research, 56*(7), 811–826. https://doi.org/10.1080/00224499.2019.1577351

Smith, D. E. (1993). The standard North American family: SNAF as an ideological code. *Journal of Family Issues, 14*(1), 50–65. https://doi.org/10.1177/0192513X93014001005

Stricker, G., & Gold, J. R. (1996). Psychotherapy integration: An assimilative, psychodynamic approach. *Clinical Psychology: Science and Practice, 3*(1), 47–58. https://doi.org/10.1111/j.1468-2850.1996.tb00057.x

van Eeden-Moorefield, B. (2018). Introduction to the special issue: Intersectional variations in the experiences of queer families. *Family Relations, 67*(1), 7–11. https://doi.org/10.1111/fare.12305

Wachtel, P. L. (1991). From eclecticism to synthesis: Toward a more seamless psychotherapeutic integration. *Journal of Psychotherapy Integration, 1*(1), 43–54. https://doi.org/10.1037/h0101201

2 IMPLICATIONS OF INCLUSION AND INTERSECTIONALITY FOR CLINICAL PRACTICE

MAYA AUTRET AND BRAD VAN EEDEN-MOOREFIELD

For the past couple of decades, various clinical disciplines (e.g., clinical psychology, counseling, social work) in the United States have increased their focus on multicultural practice. These shifts have been spurred in response not only to an increasingly diverse U.S. population but also an increasing interconnectedness between countries across the globe, both of which position clinicians in need of knowledge and skills to work across a more diverse client base. Perhaps more important, these shifts have occurred in response to (a) greater recognition of how culture informs meaning making and systemic interactions; (b) an understanding of the role culture plays when establishing a therapeutic alliance and producing outcomes, especially in relation to power dynamics; (c) an understanding of mental health disparities based on one's identities (e.g., ability status, ethnicity, race, gender, sexual orientation) and intersectional social location; and (d) the positioning of the therapist not as an objective, detached party but one with their own cultures and subjectivities. More simply, scholars now more clearly understand the importance of culture as a context in which life, interactions, and relationships occur and how these translate to one's mental health and well-being (Owen et al., 2019).

https://doi.org/10.1037/0000280-002
Treating Contemporary Families: Toward a More Inclusive Clinical Practice, S. Browning and B. van Eeden-Moorefield (Editors)

Across the past couple of decades, research and clinical scholars alike have developed approaches, terminology, and theories that aid our work. As mentioned in the previous chapter, this book is a response to these shifts and attempts to articulate a new approach to thinking about and developing clinical practices that are more inclusive, intersectional, and evidence based. Accordingly, this chapter provides a brief introduction to some of the thinking related to inclusion (e.g., American Psychological Association [APA], 2017) and intersectionality (e.g., Crenshaw, 1989) applicable to evidence-based practice in psychology (Levant, 2005). This is particularly relevant for clinicians when considering what research evidence exists, for whom that evidence applies, the quality of that research, and how that aligns (or not) with the clinician's own expertise working with a particular group, and the specific case a clinician is working with at the moment. In other words, there needs to be a balance between all of these types of information and how they inform clinical decision making when designing and implementing various interventions. Clinicians practicing inclusive evidence-based practice often find themselves navigating between the nomothetic and idiographic. We would assert this as a strength because it leads to a potentially more holistic understanding of a case and treatment.

DIVERSITY, INCLUSION, AND SOCIAL JUSTICE

Diversity, *inclusion*, and *social justice* are terms more widely used today than even a decade ago. However, there is some variation in how they are defined and used, which may result from misperceptions, overlap, and ambiguity about the meaning of each term, as well as what they represent as a whole (Thomas et al., 2010). Nonetheless, these terms collectively capture an evolution in thought and process surrounding multicultural practice, which also entail important, unique applications discussed in this section.

Diversity

For our purposes, we define diversity as a recognition of the myriad identities and group memberships one may hold at the individual (e.g., ability, age, ethnicity, gender, race, religion, sexuality), family (e.g., cohabiting, adoptive, multigenerational, stepfamily), and social levels. These represent many of the unique parts of individuals, as well as parts that allow for connections to some other individuals that share one or more of these parts (Thomas et al., 2010). Diversity is also used to report population or organizational demographics, to set targets for representation, or to report on the variety of clients we might serve. In this vein, diversity often is used primarily as a descriptive characteristic.

Historically, diversity has also been about similarity and difference between people, with an emphasis on difference, where there is an implied majority type of person or group and everyone else is considered diverse (i.e., not like the majority person or group). However, this perspective establishes an erroneous binary, or essentialist, way of thinking; emphasizes differences; and places values on such differences across those who are in the majority and minority (Thomas et al., 2010). It also easily masks variation within, or among, a particular group (i.e., a consideration of intersectionality [Crenshaw, 1989], as presented later). The need to move away from erroneous binaries helped advance thinking to focus more on inclusion.

Inclusion

Inclusion aims to move beyond "simply tolerating" differences such that people feel a sense of authentic belonging. Rather, inclusion recognizes the power differences across identities and seeks to bring diverse individuals and groups into decision-making processes and activities as part of the overarching goal of providing equal access to resources and life opportunities (Thomas et al., 2010). A commonly heard metaphor goes like this: Diversity is giving someone a seat at the table, and inclusion is giving that person a valued vote. Unfortunately, giving someone a seat at the table and a vote after years of oppression and exclusion may appear to create equality, but it is neither equitable nor just. Inequities from earlier oppressive and discriminatory practices are not undone simply by giving more people seats at the table and voting rights (or say in directing their treatment goals and interventions); more is needed. Stated differently, past injustices have cumulatively contributed to individuals' current realities and voting rights do not automatically level the playing field. Hence, inclusion also encompasses an acknowledgment of the deeper, historic grievances tied to individual and group identities. Social justice furthers such affirmations through a more active commitment to rectify these prior transgressions.

Social Justice

A primary goal of social justice is to guarantee full participation in life for everyone with access to resources and opportunities. Underlying this goal is a more fundamental recognition of the need to alleviate human suffering

(LaMantia et al., 2015) resulting from long-standing discriminatory practices. Hence, social justice also aims to challenge existing, and redress prior, institutional inequities. As such, a commitment to social justice entails seeking more equitable and fair approaches and practices that address the past, present, and future. Such commitment and activism therefore also include reassessing and reinventing existing practices to eliminate historic and embedded disadvantages for certain groups (Sharp & Weaver, 2015). In short, and oversimplified, diversity is something you have, inclusion is something you do, and social justice changes the system to create equity and fairness.

Implications for Practice

Beyond understanding and distinguishing between these concepts, there are also implications for practice when considering diversity, inclusion, and social justice. Consequently, it is important to be mindful of the aims of each of these concepts when applying them in practice. For example, a diversity approach could begin with greater awareness of one's clientele and recognizing opportunities for accepting and even attracting more diverse clients. A further step could entail adding diverse materials at the office, website, or marketing efforts. It could also mean reading diversity materials with the idea that knowledge might directly translate into a more culturally responsive practice (Sanchez et al., 2018).

Inclusion moves beyond these initial steps. A more inclusive approach involves the recognition and understanding of one's own biases, privileges, oppressions, and potential experiences with marginalization (Allen & Steed, 2016). As such, this approach encourages one to take inclusion further— to view clients as experts of their own lives and needs. In doing so, practitioners are better poised to share their knowledge and offer clients greater choice and say about their own treatment and goals. Consequently, inclusion offers opportunities for greater understanding and trust that is mutually beneficial.

Social justice could include a thorough examination of existing practice and office policies that might maintain structural inequities by recognizing and addressing specific challenges of minoritized clients in gaining access to and maintaining effective treatment (Kim-Goh et al., 2015). Another application of social justice could be to advocate deeply for historically minoritized clients at the local, state, and national levels. Such advocacy can include pushing back against one's own organization or insurance companies about unfair and unjust practices. Again, these are but a few easy examples, and we encourage readers to explore these, and other, ideas further. To sum, diversity, inclusion, and social justice represent concepts and processes that offer practitioners with the means to center culture and more effectively and equitably serve more varied and distinct needs of a wider population.

CULTURAL COMPETENCE, CULTURAL HUMILITY, AND CULTURAL RESPONSIVENESS

We have a burgeoning evidence base that suggests the importance of engaging culture when working with clients (Kim-Goh et al., 2015). Certainly diversity, inclusion, and social justice provide some entry points for doing this. Here, we discuss four concepts that can aid in incorporating culture more prominently in practice.

Cultural Competence

Most practitioners ascribe to some form of a cultural competency model, although what this means and how this work varies and has changed significantly over the past decade. The basic idea is that clinicians can read books and attend trainings related to any number of cultures and quickly gain the requisite basic knowledge and skills needed to work with people from those cultures (Yancu & Farmer, 2017). Greene-Moton and Minkler (2020) and many others (Simpkins et al., 2017) have critiqued this historical idea of cultural competence as too static and suggest that it can imply an erroneous binary (one can be competent or not). Further, there are often multiple subgroups within an ethnic group, each with its own cultural and clinical considerations (Campinha-Bacote, 2002). As such, clinicians may consider themselves culturally competent when in actuality their perspective remains limited to a subgroup or a subset of knowledge (Isaacson, 2014).

Accordingly, practitioners can better understand and support their clients' needs by centering their values and unique social locations. For example, Kim-Goh et al. (2015) examined stigma-related barriers to seeking mental health services among Asian Americans who experienced varying levels of acculturation and backgrounds. The authors highlighted the importance of not applying a single technique across all Asian American clients and groups but rather staying attuned to the unique needs of clients, their specific groups, acculturation, and relationships with other family members to address their specific needs. There are many ways of navigating the nomothetic and idiographic.

Consequently, some scholars (e.g., Campinha-Bacote, 2002) have proposed that beyond becoming more informed of clients' culture and gaining greater self-awareness of their own positionality, they should view cultural competence as an ongoing process rather than a milestone. Adopting a more continually evolving perspective promotes greater agility in practice that enables practitioners to better understand and grapple with the complexity of real life across different cultural groups in an ever-changing society (Greene-Moton & Minkler, 2020). Cultural humility and responsiveness approaches address and build on the idea of competence.

Cultural Humility

Cultural humility is an approach that is intended to be more of a dynamic process that unfolds over one's life and career. However, this approach is more introspective, involving deep intrapersonal work with the goal of engaging critical reflection and deeper understanding of the self of the therapist to increasingly understand one's attitudes, beliefs, and behaviors (Chapman, 2011; Logan et al., 2021). Through this deeper level of reflexiveness, practitioners better understand not only who they are as individuals and as therapists but also how who they are influences their interactions with clients (Logan et al., 2021; Yancu & Farmer, 2017). The greater awareness thus suggests the use of culture as a strength and facilitator of treatment. Employing such a practice helps raise awareness of and manage and work toward overcoming biases, especially those that might be implicit and could interfere with interpersonal clinical interactions.

Dee Watts-Jones (2010) highlighted the example of using uncomfortable questions that can serve to confront tacit power dynamics among White therapists working with families of color or a therapist of color working with White families. In either situation, the role of therapist is privileged, yet the race dynamic may herald unspoken influence into the treatment when unacknowledged. Starting a treatment by asking the client their thoughts on having a therapist of a different race allows space for managing such tensions, as well as an opening for the therapist to further inquire about the client's culture with the aim of becoming more informed and effective in treatment. To sum, this approach involves attending to the nature of interpersonal interactions, particularly as they relate to therapist–client power dynamics. Doing so helps reposition clients as individuals with agency and as experts of their own cultures and experiences rather than viewing the therapist as the expert and contributes to the sharing of power (Upshaw et al., 2020).

Cultural humility also recognizes people as intersectional beings who cannot be viewed simply as an additive summation of multiple cultural identities (Kolden et al., 2018). In this way, therapists must be able to work with the whole person in the context of their social location because it has a direct influence on the way clients make meaning of the world and their experiences in it.

One specific example of this approach is the multicultural orientation framework (Owen et al., 2019), which asserts that therapists must attend to cultural humility (as articulated earlier), cultural comfort (working collaboratively with the whole person and doing so with comfort), and cultural opportunities (being able to identify and clinically use markers of culture to better understand how it influences values and beliefs). Engaging each of these helps reduce the likelihood of microaggressions during therapy and supports development of stronger therapeutic alliances that are linked to stronger clinical outcomes. Hence, a more reflexive, agile practice through cultural humility can help practitioners take such complexity into account and gain greater cultural awareness in their practice.

Cultural Responsiveness

Cultural responsiveness is another highly dynamic ongoing process, although its main role is to combine the practices of cultural competence and cultural humility. It also better addresses the role of inclusion of intersectionality in clinical practice and is relational in nature (Simpkins et al., 2017). Allen and Steed (2016) explained that culturally responsive practice supports a strength-based perspective that centers culture and increases awareness and dialogue about culture. Hence, in addition to learning about others' culture, it enables reflexive examination and continual monitoring of one's own bias and adopt more mindful practices. Such a dynamic process that presses for honest introspection and open discussion of culture with clients supports practitioners in their application of the various concepts discussed here in a thoughtful way. We encourage the use of a culturally responsive approach, which is increasingly adopted for its effectiveness because it includes all the elements of competence and humility, views clients intersectionally and holistically, and equalizes power and agency.

INTERSECTIONALITY

Intersectionality remains a highly contested term with respect to its meaning and how it is referenced and applied. Aside from the label intersectionality (Butler, 2015; Davis, 2008), it is also referred to as a location of self (Dee Watts-Jones, 2010), multiculturalism (Patallo, 2019), and social justice (Chan et al., 2018), to name a few terms. Debates about intersectionality also concern its status as a paradigm, method, or theory (Few-Demo, 2014), as well as how to apply it within various realms, including research, practice, and pedagogy. Some argue that its debated ambiguity is precisely what makes it so useful and powerful (Davis, 2008). Given its multiplicity, one should take great care in intentionally identifying how they draw on the concept of intersectionality, especially in practice.

Here we define intersectionality as a concept and theoretical perspective that enables a deeper and more dynamic understanding of the complexity of people's realities as they inhabit multiple identities (Crenshaw, 1989) contextualized within a social system that entails various levels of oppression and privilege (Grzanka 2020; Shlasko, 2015). Intersectionality provides necessary tools that enable us to look beyond categories of individual identities, such as gender, race, ethnicity, sexual orientation, and religion, to better understand people's experiences at the intersection of multiple identities, inclusive of the whole person, family, and social group (Cho et al., 2013; Davis, 2008). Moreover, interpersonal relations with others are often influenced by a social context that entails embedded and interlocking systems of oppression and privilege. Such contextually charged interactions play an important role in individuals' lives and can affect them cognitively and emotionally, which is particularly clinically relevant (Clauss-Ehlers et al., 2019).

Despite intersectionality's use in other fields and its evident power in helping to get at the complexity of people's lives, it has been applied less widely within family therapy, partially due to the lack of clarity as to how it should be applied (Butler, 2015). Patallo (2019) referenced the multicultural guidelines established by the APA (2017), which he asserted is an important step but does not necessarily provide clinicians with everything they need to ensure an intersectional approach. Even with best intentions, the application of intersectionality in practice is complex, can be uncomfortable, and can result in too much comparing of group differences or trying to apply knowledge from one group to another. It can also be hard to resist falling into stereotypical notions about groups based on limited or distorted knowledge. Even individuals who share a common intersection may have very different experiences, and such differences risk being overlooked or misinterpreted (Patallo, 2019). Additionally, the clinician's understanding of themselves and their relative privilege and oppression can be overlooked yet affect the clinician–client relationship, and power dynamic (Dee Watts-Jones, 2010; Logan et al., 2022). Further, our own identities work as a lens through which we view the world, often unconsciously manifesting themselves through our interactions with others, including during clinician–client interactions. Awareness of these potential pitfalls in accounting for and contending with complex and dynamic intersecting identities can improve practitioners' application of an increasingly intersectional approach.

CONCLUSION

As scholars gain a greater understanding of the central role that culture plays in our global context and diverse relationships, the incorporation of multicultural understanding becomes increasingly necessary to incorporate into practice if we are to enhance inclusiveness and consideration of intersectionality (Kim-Goh et al., 2015). This chapter discussed three sets of key concepts that practitioners are encouraged to incorporate into their processes and that respectively build on each other.

- Diversity, inclusion, and social justice
  - Diversity enables recognition of individual and group identities with a focus on inclusion, not emphasizing differences or reinforcing historic power differentials.
  - Inclusion underscores the importance of involving diverse individuals and groups in decision-making processes with the aim of securing equal resources and opportunities.
  - Social justice endorses systemic and institutional change that supports more equitable access to resources and opportunities and redresses historic injustices.
  - Incorporating these concepts into practice entails greater awareness of one's own biases, privileges, and oppressions and taking actions that account for such realizations.
- Cultural competence, cultural humility, and cultural responsiveness
  - Cultural competence enables practitioners to inform themselves about clients' culture through research and discussion with clients and making clients' values and needs central.
  - Cultural humility is an introspective process for practitioners to reflexively examine how their identities can affect their perspectives and interactions with clients.
  - Cultural responsiveness is the dynamic merging of cultural competence, humility, and intersectionality and is strengths-based.

- Intersectionality is a lens that centers on location of multiple identities as a dynamic rather than summative form of individuality; it engenders greater understanding of the complexity of life and the interlocking systems of oppression of individual's multiple identities.

Taken together, we believe there is great merit in using a culturally responsive approach to practice that uses techniques of cultural competency and cultural humility while highlighting intersectionality and the whole person. We see this as being a dynamic, inclusive, and intersectional practice. Additionally, we encourage practitioners to continually inform themselves on these and other related concepts on an ongoing basis to enhance their efforts in becoming more inclusive, understanding, and effective in their practice (Allen & Steed, 2016). At the same time, it is important to keep in mind that these are ideas that should remain fluid and continue to develop over time and that introspective work should always accompany such readings to continually improve awareness and understanding of clients' realities and needs. In the chapters that follow, much of what is written in research sections provides insight into diversity and cultural competence knowledge and its quality. The clinical sections demonstrate how clinical experience combines with research evidence to inform clinical decision making and intervention implementation. This leads to more inclusive and socially just interventions. Accordingly, it is important not simply to read the chapters but to consider the process going on between and behind the words, sentences, and "scenes." Importantly, the chapters do not have space allocated for a thorough discussion of how one's own intersectionality influenced the clinical decision-making process. Stated another way, although much of the practice detailed in the following chapters uses cultural responsiveness, parts of that process (i.e., reflexivity) are not explicitly included in this text, and we refer readers to Logan and colleagues (2021) for an in-depth discussion of those strategies.

REFERENCES

Allen, R., & Steed, E. A. (2016). Culturally responsive pyramid model practices: Program-wide positive behavior support for young children. *Topics in Early Childhood Special Education*, *36*(3), 165–175. https://doi.org/10.1177/0271121416651164

American Psychological Association. (2017). *Multicultural guidelines: An ecological approach to context, identity, and intersectionality*. https://www.apa.org/about/policy/multicultural-guidelines.pdf

Butler, C. (2015). Intersectionality in family therapy training: Inviting students to embrace the complexities of lived experience. *Journal of Family Therapy*, *37*(4), 583–589. https://doi.org/10.1111/1467-6427.12090

Campinha-Bacote, J. (2002). The process of cultural competence in the delivery of healthcare services: A model of care. *Journal of Transcultural Nursing, 13*(3), 181–184. https://doi.org/10.1177/10459602013003003

Chan, C. D., Cor, D. N., & Band, M. P. (2018). Privilege and oppression in counselor education: An intersectionality framework. *Journal of Multicultural Counseling and Development, 46*(1), 58–73. https://doi.org/10.1002/jmcd.12092

Chapman, C. (2011). Resonance, intersectionality, and reflexivity in critical pedagogy (and research methodology). *Social Work Education, 30*(7), 723–744. https://doi.org/10.1080/02615479.2010.520120

Cho, S., Crenshaw, K., & McCall, L. (2013). Toward a field of intersectionality studies: Theory, applications, and praxis. *Signs: Journal of Women in Culture and Society, 38*(4), 785–810. https://doi.org/10.1086/669608

Clauss-Ehlers, C. S., Chiriboga, D. A., Hunter, S. J., Roysircar, G., & Tummala-Narra, P. (2019). APA Multicultural Guidelines executive summary: Ecological approach to context, identity, and intersectionality. *American Psychologist, 74*(2), 232–244. https://doi.org/10.1037/amp0000382

Crenshaw, K. (1989). Demarginalizing the intersection of race and sex: A Black feminist critique of antidiscrimination doctrine, feminist theory and antiracist politics. *University of Chicago Legal Forum, 1989*, 139–167. https://chicagounbound.uchicago.edu/uclf/vol1989/iss1/8

Davis, K. (2008). Intersectionality as buzzword: A sociology of science perspective on what makes a feminist theory successful. *Feminist Theory, 9*(1), 67–85. https://doi.org/10.1177/1464700108086364

Few-Demo, A. (2014). Intersectionality as the "new" critic approach in feminist family studies: Evolving racial/ethnic feminisms and critical race theories. *Journal of Family Theory & Review, 6*(2), 169–183. https://doi.org/10.1111/jftr.12039

Greene-Moton, E., & Minkler, M. (2020). Cultural competence or cultural humility? Moving beyond the debate. *Health Promotion Practice, 21*(1), 142–145. https://doi.org/10.1177/1524839919884912

Grzanka, P. R. (2020). From buzzword to critical psychology: An invitation to take intersectionality seriously. *Women & Therapy, 43*(3–4), 244–261. https://doi.org/10.1080/02703149.2020.1729473

Isaacson, M. (2014). Clarifying concepts: Cultural humility or competency. *Journal of Professional Nursing, 30*(3), 251–258. https://doi.org/10.1016/j.profnurs.2013.09.011

Kim-Goh, M., Choi, H., & Yoon, M. S. (2015). Culturally responsive counseling for Asian Americans: Clinician perspectives. *International Journal for the Advancement of Counseling, 37*(1), 63–76. https://doi.org/10.1007/s10447-014-9226-z

Kolden, G. G., Wang, C. C., Austin, S. B., Chang, Y., & Klein, M. H. (2018). Congruence/genuineness: A meta-analysis. *Psychotherapy: Theory, Research, & Practice, 55*(4), 424–433. https://doi.org/10.1037/pst0000162

LaMantia, K., Wagner, H., & Bohecker, L. (2015). Ally development through feminist pedagogy: A systemic focus on intersectionality. *Journal of LGBT Issues in Counseling, 9*(2), 136–153. https://doi.org/10.1080/15538605.2015.1029205

Levant, R. (2005). *Report of the 2005 Presidential Task Force on Evidence-Based Practice.* American Psychological Association. https://www.apa.org/practice/resources/evidence/evidence-based-report.pdf

Logan, J., van Eeden-Moorefield, B., & Browning, S. (Eds.). (2022). *Constructing authentic relationships in clinical practice: Working at the intersection of therapist and client identities*. Routledge.

Owen, J., Tao, K., & Drinane, J. (2019). Microaggressions: Clinical impact and psychological harm. In G. Torino, D. Rivera, C. Capodilupo, K. Nadal, & D. Sue (Eds.), *Microaggression theory: Influence and implications* (pp. 67–85). John Wiley & Sons.

Patallo, B. J. (2019). The multicultural guidelines in practice: Cultural humility in clinical training and supervision. *Training and Education in Professional Psychology*, *13*(3), 227–232. https://doi.org/10.1037/tep0000253

Sanchez, J. E., DeFlorio, L., Wiest, L. R., & Oikonomidoy. (2018). Student perceptions of inclusiveness in a college of education with respect to diversity. *College Student Journal*, *52*(3), 397–409.

Sharp, E. A., & Weaver, S. E. (2015). Feeling like a feminist fraud: Theorizing feminist accountability in feminist family studies research in a Neoliberal, postfeminist context. *Journal of Family Theory & Review*, *7*(3), 299–320. https://doi.org/10.1111/jftr.12080

Shlasko, D. (2015). Using the five faces of oppression to teach about interlocking systems of oppression. *Equity & Excellence in Education*, *48*(3), 349–360. https://doi.org/10.1080/10665684.2015.1057061

Simpkins, S. D., Riggs, N. R., Ngo, B., Ettekal, A. V., & Okamoto, D. (2017). Designing culturally responsive organized after-school activities. *Journal of Adolescent Research*, *32*(1), 11–36. https://doi.org/10.1177/0743558416666169

Thomas, K. M., Tran, N. M., & Dawson, B. L. (2010). An inclusive strategy of teaching diversity. *Advances in Developing Human Resources*, *12*(3), 295–311. https://doi.org/10.1177/1523422310375035

Upshaw, N. C., Lewis, D. E., & Nelson, A. L. (2020). Cultural humility in action: Reflective and process-oriented supervision with Black trainees. *Training and Education in Professional Psychology*, *14*(4), 277–284. https://doi.org/10.1037/tep0000284

Watts-Jones, T. D. (2010). Location of self: Opening the door to dialogue on intersectionality in the therapy process. *Family Process*, *49*(3), 405–420. https://doi.org/10.1111/j.1545-5300.2010.01330.x

Yancu, C., & Farmer, D. (2017). Product or process: Cultural competence or cultural humility. *Palliative Medicine and Hospice Care*, *3*(1), e1–e4. https://doi.org/10.17140/PMHCOJ-3-e005

3

STRESS FROM MICROAGGRESSIONS AND DISCRIMINATION

A Focus on Asian American, African American, Latina/o/x, and Queer Families

RESEARCH: LINDSEY SANK DAVIS
CLINICAL APPLICATIONS: CLAUDIA GARCÍA-LEEDS, YIQING YOUNGMAN, CHERYLL ROTHERY, AND ERIKA GRAFSKY

RESEARCH: LINDSEY SANK DAVIS

Marginalized groups in the United States have historically been subjected to legalized exclusion, such as the denial of education, marriage, medical care, immigration status, housing, and employment. Although Asian American, Black, Latinx, and lesbian, gay, bisexual, transgender, and queer (LGBTQ+) families have more legal protections than they did a few decades ago, they are still exposed to the toxic effects of biases held against them based on their marginalized identities. Expressions of bias and prejudice include two broad categories: **overt** and **covert**. For the better part of the past decade, researchers in this field (e.g., Nadal et al., 2016) have frequently commented on a general decline in public acceptance of overt prejudice in American society; this apparent decline led to an increased interest in studying covert forms of prejudice, including **microaggressions**—subtle, everyday denigrations and expressions of bias directed toward individuals with marginalized identities (Sue & Sue, 2013). This new interest exposed the nature, frequency, and impact of microaggressions, but considerable evidence now suggests that

https://doi.org/10.1037/0000280-003
Treating Contemporary Families: Toward a More Inclusive Clinical Practice, S. Browning and B. van Eeden-Moorefield (Editors)

the downward trend in overt prejudice and discrimination has reversed course. It has become evident that experiences of both overt and covert prejudice have detrimental impacts on individuals and, by extension, their families.

Meyer (2003) connected social psychological research to clinical observations and coined the term **minority stress** to describe "the excess stress to which individuals from stigmatized social categories are exposed as a result of their social, often a minority, position" (p. 675). Although the term was originally coined to describe the experiences of LGB individuals, racial, ethnic, and gender minority individuals are also likely to experience key components of minority stress: (a) acute and chronic events that are objectively stressful (e.g., exposure to hateful language or violence); (b) vigilance for the possibility that such an event is nearing (e.g., discomfort in predominantly White settings, anxiety in the presence of law enforcement); and (c) internalization of stereotypes and attitudes toward one's own identity group (e.g., preferring fairer skinned partners, using homophobic slurs toward others despite having same-sex attractions). A fourth component, concealment of concealable aspects of identity, is most applicable to LGBTQ+ individuals but may also apply to "passing" as White and to concealment of immigration status. Just as marginalized individuals are exposed to this minority stress, marginalized families are also exposed. All families experience intrafamilial stressors (e.g., distribution of parenting responsibilities), but marginalized families experience additional externally imposed stressors related to prejudice, including systemic prejudice. This chapter synthesizes research on discrimination and microaggressions with marginalized families (see Table 3.1). For each of the four types of families included here, we also present a clinical case with an intervention informed by the research.

Research Evidence on Overt Expressions of Prejudice

Overt expressions of prejudice include hate speech, hate crimes, and other visible or spoken forms of discrimination. Whereas public displays of hate, such as cross-burning and lynching, were once common in the United States, these displays became less visible after the specter of punishment was raised by law aimed at these offenses but have increased steadily since 2015 (e.g., Center for the Study of Hate and Extremism, 2017; D'Onofrio, 2019). Starting with the Civil Rights Act of 1964 (a response to the violent reaction to racial desegregation and the murder of Black Civil Rights leader Medgar Evers) and continuing through the Matthew Shepard and James Byrd, Jr. Hate Crimes Prevention Act of 2009 (named after two young men who were brutally murdered for their sexual orientation and race, respectively), the federal

TABLE 3.1. Stress From Microaggressions and Discrimination

Evidence-based area of clinical focus	Type of factor	Appropriateness for use across families	Selected references indicating evidence base
Overt and covert bias	General	All[a]	Nadal et al., 2016; Sue & Sue, 2013
Minority stress	General	All[a]	Meyer, 2003
Model minority	Unique	Asian American families	Gupta et al., 2011
Inequality in the criminal justice system	Unique	Black families	Huq, 2017
Health disparities	Unique	Black, Latinx, and queer families	FitzGerald & Hurst, 2017
Immigrant experiences in school	Unique	Latinx families	Crosnoe, 2005
Invalidation of familial relationships	Unique	Queer families	Meyer, 2003
Gender-based bullying	Unique	Queer families	Kosciw et al., 2020

[a]The general factor could work for other family types included in this chapter but needs a small adaptation to ensure cultural relevance. Information about potential adaptations is included in the text.

government has become more aggressive in punishing bias-motivated behavior. Although many hateful expressions moved into the private sphere to avoid public scrutiny, many now occur on social media and Internet forums and in televised events; policy should therefore attend to these more.

Hate crimes serve both instrumental and symbolic functions, not only injuring and denigrating their victims but also sending messages to intimidate and humiliate their families and communities (Bell & Perry, 2015). The courts (e.g., *Wisconsin v. Mitchell*, 1993) have recognized that hate crimes inflict psychological trauma, creating an *in terrorem* effect on their victims in which there is a fear of retaliatory violence from family and community members. Furthermore, hate crimes have low clearance rates (solved crimes) compared with other crimes (Lyons & Roberts, 2014).

Research on Covert Expressions of Prejudice

Microaggressions, a burgeoning area of psychological research, are defined as "brief and commonplace daily verbal, behavioral, and environmental indignities, whether intentional or unintentional, that communicate hostile, derogatory, negative racial [or ethnic, sexist, homophobic, transphobic, anti-Semitic, etc.] slights and insults to the target person or group" (Sue et al.,

2007, p. 273). Microaggressions include *microassaults*, consciously discriminatory behavior that may not be intended to harm the recipient (e.g., using racial slurs, exhibiting lower expectations of Latinx students); *microinsults*, degrading comments or behaviors based on identity (e.g., suggesting that a Black student gained admission to an elite school because of affirmative action or athletic recruitment, telling a bisexual person that they are "just confused"); and *microinvalidations*, statements that deny or question a marginalized person's feelings or lived experience (e.g., denying the existence of racism, telling someone who is upset about a microaggression that they are being "too sensitive"). It is worth noting that these categories are not mutually exclusive, and some conflict exists about the precise definitions of these terms. For example, Sue and Sue (2013) indicated that microassaults are blatant and *intended* to express a bias, whereas Nadal et al. (2014) indicated they may not be intentionally hurtful yet still convey a bias. The intent and the cause of the behavior are not immediately clear to the person experiencing the microaggression; the recipient can never be sure whether they were treated in such a way due to one of their identities or due to some other reason (e.g., an unrelated bad mood). This feature of microaggressions makes them particularly pernicious, as the recipients of the hurtful behaviors may come to question their own sense of reality (Sue et al., 2007).

Research Evidence on the Detrimental Impact of Discrimination

In his seminal 1954 work *The Nature of Prejudice*, psychologist Gordon Allport surmised: "One's reputation, whether false or true, cannot be hammered, hammered, hammered, into one's head without doing something to one's character" (p. 142). As Allport predicted, research has demonstrated that discrimination takes its toll on both individuals and families, with immediate, ongoing, and compounding effects. Table 3.1 demonstrates themes of discrimination and **microaggressions** that frequently affect Asian American, Black, Latinx, and LGBTQ+ Americans; these themes are described in further detail in what follows.

Individual Level

Although Asian, Black, Latinx, and LGBTQ+ Americans have been historically oppressed and their opportunities have been systematically limited, youth from these marginalized groups are rarely exposed to this history in the heteronormative, Eurocentric American educational curriculum. For example, only about 20% of LGBTQ+ students report learning anything positive about queer people or history in school, despite evidence that inclusive curriculum improves their safety and well-being (Kosciw et al., 2020). As a result, marginalized youth may come to question their own abilities when they experience rejection from biased systems or fail to achieve on par with their more privileged peers. These doubts start to affect children early and can last until adulthood (Adair, 2015). This is one path whereby oppression is internalized (Speight, 2007), which can lead to increased stress (Tull et al., 2005), poor academic performance (Steele & Aronson, 1995), and eventual disengagement from school (Perez Huber et al., 2006).

Furthermore, discrimination is associated with a variety of mental health symptoms and disorders. In a study of Asian American and Latinx individuals (Hwang & Goto, 2008), perceived discrimination was positively correlated with suicidal ideation, depression, anxiety, and general distress. Similarly, Davis and Stevenson (2006) found an association between perceived discrimination and depressive and stress-related symptoms among Black youth. **Microaggressions** have been specifically implicated because research (Nadal et al., 2014) demonstrates a negative correlation between mental health and well-being and the number of racial/ethnic microaggressions an individual experience. Sexual orientation and gender minority microaggressions produce similar effects (for a review, see Nadal et al., 2016). Microaggressions have also been linked to an increased likelihood of role limitations due to physical symptoms, including pain and fatigue (Nadal et al., 2017).

Family Level

Individual-level struggles may affect one or more family members, causing a variety of strains on family functioning as stress is magnified and spread throughout the family unit. For example, Fischer (2007) defined *emotional contagion* as a form of social influence in which an individual's own emotions are affected by observing another's emotions, thereby altering their own mood state to mimic the person they are observing. Qualitative research on trauma (e.g., Goff et al., 2006) suggests that when one member of a family experiences a traumatic event (which may include bias-related incidents), this often leads to other difficulties within the family, such as decreased communication and cohesion.

Additionally, the downstream physical and mental health problems caused or exacerbated by discrimination can affect family functioning. Health care costs and work absenteeism associated with physical health problems can cause financial strain. Parental health problems are also associated with poor health in children (Waters et al., 2000), ineffective parenting (Mulder et al., 2018), and internalizing and externalizing symptoms in children (Hardie & Turney, 2017). Untreated mental health and substance abuse problems can contribute to intimate partner violence (Cafferky et al., 2018) and ineffective parenting (Mulder et al., 2018). Mood disorders, especially depression, have also been linked to greater health care costs and lost wages (Simon, 2003), which can cause financial strain on the family.

Research Evidence on Asian American Families

Asians and Asian Americans are in the unusual position of being identified by the dominant culture as the "**model minority**." This label came into use in the 1960s and entails many positive stereotypes, such as being well-educated, successful, financially well-off, hardworking, and intelligent (e.g., Gupta et al., 2011). Although these are positive qualities, they do not reflect the reality of a heterogeneous Asian American population; as a result, these stereotypes can laden Asian Americans (particularly youth) with additional pressure to succeed. Furthermore, because Asian cultures often do not encourage the seeking of psychological services, many Asian Americans who internalize the model minority stereotype experience higher rates of distress while simultaneously failing to seek mental health services (Gupta et al., 2011). Asian American youth are especially at risk for depression, anxiety disorders, eating disorders, substance abuse, and suicide (e.g., Nadal et al., 2015), with young women at particularly high risk (e.g., Arora et al., 2017). These trends vary by specific ethnicity, with Filipino youth experiencing higher rates of depression, suicidal ideation, and substance abuse than do their peers of other Asian ethnicities (Javier at al., 2010).

Research also indicates that experiencing racial or ethnic **microaggressions** is associated with anger, anxiety, depression, stress, and somatic symptoms in Asian American adolescents and young adults (Wong-Padoongpatt et al., 2017). These are often centered on themes of being a "perpetual foreigner" (Liang et al., 2004) or an "alien in one's own land" (Sue et al., 2007) and include presuming nonnative status of any Asian-appearing person or expecting an Asian-appearing person to speak English poorly. A salient example of large-scale discrimination against Asian Americans appeared amid the COVID-19 pandemic, which was believed to have originated in China (Jeong & Nham, 2020). Most (70.6%) were instances of verbal harassment that might range from more subtle microaggressions to violent hate speech; however, more than 200 instances of physical assault were reported during this brief window.

Research Evidence on Black Families

Although federal law has attempted to address employment discrimination, it continues to be a significant issue for Black Americans. Experimental research (e.g., Pager & Western, 2012) has established that Whites are more likely to be hired than are equally qualified Blacks. Combined with unequal educational opportunity, discrimination perpetuates an employment gap such that Blacks are almost twice as likely to be unemployed compared with Whites (U.S. Department of Labor, 2019). Furthermore, among those with full-time employment, Blacks still earn about 22% less per week than Whites, on average.

Research (e.g., Pickett et al., 2012) indicates that Americans continue to view Blacks as the most violent racial or ethnic group in the United States; given this view, it is not surprising that Blacks face considerable **inequality in the criminal justice system**. Policies such as stop-and-frisk have exposed Blacks, especially Black male youth, to increased contact with law enforcement, even when they have not committed any criminal offense (e.g., Huq, 2017). Furthermore, law enforcement officers kill a disproportionate number of Blacks compared with other races (e.g., Sadler et al., 2012). The courts further contribute to the mass incarceration of Black men, separating them from their families. Research indicates that jurors are more likely to sentence Black defendants to death compared with White defendants (Baldus et al., 1998) and more likely to impose the death penalty in capital murder cases in which the defendant has "stereotypically black features" (Eberhardt et al., 2006). The impact of these inequities on Black families is vast, including increased parenting pressure on Black mothers, increased aggressive behaviors in sons of incarcerated men, and more (for a review, see Western & Lopoo, 2004).

There are significant physical **health disparities** between Whites and Blacks, many of which are attributable in part to structural inequalities, including those just described. Additionally, research indicates that different diagnostic and treatment decisions are made between racial groups, suggesting that the quality of care is affected by biases held by medical practitioners (for a review, see FitzGerald & Hurst, 2017). Furthermore, many Black Americans are distrustful or avoidant of medical and mental health professionals due to their own experiences and historical examples of unethical treatment (e.g., the Tuskegee study).

The COVID-19 pandemic brought these disparities into stark relief, as it became clear that Black Americans were significantly more likely than White Americans to contract and die from the virus. The Centers for Disease Control and Prevention (2020) reported that in a sample of 580 patients hospitalized with COVID-19, 33% were Black despite only 18% of residents in the catchment area being Black, as but one example of many. Clinicians should be aware that Black Americans are a diverse group, encompassing families with recent histories in the United States, the Caribbean, Africa, and elsewhere. In some regards, Black individuals share common experiences of racism and discrimination; however, research (Nadal et al., 2021) also indicates that Black Americans experience different types of **microaggressions** depending on their particular heritage, as well as their gender, education level, and other factors.

Research Evidence on Latinx Families

Research (e.g., Ayón & Philbin, 2017) indicates that schools are a site of frequent ethnic **microaggressions** towards Latinx youth. Adair (2015) reported that young children of **immigrants experience** microaggressions from teachers, such as comments about their accents, devaluation of their home language and culture, harsher discipline, and low academic expectations. Children of Mexican immigrant families appear to begin school on par socially and emotionally with their American-born peers but quickly fall behind academically (Crosnoe, 2005). Martínez (2013) found that bilingual Latinx youth often felt their *Spanglish*—a hybrid of Spanish and English—made them deficient, suggesting they had absorbed the dominant cultural narrative; however, they were also able to conceptualize their Spanglish as a way of remaining connected to their Latinx heritage. The way educators respond to language-related struggles in the classroom, and whether they demonstrate respect for Latinx culture, will determine much of what children think and feel about themselves and their families.

Although most Latinx individuals living in the United States are natural-born or legalized U.S. citizens, many have a loved one whose immigration status is not as secure; thus, threats of deportation are likely to evoke broad anxiety among Latinx individuals. Additionally, research on group-level emotions (Smith & Mackie, 2016) has suggested that members of stigmatized groups often experience negative emotions when other ingroup members are confronted with discrimination. Jones et al. (2021) found that Latinx individuals experienced deportation-related anxiety when exposed to images of Donald Trump and information pertaining to his stance on immigration, particularly if they identified strongly with their Latinx heritage or possessed stigmatized Latinx attributes (e.g., darker skin, limited English proficiency).

During the COVID-19 pandemic, this stress was undoubtedly heightened as hundreds of children were expelled and deported from the United States after arduous trips to the border (Semple, 2020). Whereas migrant children arriving at the southern border had historically been provided with basic protections of safety and legal rights, these provisions have been all but abandoned in 2020. Clinicians should be aware that most individuals from

Latin American countries prefer to identify themselves by their nation of origin (Pew Research Center, 2020). Although few individuals in this diverse and growing group of American residents refer to themselves as *Latinx*, the term has been gaining popularity, particularly among young and queer individuals, as well as in academia, due to its gender-inclusive, pan-ethnic nature. Clinicians also should be aware that intrafamilial microaggressions also occur within Black, Asian, Latinx, and multiracial families, often with regard to *colorism*, the preference for and privileging of those with stereo-typically "whiter" physical features, or levels of *acculturation*, the incorporation of aspects of the dominant American culture into one's ethnic identity (e.g., Nadal et al., 2013).

Research Evidence on Queer Families

Despite a landmark decision in *Obergefell v. Hodges* (2015) granting marriage rights to same-gender couples, research (Farr et al., 2016; Haines et al., 2018) indicates that queer families continue to experience **microaggressions**. These include questions about the legitimacy of their families, **invalidation of their familial relationships** (e.g., calling a woman's wife her "friend"), and con-demnation for perceived violations of traditional family values and gender norms. Many members of the queer (used here as an umbrella term) com-munity develop *chosen families*, which are groups of individuals who are not biologically related but who understand and accept one another in a way many queer individuals' biological families have not. Haines and colleagues (2018) found that these chosen families are often considered illegitimate; similarly, the law does not recognize these relationships as familial. There also continue to be barriers to queer adoption (e.g., Goldberg, 2012) and discrimination in family planning services for queer individuals who were assigned female at birth (e.g., Wingo et al., 2018).

Research on planned families with lesbian parents (Bos et al., 2004) shows that lesbian parents report low levels of social rejection overall; however, when they *do* experience rejection, they are more likely to report parenting-related stress and problem behaviors in their children. Most lesbian mothers reported experiencing **microaggressions**, such as being questioned about their parenting or their relationships. A smaller portion reported hearing gossip or disparaging remarks about their families. Experiences of rejection were associated with increased doubt of one's parenting competence and increased drive to demonstrate parenting competence to others.

Children of queer parents experience microaggressions, bullying, and rejec-tion as well. In a study of children with queer parents (Farr et al., 2016), most reported microaggressions related to their parents, typically from peers.

Themes included heterosexist assumptions about their families, outing of their parents as queer, and hearing derogatory remarks about queer people. Fortunately, although these children often felt different from their peers, they also typically had positive feelings about their families and demonstrated resilience in the face of prejudice.

Additionally, experiences of sexual orientation and **gender-based bullying** and microaggressions are common among queer youth and are associated with a host of negative psychological and behavioral outcomes (e.g., Kosciw et al., 2020), some of which continue into adulthood (Toomey et al. 2010). Although the prevalence of verbal harassment based on sexual orientation or gender expression occurring in schools has declined significantly over the past 10 years, physical harassment and assault have shown only a modest decline over the same period (Kosciw et al., 2020). Those youth who experienced microaggressions, discrimination, and violence at school were more likely to have issues with problematic attendance and academic performance, were more likely to be disciplined by school officials, and had poorer self-esteem and increased depressive symptomology compared with their queer peers who did not experience such discrimination. Although most youth could identify one or more adults in their school who were affirming of their identities, more than half of queer students reported that their schools enacted policies or practices that were discriminatory, including obstructing the use of restrooms and locker rooms consistent with their gender identity (Kosciw et al., 2020).

Not only do queer youth struggle to find appropriate support at school, they often struggle to find support and acceptance at home. Research has indicated that queer youth experience high levels of physical, emotional, and sexual abuse from family members (e.g., Friedman et al., 2011), as well as heteronormative and cisnormative microaggressions asserting that heterosexual and cisgender identities are more desirable and therefore superior to queer identities (e.g., Gartner & Sterzing, 2018). Sadly, parental rejection on the basis of sexual orientation or gender identity is not an uncommon experience among queer youth (e.g., Gartner & Sterzing, 2018; Koken et al., 2009); therefore, queer youth are overrepresented among youth in foster care or unstable housing conditions (e.g., Baams et al., 2019).

CLINICAL APPLICATIONS: CLAUDIA GARCÍA-LEEDS, YIQING YOUNGMAN, CHERYLL ROTHERY, AND ERIKA GRAFSKY

Clinical Expertise and Interpretation of Evidence: An Overview

As Davis points out in the research section of this chapter, it is common for all families to experience some degree of intrafamilial and externally based stress. This can include anything from neglected household chores or disagreements over parenting styles (intrafamilial) to the stress experienced through the loss of a job (external). However, some families—those belonging to marginalized social groups—face additional stressors and challenges that are firmly rooted in prejudice. This prejudice, which manifests itself through discriminatory acts and instances of **microaggressions**, can have a devastating impact on individuals and families. In some cases, prejudice and its resulting stress is interfamilial in nature (Nadal et al., 2013). For example, an African American woman might be subjected to constant microaggressions from her White stepchildren. In other cases, prejudice is externally based, as the entire family is stigmatized by virtue of their inclusion in a specific group. Although this section focuses on the latter, it is important to point out that many individuals may experience both intrafamilial and externally based prejudice.

In addition to being possible targets of hate crimes, families experiencing **minority stress** are more likely to have physical and mental health problems, greater financial challenges, and intrafamilial conflict. Minority stress (and its effects) resulting from discrimination and microaggression poses an uncommon challenge both for the therapist and for the family in treatment. Unlike many—although certainly not all—stressors, minority stress is the result of externally imposed, long-lasting discrimination and microaggression that is unlikely to abate or disappear. It is essential, then, for the therapist to help the family build and maintain a sense of resilience. To do this, the therapist must first recognize and understand the particular stressors unique to that family's particular context. For some marginalized groups, these stressors include those resulting not only from discrimination and microaggression but also from conflicting values between the majority culture and their own culture of origin. This can lead to intrafamilial conflict, especially between older and younger generations, and impede communication among family members, which is crucial for strengthening the family's resilience as a unit. Recognizing and understanding the true causes and effects of these stressors, the therapist will be in a better position help the family gain insight into the nature of their struggles and conflicts—both internal and external. This can be achieved using psychoeducation, along with other techniques.

This section of the chapter translates the research described by Davis into clinical practice. Each clinical section focuses on a specific marginalized family context and explores challenges such families commonly face. The clinical experts share their knowledge, corroborated by research, along with their clinical experience. An essential aspect highlighted by all is the importance of gaining the family members' trust and confidence. Families who experienced discrimination and microaggression will be more likely to take longer in opening up or accepting assistance. Therefore, what appears as a lack of motivation or resistance is a healthy protective reaction on their part.

Although a variety of interventions are used, a common theme evident across all the families is that there is a dominant narrative that dictates (among many other variables) which races, nationalities, and gender identities are valued and which are not. Ultimately—regardless of their theoretical inclinations—the therapist's continuous task is to explore the extent to which this dominant narrative has been internalized and how this internalization has affected not only the members of the family but the therapist as well.

Clinical Expertise and Interpretation of Evidence: Asian American Families

A discussed by Davis, Asian Americans are often labeled a "model minority," characterized as being well-educated, financially well-off, hardworking, and intelligent. These positive stereotypes can lead to both **overt and covert expressions of prejudice** (discrimination and **microaggression**, respectively), which in turn result in increased minority stress within the Asian American community. Asian American families may perceive their symptoms as an isolated phenomenon, failing to see the cultural context in which they are embedded, the collision of cultural differences, and the systemic consequences of such collision. Clinicians who work with Asian American families may also overlook the subtlety and insidiousness of the effects of bias on these families. This section explores the effects of microaggression and discrimination on Asian American families and how these expressions of bias are often internalized, and also illustrates specific interventions that can be used to help families in distress.

Clinical Experience: Observations of Common Interactional Patterns
Davis introduced two concepts that summarize the most common forms of **microaggression** and discrimination experienced by Asian Americans. The first centers on the theme of being a "perpetual foreigner," an "alien in one's own land," which leads to a sense of exclusion and isolation. This theme of exclusion finds its historical origins in a number of governmental policies, such as the Naturalization Act of 1790, the 1882 Chinese Exclusion Act, the Asian Exclusion Act of 1924, and so on. This, in turn, creates a cyclical pattern whereby the more excluded Asian Americans feel, the more they withdraw from the larger American culture; the more they withdraw from the larger American culture, the more they are, in turn, excluded by that very culture. To combat the stress of exclusion and isolation and to find and maintain a sense of belonging, the Asian American community fortifies its own subculture and identity by strictly adhering to traditional Asian values. These traditional values, which are passed down through multiple generations

in the United States are expressed within individual families and are often manifested in the parents' expectations of their children. These values include the expectation to marry within one's race/ethnicity, the importance of sticking together regardless of the need for individuality, high academic and professional achievement, and financial success.

The second concept highlighted by Davis is that of the "**model minority**," which pressures Asian Americans to behave and excel, regardless of circumstance or the stress it creates to do so. When experiencing discrimination or microaggression, it is expected that Asian Americans will "keep their heads down" and "keep quiet." This too, creates a cyclical pattern that reinforces the community's separation and isolation: The more Asian Americans passively accept the abuse, the easier of a target they are, and thus they retreat into their own community, reinforcing the concept of the "perpetual foreigner." Additionally, to compensate for the lack of acceptance and respect, Asian Americans typically work extra hard to achieve professional and financial success, which reinforces the stereotype of the model minority. This, in turn, perpetuates the pressure of having to excel.

Davis highlighted the harmful effects of the internalization of discrimination and microaggression not only within the individual but within the family unit as well.

Within Asian American families, the effects of microaggression and discrimination are commonly expressed in disturbances in family structure or hierarchy, which frequently manifests in the form of parent–child or intergenerational relationship conflict. Younger generations are generally highly exposed to mainstream U.S. culture and might often feel pressure to conform to the norms and values of the majority culture to be accepted.

Older family members adhere more closely to traditional Asian values, which creates a conflict between parental expectations and their children's behavior. This dynamic challenges the traditionally respected family hierarchy and leads to disturbances in the family structure. In families with younger children, parents often describe children's behavioral problems as talking back, being disrespectful, shutting them out, and so on. In families with adult children, the problems presented often include children being undutiful (as opposed to filial), disloyal, losing face for the family, and parents being controlling, outdated, or narrow-minded. Nevertheless, although family members may reach a level of communication about the good intentions underlying each other's behavior, they may not understand the driving force behind the intentions. Such intellectual understanding without empathy is fragile and breaks down easily, leading to increasingly conflictive rounds of interaction, which gradually threaten the togetherness of the family unit.

Case Context: Characteristics, Culture, and Preferences

Amy is a 22-year-old, Chinese American woman, born in the United States. She withdrew from school during her senior year in college and has been living at home with her parents. Her parents, Alan and Sue, were born in China and immigrated to the United States in their 20s. Both parents hold multiple postgraduate degrees and work in senior positions in IT. The family has a prominent status within the Chinese community. Assessment is done with the whole family at intake to retrieve typical information needed before therapy. In addition, special attention is paid to observing the family's level(s) of acculturation and subtle differences of values expressed. Since Amy's withdrawal from school, Sue has become "somewhat depressed" and feels "ashamed to show her face at her community activities." Alan is angry at Amy and has "exploded at Amy before," at times "taking it out" on his wife, Sue, as well. Alan and Sue have taken Amy to see a therapist, a psychiatrist, and an acupuncturist in their attempts to motivate her to go back to school. However, Amy seems to have withdrawn even more, abandoning various treatments, stopping medications, and staying in her room. Recently she changed her sleep schedule to be the opposite of her parents. During a parental subsystem session, Alan and Sue express the belief that Amy is "just being lazy." "She knows that we won't have the heart not to care for her, so she's just going to stay this way." They believe she views them as "invalidating and controlling and that she's failing to meet their expectations," which contributes to her low self-esteem and depression. Sue and Alan state that they are trying to "be more American" and praise Amy and are trying to be mindful about not being "harsh and critical Chinese parents." "We encourage her and tell her that she is smart. She is capable of achieving great success in life. All she has to do is put in the work, she'll definitely do great." They express that the more they try to "help and motivate Amy," the more she feels invalidated and controlled, the more resistant and rebellious she becomes, and the more she distances herself from her family. In a way, they believe, Amy is trying harder to stay depressed.

Clinical Decisions: Intervention Implementation

As Davis points out, Asian culture discourages mental health treatment. In this case, using a strength-based approach is essential not only to destigmatize mental health treatment but also to relieve the shame Asian Americans experience when seeking treatment. This can be achieved by reframing the seeking of treatment to reflect values that Asian American families regard highly, such as highlighting their ability to utilize resources, their wishes to improve family life, their motivation to strive for growth.

Amy, Sue, and Alan are invited to share their experiences as a minority family in the United States and the discrimination they have encountered. Having the clinical impression about this family's levels of acculturation and differences in values from the initial assessment, brief psychoeducation is provided on discrimination and **microaggression**. Specific examples are given to help the family (more so with the parents, in this case) detect such experiences in their lives. Amy is more readily able to share her experiences. She recalls classmates saying to her, "aren't you supposed to be good at math?" Amy is invited to talk about her thoughts and feelings about this experience. She feels as though something is wrong with her, that she is the dumb Asian, and that it makes her feel depressed. At this point, her parents eagerly jump in, and her mother says, "Oh, why didn't you tell us? Had we known, I would have comforted you and told you to not listen to them. You're smart and you can prove them wrong." This is an opportunity for the parents to understand Amy's depression. "Mom, it's endearing to see your strong belief in Amy. I can see that it means a lot to Amy, to the point that she is so depressed about being the dumb Asian." "But she is not," her parents quickly reply. "But what if she is, for she does not do well in school to prove it?" For the first time, the parents start to see the effect of microaggression on Amy's well-being and how their own "words of encouragement" serve not to deflect but to enhance that effect. Amy now feels more encouraged to open up to her parents and continues to talk, but this time about her relationship with them. She recalls instances when she did well in school, the achievement was celebrated, but her efforts were minimized. To her parents, her hard-earned achievements are something predictable and expected. "See? I knew you could do it!"— even when said with a proud smile—causes Amy to feel pressured. Upon realizing this, Sue and Alan feel immense guilt for having unknowingly colluded with the exact forces from which they feel they have been trying to protect their daughter, thus causing her pain. For once, Amy feels genuinely heard and understood; at the same time, she feels sorry for her parents for feeling guilty.

Reframing is used here again to ease the parents' guilt. "I wonder what has motivated your parents to be so protective of you?" This gives Amy an opportunity to come up with a few answers that show she *does* see the good intentions behind her parents' actions. More important, Sue and Alan start sharing their own historical encounter with microaggression and discrimination. They share how hard they had to work, with no help, to establish themselves in this country, how much extra effort they had to put in to compete with "real Americans" for the same opportunities. Amy's mother breaks down in tears, "I worry that if Amy doesn't do well and do better than others, she won't be able to have a good life. We will always take care of her, but no one will after we are gone." Amy now understands that her parents' pressure on her stems from the anxiety from their own experiences of being part of a marginalized group. She gains a sense of respect and empathy for them, which she expresses along with her appreciation.

Clinical Expertise and Interpretation of Evidence: African American Couples

Microaggressions are a major contributor to the phenomenon of **minority stress** (Meyer, 2003). Although African American males and females share many common experiences of microaggression consequent to systemic racism and oppression, there are unique aspects of these experiences that are **gender based**. This may seem obvious, but an exploration of the sometimes nuanced, sometimes overt encounters that African American men and women experience has been found to be an important component of their therapy, whether treatment is for the individual, couple, or family system.

Conversations that promote insight and awareness, empathy and compassion, and greater understanding of microaggressions and their impact on the loved but sometimes judged other are often a focal point in helping clients resolve conflicts and areas of misunderstanding between themselves and loved ones of a different gender. A lack of understanding and appreciation for the impact of gendered microaggressions can add salt to the wounds of racially traumatic experiences by the very individual who has the potential to be the greatest source of comfort, compassion, understanding, and support. Further, consequent displaced or internalized anger, frustration, confusion, or self-blame can compound the stress of microaggressions and be even further destructive to the individual or their partner, thereby eroding relationship quality.

Clinical Experience: Observations of Common Interactional Patterns

All couples comprise individuals of diverse and intersecting identities. For African American couples, their individual and shared identities, in combination with other factors, inform significant aspects of their exposure to gendered racial **microaggressions**, as well as the frequency, content, impact, and the individual's response. When one's partner is unable to recognize and acknowledge the occurrence and impact of gendered racial microaggressions, the opportunity is lost for them, and the context of their relationship to serve as a source of reality testing, validation, affirmation, and proactive coping and problem-solving for their loved one.

Beyond the cumulative physiological and physical health consequences of microaggressions for African Americans an African American couple's individual identity factors and experiences affect how each respond to micro-aggressions. A lack of appreciation of the influence of gender, personality, and perspective can make it challenging for one member of the couple to understand their partner's responses to microaggressions, especially if they are dramatically different from their own. In treatment, this may lead to a premature and judgmental focus on their partner's response to a micro-aggression, as well as statements that inadvertently serve to support the microaggression because of how they feel about their partner's response to this psychological assault. Just as the cumulative impact of microaggressions toward African Americans erodes their mental and physical health, it can erode the African American couple's relationship. The encouragement of an emic perspective of each other's experiences of microaggressions, their impact, and outcome is a critical intervention for the African American couple strug-gling to be a salve of healing for one another in a country where micro-aggressions toward African Americans is often not the exception but the norm of their lived experience.

Case Context: Characteristics, Culture, and Preferences
The following case was a collaboration with a colleague. I worked with the woman in the couple, and my colleague worked with her husband. The couple consented to regular consultation between the therapists, as well as joint couple's sessions with me approximately once a month. This approach to the couple's treatment was based on the couple's primary personal treatment goals coupled with their desire to address any related or consequent couple's issues that might be uncovered in the work. "Cassandra" is a 33-year-old, African American woman, married to "Anthony," age 35. Cassandra has a master's degree and works for a Fortune 500 company. Her career trajectory has gone well for her, and she has received two promotions since starting at her company 3 years ago. Cassandra met Anthony through mutual friends, and the couple has been married for the past 5 years. Cassandra described Anthony as the love of her life and her "rock." She reported that Anthony was less professionally accomplished because he could not seem to "catch a break" but was very intelligent, "kind of a nerd," and a wonderful man. Cassandra elaborated that Anthony had been struggling for some time to make the transition to a more professional position that would be a better fit for his intellect and ability. Although Anthony was often successful in securing interviews, and even in making it to finalist status in searches, he was never the ultimate choice for the positions to which he applied.

Over the course of several months, Anthony's near-hire experiences were starting to weigh on the couple. As Anthony grew more discouraged and depressed, Cassandra grew more disappointed in and frustrated with him. Although she had an acute awareness of systemic racism and its impact on hiring practices, as well as the impact of racial microaggressions, which she experienced all day at work in her mostly White corporate setting, Cassandra began to internalize a perception of Anthony as weak and ineffectual. She attributed her feelings to Anthony's lack of success in securing a better position, as well as his inability to deal effectively with his boss.

Clinical Decisions: Intervention Implementation

Two experiences reported by Cassandra provided the opportunity to enhance her ability to better understand her husband's reaction to his unsuccessful job searches and related depressive and other symptoms. Cassandra reported that she and Anthony were out for a walk at dusk one evening. As they encountered a White woman who appeared to be of similar age walking in their direction, Anthony quickly took Cassandra's hand and started leading her to move the two of them into the street. Cassandra was shocked and insulted when she realized that Anthony was leading her into the street so that the woman would not have to share the sidewalk or "have to walk by two Black people." As Cassandra was accustomed to feeling protected and cherished by her husband, she was wounded by what she experienced as his attending to the "comfort" of the White stranger over her.

Soon after this experience, Cassandra and Anthony were on their way to her aunt's house to drop off money to contribute to a large family gathering that was being planned for the holidays. After driving around the block several times, Anthony finally parked about a block away from her aunt's home, which was in a predominantly Black neighborhood in the city. Cassandra was already frustrated, unable to understand Anthony's multiple trips around the block, only to end up in the parking space that was available the whole time. Cassandra concluded that Anthony was just "too lazy to walk the block" to her aunt's house. Cassandra became further frustrated when Anthony hesitated after getting out of the car, then walked quickly ahead of her, reaching her aunt's house when she was still about a half a block away. When Cassandra angrily confronted her husband for his "bizarre" behavior, especially since they were familiar with her aunt's neighborhood and it was broad daylight, Anthony reminded her that he was carrying the large sum of money and that a few young adult males were "hanging out" on the block. This explanation infuriated Cassandra. As they were both subjected to **microaggressions** on a daily basis, she felt that Anthony's assumption that he would be robbed in her aunt's neighborhood was an act of microaggression toward the young men who lived on the block. She also felt it was a cowardly act and reported that she had to restrain herself from screaming at him to "man up!" Finally, Cassandra was also disheartened by what she again experienced as Anthony's total disregard for her. "If you felt so unsafe, then why did you just run off and leave me?!" she inquired.

The couple's session that followed built on the work that had been done with Cassandra around the microaggressions she experienced, to help her put her husband's experiences and reactions in context. Starting with the session's presenting concerns of the couple, which for Cassandra was Anthony's lack of resilience and perseverance and for Anthony was Cassandra's lack of compassion and understanding, the concept of the emic (insider) versus etic (outsider) perspective was introduced. Anthony was then invited to share his job search experiences and Cassandra was asked to try to walk alongside him to hear Anthony's lived experience from his unique perspective as an African American male. Hardy's (2013) model for racial healing was used to facilitate Anthony's sharing the wounds of racial oppression (internalized devaluation, assaulted sense of self, and internalized voicelessness) he experienced as a result of various gendered racial microaggressions he encountered, both in his current position and on every job search—this, in addition to the daily experiences he had "breathing while Black."

Although Cassandra was able to recognize and acknowledge her husband's experiences, she continued to have difficulty understanding why he was not more resilient and persevering in his efforts to find a new job. She was further irritated that he had not stood up to and filed a complaint against his current White female supervisor, who was **overt** in her differential treatment of him and had engaged in a number of gendered microaggressions against him, the only African American male on her team. It was clear from Anthony's response that he had made a conscious decision not to act against his supervisor. Nadal (2011) recommended a three-step process that involves assessing the occurrence of a microaggression, deciding whether to respond, and deciding how to respond. Seeing this reflective process through Anthony's eyes helped Cassandra realize that Anthony's gender, size, complexion, prior life experiences, racial socialization, and personality were factors that resulted in decisions that were different from hers. It was also sobering for Cassandra to realize that qualities she found so attractive in Anthony were qualities that he had been taught to downplay in certain situations to be perceived as "less threatening." Cassandra was proud to have a "big, Brown, teddy bear" husband, as he made her feel protected, and she looked forward to the "beautiful brown babies" they would make together. Even though Cassandra recognized that many in mainstream society likely had a very different perception of Anthony when they saw him, she had failed to take into consideration the fact that prospective and current employers might see what strangers saw: a big, Black, potentially dangerous man.

The next intervention for the couple was to revisit the two recent experiences that Anthony and Cassandra had when out together. Anthony's experiences and responses reflect two more powerful consequences of microaggressions: anticipatory anxiety and compensatory behaviors, and internalized racism and its external manifestations. Anthony was able to share how his work and job search experiences had fueled his internalized self-devaluation and negative self-esteem. These and similar experiences caused Anthony to experience anxiety during both actual and anticipated interactions with White people, leading to compromised performance in his interviews, despite his qualifications. These experiences also led Anthony to (unsuccessfully) minimize the way he was being treated at his job in an effort not to react in a way that could be interpreted as aggressive or perceived as a problem. From here, Cassandra was able to gently interpret Anthony's actions during their recent walk as a desire to move away to avoid another potential encounter of being perceived as dangerous by a White person. She could also now see that Anthony's instinct was to protect her as well. Cassandra also listened intently as Anthony shared what was happening for him the day they went to her aunt's house. The couple was then able to benefit from an exploration of the internalized racism that caused Anthony to judge the young African American men in the neighborhood (scary, dangerous, threatening) in the same way that he was judged by White people and had internalized. Anthony was also able to share with Cassandra that his walking ahead of her was not an act of disregard for her safety—rather the opposite: If someone saw the bulge of the money in his pocket and tried to rob him, Cassandra would be out of harm's way.

Exploration of racial wounds and their consequences and an increased understanding of the ways in which gender, size, complexion, and other personal attributes and experiences can influence the types and content of microaggressions that individuals experience can increase a couple's ability to serve as vital resources of support, understanding, and healing for one another.

Clinical Expertise and Interpretation of Evidence: Latinx Families

Latinx families' experiences of discrimination, **microaggression**, and the resulting stress can be both debilitating and destructive, leaving broken individuals and families in their wake. In her research, Davis highlights several mental health symptoms associated with discrimination against Latinx individuals including suicidal ideation, depression, anxiety, and general distress.

These individual struggles can spread throughout the entire family unit through *emotional contagion* (Fischer, 2007), which poses a particular threat to Latinx families, given the highly cherished cultural value of family identity above individual identity. This emotional contagion is often extended beyond the family unit to include the Latinx community as a whole, as even those who are of legal status (citizens or legal residents) often experience the stress of those at risk of deportation, confined to detention centers, or separated at the border from their loved ones. A primary source of **minority stress** for Latinx individuals and their families results from discrimination and micro-aggressions occurring in schools. Such experiences often lead to truancy, encounters with the justice system, and existential threats to the family unit. The case study that follows and the accompanying therapeutic intervention focus one such example.

Clinical Experience: Observations of Common Interactional Patterns
Although many Latinx individuals and families are fluent in English, there are many families in which some or all members either speak only Spanish or have a limited knowledge of English. In many cases, this occurs along generational lines, where parents, grandparents, and other elders primarily speak Spanish and younger adults and children are proficient, if not fluent, in English and Spanish (or "Spanglish," as Davis mentioned). In first-generation immigrant families, however, there may be no one family member with any knowledge of English. As Davis indicated, in the United States there is extensive use of English-only signage and written materials (even though one in six Americans speak Spanish). This form of **microaggression** makes it even more challenging for Latinx families not only to navigate the challenges of everyday life in the majority culture but to access resources and essential information as well. As a result, like other marginalized groups. Latinx families gravitate toward their own isolated communities.

This is a prime example of what Davis referred to as the process of being "subjected to legalized exclusion" and systemic discrimination, and it ultimately creates a sense of invisibility and voiceless. Although Latinx families might in one sense perceive this invisibility as a protection against being targeted by powerful others who could hurt them in a multitude of ways, this invisibility ultimately becomes disempowering: The more one sacrifices their voice for protection, the less they can use it to demand their rights and to advocate for themselves, their loved ones, and their community.

The effects of this legalized exclusion and systemic discrimination, along with the experience of disempowerment, is often seen in Latinx individuals and families either seeking or referred for mental health treatment and other related services. In many cases, especially where teenagers are concerned, the referral is the result of negative interactions with the educational or criminal justice systems. In many cases, treatment has been mandated by the courts. Often, this path to mandated treatment begins at school where the teenager has faced both discrimination (e.g., ethnically based bullying by peers) or (more commonly) a pervasive pattern of microaggressions that is reflected in a lack of bilingual classrooms, English-only signage and textbooks, and little, if any, attention from the English-only speaking faculty. As a result, the student feels lost academically, experiences boredom, and ultimately perceives school as aversive. In addition to poor grades and a sense of failure, the student often internalizes the negative ethnic stereotypes directed at them by others. Seeking an escape from these negative feelings and experiences, looking for a way out, the student may begin skipping school and gravitate toward antisocial behaviors, such as gang involvement or drug use. Eventually, this leads to involvement with the criminal justice system and family courts. At this point, the family is brought into the picture. However, they often feel helpless and unable to advocate for their child, as they too are subjected to systemic, pervasive microaggressions, and discrimination in the justice system. When the student is sentenced to a juvenile criminal facility or residential treatment center, the family is torn apart: The teenager feels abandoned by their parents, and the parents feel a sense of failure and hopelessness.

Case Context: Characteristics, Culture, and Preferences

Maria and Juan came to the agency seeking services for their 16-year-old son Carlos, who was about to be released from a court-ordered 4-month stay in a residential treatment center for substance abuse. The family had only moved to the United States from Puerto Rico 8 months earlier, had little English proficiency, and appeared very distressed and unsure about "the right thing to do." Maria and Juan explained in Spanish that they were confused and anxious about the situation, including the court hearing that had led to Carlos being placed in an inpatient setting. They expressed shock at the memory of seeing their son physically removed at the end of the hearing without any explanation. The court proceedings had been conducted in English, with no interpreter, and they could not understand what was taking place. They explained that Carlos had been a "regular" kid in Puerto Rico. There, he had been close to his family, had always maintained average grades, had lots of friends, and was never involved in serious trouble—including any use of illegal substances.

During the initial sessions, which consisted of both family and individual sessions with Carlos, it became clear that the family had a strong, healthy emotional connection with one another. However, Maria and Juan expressed uncertainty about how to parent Carlos in their new environment. They felt they had failed in their parental duties and were responsible for "losing" him during the court proceeding. Carlos said, "I'm ashamed I caused my parents pain and stress" and that he was confused about how to behave as an adolescent in north Philadelphia.

At this point in the session, the family was asked to recount the events leading up to Carlos's court appearance. As the story unfolded, it became clear that both the educational system and judicial systems failed them on a number of fronts. The family explained that several months before Carlos's arrival at high school, the school administration had discontinued bilingual courses due to a lack of funding. These classes were essential for Spanish-speaking students such as Carlos, who would not be able to understand the material in mainstream, English-language classes. As time went by, he grew bored and felt embarrassed when the teachers called on him because he could not understand what they were saying. Eventually, the teachers began to ignore him. In other words, they lowered their expectations of him. As pointed out by Davis, "low expectations" in this context are a form of micro-aggression. As a result, Carlos felt invisible and that he "didn't matter."

It is apparent from this recounting of events that Carlos and his family had faced systemic discrimination and microaggressions. In the educational context, Carlos was prevented from having an opportunity to be taught in a language he could understand. In addition, the school failed to contact his parents during Carlos's absences, thus preventing them from exercising their parental roles. During the subsequent court proceedings, no interpreter was provided, which left Maria and Juan unable to understand what was happening or provide any input during the hearing. In other words, their voices were silenced. Carlos and his parents described the experience in court as a traumatic event, especially when he was forcibly taken away with no explanation that they could understand.

Clinical Decisions: Intervention Implementation

It was clear the family's experiences with the educational and judicial systems had severely damaged their sense of identity and value, both individually and as a whole. Because they would continue to exist as a marginalized family, most likely encountering future instances of discrimination and **micro-aggression**, an immediate goal in therapy was to help them become more resilient. Toward this end, Davis pointed out the importance of family members viewing "themselves as a team facing a common obstacle." Thus, it was essential to help them rediscover and reconnect with the experiences that had previously formed their identities.

Narrative therapy approaches by White and Epston (1990) were instrumental in identifying the family members' needs and ultimately guiding the interventions used in the family work. A modified reauthoring process was used to help the family reconnect with their identities in Puerto Rico before the discrimination and microaggression they had experienced after coming to Philadelphia. Carey and Russel (2003) explained this process as taking the form of dialogues between therapists and clients. It comprises the naming and cocreation of alternative identity stories. Ultimately, the reauthoring process involves the coauthoring of storylines that will help clients address the presenting problem.

Family members were invited to bring photographs of themselves to help convey how different their lives had been in Puerto Rico. They brought pictures of various celebrations, birthdays, and holidays. Using the process prescribed by narrative therapy, they were asked to describe the different events in terms of a story—their story as a family. They appeared happy, engaged, and easily interacted with one another. To help them reconnect with their previous identities, the therapist highlighted instances of good parenting, affection toward one another, and resiliency. It was crucial that each family member reconnect with and appreciate who they were and, most importantly, who they continue to be. The trauma caused by their experiences of discrimination and microaggressions separated them from each other and from their own identities, but shared life experiences recorded in their photos brought them back together.

Davis also mentioned that marginalized youth, after experiences of discrimination, start to doubt their abilities. Given Carlos's developmental stage, he needed to find his own unique identity, which was at the same time separate, yet still connected, to his family. He talked about his previous interest in writing lyrics to *boleros*—slow-tempo romantic music that has been popularized throughout Latin America for decades. He also disclosed that he had given up on writing songs, saying, "I felt so dumb for not being able to learn English fast enough and understand classes." In therapy, he worked on *externalizing* his perceived challenges and correctly placing them in the school system. This process helped Carlos realize that he did not fail; rather, the school system failed *him* by not providing essential resources to succeed. He began to truly recognize that it was not he who had failed, but rather the school and judicial systems. Soon after, he began to write boleros again and use his voice to talk about a brighter future.

Clinical Expertise and Interpretation of Evidence: Queer Families

As Davis indicated in the research section, an important foundation for clinicians and other service providers working with queer families is to understand both the within-group diversity of queer families and the larger sociopolitical and historical contexts of heteronormativity and cisnormativity that fuel the **microaggressions** and discrimination that queer families experience. The term *queer family* can be used to refer to a variety of individuals who identify with a minority sexual or gender identity and or gender minority, along with their partner(s), child(ren), parent(s), or other family members. Queer families are constructed through diverse representations of gender, sexual orientation and identity, and family structure. Consider these four examples, which are just a subset of the myriad constellations of queer families that clinicians and service providers may encounter: An adolescent who has recently disclosed their bisexual identity to their heterosexual, cisgender parents presents with their parents and sibling; a male-identified couple comes in seeking to enhance their communication; a lesbian-identified female seeks services to better support her transgender partner who is exploring gender-confirming surgeries; and a cisgender male, his wife, and their girlfriend enter therapy to discuss concerns that have emerged among them about how they can all be involved in raising their three school-age children.

Clinical Experience: Observations of Common Interactional Patterns
It is impossible to understand how the stress from **microaggressions** and discrimination impacts queer clients without recognizing how such acts are supported by the larger social context. *Heteronormativity* is the belief that heterosexuality is the norm, or expected, sexual orientation. That is, everyone is heterosexual unless otherwise stated. *Cisnormativity* involves the assumption that one's gender identity is aligned with one's assigned gender at birth (i.e., everyone is cisgender unless otherwise stated). These belief systems perpetuate marginalization, which in turn fuels prejudice and even unconscious or implicit bias about such identities. The historical legacy of discriminatory laws and policies have an impact on queer individuals and their families on a daily basis. Same-sex marriage has only been legal at the national level since 2015, there are no federal nondiscrimination protections for sexual orientation and gender identity; 2019 and 2020 saw the largest number of antitransgender law bills being considered in state legislatures across the country.

There are several ways clinicians working with queer families can convey an understanding of the impact of stress from microaggressions and discrimination. First, an ecological systems framework can assist the clinician in recognizing how bidirectional influences between multiple systems can shape clients' experiences, including the presenting problem. Heteronormativity and cisnormativity are macrosystemic influences that shape interactions between individuals, couples, families, and other microsystems in which queer families interact, such as schools, places of work, religious institutions. An ecological systems framework can guide assessment to explore experiences of discrimination in various contexts and how these experiences are affecting the presenting problem. Second, the **minority stress** model (Meyer, 2003) encourages clinicians to understand the ways in which proximal and distal stressors influence negative health outcomes. Acknowledging the potential role of this stress explicitly with queer clients communicates an affirming clinical stance that realizes a minority identity status does not cause **health disparities**. Further, the model posits that community and social support can provide a buffer against this stress. Exploring these factors can provide opportunities to build coping strategies to reduce the impact of this stress on queer families.

There are no evidence-based clinical interventions for queer families that specifically target discrimination and microaggressions. However, LGBTQ+ affirmative therapy practice is a more general approach for working with LGBTQ+ individuals and their families that recognizes that a sexual or gender minoritized identity is not a mental illness and implores clinicians to acknowledge the influence of a heteronormative and cisnormative society on the lives of our queer clients. The case described here is situated within this approach.

Case Context: Characteristics, Culture, and Preferences

Hailey and Sky present to couples therapy for help in decision making about parenthood. Hailey uses she/her/hers pronouns and identifies as a Black, bisexual, cisgender woman. Sky uses they/them/theirs pronouns and identifies as White, queer, and gender nonbinary and was assigned female at birth. The couple has been together for 6 years and has always planned on raising children together. Hailey grew up in a large, accepting family and enjoyed being surrounded by many family members throughout her adolescent years. Sky has only one sister and is somewhat disconnected from their mother and father. The information from the intake paperwork tells the therapist the couple's names and that they are coming to therapy for help with parenting decisions. On the basis of their names, the therapist assumes that they are a cisgender, lesbian couple. During the first session, the therapist asks the couple about their experiences being a lesbian couple who are pursuing parenthood. Although the couple is able to correct the therapist, they have experienced this with other providers and feel uncomfortable about having to correct others. Sky expresses that one of the options they have talked about is Sky carrying a child for them but is worried about being misgendered throughout their pregnancy. Every time the couple discusses this issue, Hailey reports that she struggles with how to respond to Sky's concerns.

Clinical Decisions: Intervention Implementation

The therapist realized her mistake and was able to begin the next session by socially locating herself and saying to the clients, "I'd like to start again. My pronouns are she/her/hers, I am cisgender and straight. Could you tell me about your identities and pronouns?" This spurred a conversation about the clients' intersecting identities and how each of their identities influenced the other's. The therapist was able to ask gender neutral questions about each partner's dating history and provide space to allow the couple to talk about past experiences. Throughout this process, the therapist made sure to immerse herself in literature around LGBTQ-affirmative therapy practices.

The therapist asked the clients about what each hoped for and was concerned about in terms of parenting. The therapist also asked about their experiences with **microaggressions** and discrimination in the past. Sky explained that they had experienced being misgendered at the doctor's office and was particularly concerned about how much they would be able to feel affirmed in their gender, given the very gendered atmosphere surrounding pregnancy. At that point, the therapist stated, "These events occur so quickly that it is best to have practiced a response so that you are able to respond naturally and without excess emotions." Thus, examples of possible comments were generated, and Sky and Hailey practiced possible responses to confront, in a healthy manner, moments of being misgendered. The couple also discussed concerns around who will help them in the pregnancy and birthing process. The therapist made a point of asking "who is important in your lives?" along with other questions that allowed the clients to discuss both their chosen family as well as the support of Hailey's birth family.

Conclusion

A major contributor to a family's experiencing minority stress is the presence of microaggressions and discrimination. When one or multiple members of a family unit experience legalized exclusion, disempowerment, and systemic injustices, the functioning of the entire family system suffers. When a clinician is unable to fully grasp the impact of microaggressions aimed at a family, the family is retraumatized. To avoid retraumatizing already marginalized families, it is paramount that clinicians be aware of their own bias and become highly attuned to microaggressions, macroaggressions, and societal prejudice that impact the families with whom they work. To effectively treat and support marginalized families, proximal and distal stressors must be incorporated in the clinical space and targeted efforts to support these families through systemic injustices must be at the forefront of the work.

REFERENCES

Adair, J. K. (2015). *The impact of discrimination on the early schooling experiences of children from immigrant families*. Migration Policy Institute.

Allport, G. W. (1954). Traits due to victimization. In *The nature of prejudice* (pp. 142–162). Basic Books.

Arora, P. G., Wheeler, L. A., Fisher, S., & Barnes, J. (2017). A prospective examination of anxiety as a predictor of depressive symptoms among Asian American early adolescent youth: The role of parent, peer, and teacher support and school engagement. *Cultural Diversity & Ethnic Minority Psychology, 23*(4), 541–550. https://doi.org/10.1037/cdp0000168

Ayón, C., & Philbin, S. P. (2017). "Tu no eres de aqui": Latino children's experiences of institutional and interpersonal discrimination and microaggressions. *Social Work Research, 41*(1), 19–30. https://doi.org/10.1093/swr/svw028

Baams, L., Wilson, B. D. M., & Russell, S. T. (2019). LGBTQ youth in unstable housing and foster care. *Pediatrics, 143*(3), 1–9. https://doi.org/10.1542/peds.2017-4211

Baldus, D. C., Woodworth, G., Zuckerman, D., & Weiner, N. A. (1998). Racial discrimination and the death penalty in the post-Furman era: An empirical and legal overview with recent findings from Philadelphia. *Cornell Law Review, 83*(6), 1638–1770. https://scholarship.law.cornell.edu/clr/vol83/iss6/6/

Bell, J. G., & Perry, B. (2015). Outside looking in: The community impacts of anti-lesbian, gay, and bisexual hate crime. *Journal of Homosexuality, 62*(1), 98–120. https://doi.org/10.1080/00918369.2014.957133

Bos, H. M. W., van Balen, F., van den Boom, D. C., & Sandfort, T. G. M. (2004). Minority stress, experience of parenthood and child adjustment in lesbian families. *Journal of Reproductive and Infant Psychology, 22*(4), 291–304. https://doi.org/10.1080/02646830412331298350

Cafferky, B. M., Mendez, M., Anderson, J. R., & Stith, S. M. (2018). Substance use and intimate partner violence: A meta-analytic review. *Psychology of Violence, 8*(1), 110–131. https://doi/org/10.1037/vio0000074

Carey, M., & Russell, S. (2003). Re-authoring: Some answers to commonly asked questions. *The International Journal of Narrative Therapy and Community Work, 2003*, 60. https://narrativepractices.com.au/attach/pdf/Re-Authoring_Commmonly_asked_questions.pdf

Center for the Study of Hate and Extremism. (2017). *Final U.S. status report: Hate crime analysis & forecast for 2016/2017*. California State University.

Centers for Disease Control and Prevention. (2020). *Demographic trends of COVID-19 cases and deaths in the US reported to CDC*. https://covid.cdc.gov/covid-data-tracker/#demographics

Civil Rights Act of 1964, Pub. L. 88–352, 78 Stat. 241 (1964).

Crosnoe, R. (2005). The diverse experiences of Hispanic students in the American educational system. *Sociological Forum, 20*(4), 561–588. https://doi.org/10.1007/s11206-005-9058-z

Davis, G. Y., & Stevenson, H. C. (2006). Racial socialization experiences and symptoms of depression among Black youth. *Journal of Child and Family Studies, 15*(3), 293–307. https://doi.org/10.1007/s10826-006-9039-8

D'Onofrio, M. (2019, March 3). Hate incidents in Philadelphia on the rise. *The Philadelphia Tribune*. https://www.phillytrib.com/news/local_news/hate-incidents-in-philadelphia-on-the-rise/article_c00cd65b-df7b-5ca1-a55d-d7dfb868f0ad.html

Eberhardt, J. L., Davies, P. G., Purdie-Vaughns, V. J., & Johnson, S. L. (2006). Looking deathworthy: Perceived stereotypicality of Black defendants predicts capital-sentencing outcomes. *Psychological Science, 17*(5), 383–386. https://doi.org/10.1111/j.1467-9280.2006.01716.x

Farr, R. H., Crain, E. E., Oakley, M. K., Cashen, K. K., & Garber, K. J. (2016). Microaggressions, feelings of difference, and resilience among adopted children with sexual minority parents. *Journal of Youth and Adolescence, 45*(1), 85–104. https://doi.org/10.1007/s10964-015-0353-6

Fischer, A. (2007). Emotional contagion. In R. F. Baumeister & K. D. Vohs (Eds.), *Encyclopedia of social psychology* (Vol. 1, pp. 292–293). SAGE Publications. https://doi.org/10.4135/9781412956253.n176

FitzGerald, C., & Hurst, S. (2017). Implicit bias in healthcare professionals: A systematic review. *BMC Medical Ethics, 18*(1), 19–36. https://doi.org/10.1186/s12910-017-0179-8

Friedman, M. S., Marshal, M. P., Guadamuz, T. E., Wei, C., Wong, C. F., Saewyc, E., & Stall, R. (2011). A meta-analysis of disparities in childhood sexual abuse, parental physical abuse, and peer victimization among sexual minority and sexual non-minority individuals. *American Journal of Public Health, 101*(8), 1481–1494. https://doi.org/10.2105/AJPH.2009.190009

Gartner, R. E., & Sterzing, P. R. (2018). Social ecological correlated of family-level interpersonal and environmental microaggressions toward sexual and gender minority adolescents. *Journal of Family Violence, 33*(1), 1–16. https://doi.org/10.1007/s10896-017-9937-0

Goff, B. S. N., Reisbig, A. M., Bole, A., Scheer, T., Hayes, E., Archuleta, K. L., Henry, S. B., Hoheisel, C. B., Nye, B., Osby, J., Sanders-Hahs, E., Schwerdtfeger, K. L., & Smith, D. B. (2006). The effects of trauma on intimate relationships: A qualitative study with clinical couples. *American Journal of Orthopsychiatry, 76*(4), 451–460. https://doi.org/10.1037/0002-9432.76.4.451

Goldberg, A. E. (2012). *Gay dads: Transitions to adoptive fatherhood.* New York University Press. https://doi.org/10.18574/nyu/9780814732236.001.0001

Gupta, A., Szymanski, D. M., & Leong, F. T. (2011). The "model minority myth": Internalized racialism of positive stereotypes as correlates of psychological distress, and attitudes toward help-seeking. *Asian American Journal of Psychology, 2*(2), 101–114. https://doi.org/10.1037/a0024183

Haines, K. M., Boyer, C. R., Giovanazzi, C., & Galupo, M. P. (2018). "Not a real family": Microaggressions directed toward LGBTQ families. *Journal of Homosexuality, 65*(9), 1138–1151. https://doi.org/10.1080/00918369.2017.1406217

Hardie, J. H., & Turney, K. (2017). The intergenerational consequences of parental health limitations. *Journal of Marriage and the Family, 79*(3), 801–815. https://doi.org/10.1111/jomf.12341

Hardy, K. V. (2013). Healing the hidden wounds of racial trauma: Enhancing professional and research training. *Reclaiming Children and Youth, 22*, 24–28

Huq, A. Z. (2017). The consequences of disparate policing: Evaluating stop and frisk as a modality of urban policing. *Minnesota Law Review, 178*, 2397–2480. https://scholarship.law.umn.edu/mlr/178

Hwang, W. C., & Goto, S. (2008). The impact of perceived racial discrimination on the mental health of Asian American and Latino college students. *Cultural Diversity & Ethnic Minority Psychology, 14*(4), 326–335. https://doi.org/10.1037/1099-9809.14.4.326

Javier, J. R., Lahiff, M., Ferrer, R. R., & Huffman, L. C. (2010). Examining depressive symptoms and use of counseling in the past year among Filipino and non-Hispanic white adolescents in California. *Journal of Developmental and Behavioral Pediatrics, 31*(4), 295–303. https://doi.org/10.1097/DBP.0b013e3181dbadc7

Jeong, R., & Nham, K. (2020). *Incidents of coronavirus-related discrimination: A report for A3PCON and CAA.* Asian Pacific Policy & Planning Council.

Jones, B. S., Sherman, J. W., Rojas, N. E., Hosek, A., Vannette, D. L., Rocha, R. R., García-Ponce, O., Pantoja, M., & García-Amador, J. M. (2021). Trump-induced anxiety among Latina/os. *Group Processes & Intergroup Relations, 24*(1), 68–87. 10.1177/1368430219889132

Koken, J., A., Bimbi, D. S., & Parsons, J. T. (2009). Experiences of familial acceptance–rejection among transwomen of color. *Journal of Family Psychology, 23*(6), 853–860. https://doi.org/10.1037/a0017198

Kosciw, J. G., Clark, C. M., Truong, N. L., & Zongrone, A. D. (2020). *The 2019 National School Climate Survey: The experiences of lesbian, gay, bisexual, transgender, and queer youth in our nation's schools.* GLSEN. https://www.glsen.org/sites/default/files/2021-04/NSCS19-FullReport-032421-Web_0.pdf

Liang, C. T., Li, L. C., & Kim, B. S. (2004). The Asian American racism-related stress inventory: Development, factor analysis, reliability, and validity. *Journal of Counseling Psychology, 51*(1), 103–114. https://doi.org/10.1037/0022-0167.51.1.103

Lyons, C. J., & Roberts, A. (2014). The difference "hate" makes in clearing crime: An event history analysis of incident factors. *Journal of Contemporary Criminal Justice, 30*(3), 268–289. https://doi.org/10.1177/1043986214536663

Martínez, R. A. (2013). Reading the world in Spanglish: Hybrid language practices and ideological contestation in a sixth-grade English language arts classroom. *Linguistics and Education, 24*(3), 276–288. https://doi.org/10.1016/j.linged.2013.03.007

Meyer, I. H. (2003). Prejudice, social stress, and mental health in lesbian, gay, and bisexual populations: Conceptual issues and research evidence. *Psychological Bulletin, 129*(5), 674–697. https://doi.org/10.1037/0033-2909.129.5.674

Mulder, T. M., Kuiper, K. C., van der Put, C. E., Stams, G. J. M., & Assink, M. (2018). Risk factors for child neglect: A meta-analytic review. *Child Abuse & Neglect: The International Journal, 77*, 198–210. https://doi.org/10.1016/j.chiabu.2018.01.006

Nadal, K. L. (2011). Responding to racial, gender, and sexual orientation microaggressions in the workplace. In M. A. Paludi, E. R. DeSouza, & C. A. Paludi Jr. (Eds.), *The Praeger handbook on understanding and preventing workplace discrimination: Legal, management, and social science perspectives* (pp. 23–32). Praeger/ABC-CLIO.

Nadal, K. L., Davidoff, K. C., Davis, L. S., Wong, Y., Marshall, D., & McKenzie, V. (2015). A qualitative approach to intersectional microaggressions: Understanding influences of race, ethnicity, gender, sexuality, and religion. *Qualitative Psychology, 2*(2), 147–163. https://doi.org/10.1037/qup0000026

Nadal, K. L., Davis, L. S., Stephens, A., & McLean, K. (2019). *How gender, sexual orientation, and education influence racial microaggressions among Black Americans: An exploratory study.* Manuscript submitted for publication.

Nadal, K. L., Griffin, K., Wong, Y., Davidoff, K., & Davis, L. S. (2017). The injurious relationship between racial microaggressions and physical health: Implications for social work. *Journal of Ethnic & Cultural Diversity in Social Work, 26*(1–2), 6–17. https://doi.org/10.1080/15313204.2016.1263813

Nadal, K. L., Griffin, K., Wong, Y., Hamit, S., & Rasmus, M. (2014). The impact of racial microaggressions on mental health: Counseling implications for clients of color. *Journal of Counseling and Development, 92*(1), 57–66. https://doi.org/10.1002/j.1556-6676.2014.00130.x

Nadal, K. L., King, R., Sissoko, D. R. G., Floyd, N., & Hines, D. (2021). The legacies of systemic and internalized oppression: Experiences of microaggressions, imposter phenomenon, and stereotype threat on historically marginalized groups. *New Ideas in Psychology, 63*, 1–9. https://doi.org/10.1037/cdp0000161

Nadal, K. L., Sriken, J., Davidoff, K. C., Wong, Y., & McLean, K. (2013). Microaggressions within families: Experiences of multiracial people. *Family Relations, 62*(1), 190–201. https://doi.org/10.1111/j.1741-3729.2012.00752.x

Nadal, K. L., Whitman, C. N., Davis, L. S., Erazo, T., & Davidoff, K. C. (2016). Microaggressions toward lesbian, gay, bisexual, transgender, queer, and genderqueer people: A review of the literature. *Journal of Sex Research, 53*(4–5), 488–508. https://doi.org/10.1080/00224499.2016.1142495

Obergefell v. Hodges, 576 U.S. 644 (2015).

Pager, D., & Western, B. (2012). Identifying discrimination at work: The use of field experiments. *Journal of Social Issues, 68*(2), 221–237. https://doi.org/10.1111/j.1540-4560.2012.01746.x

Perez Huber, L., Huidor, O., Malagon, M. C., Sanchez, G., & Solórzano, D. G. (2006). *Falling through the cracks: Critical transitions in the Latina/o educational pipeline, 2006 Latina/o Education Summit Report.* UCLA Chicano Studies Research Center. https://files.eric.ed.gov/fulltext/ED493397.pdf

Pew Research Center. (2020, August 8). *About one-in-four U.S. Hispanics have heard of Latinx, but just 3% use it.* https://www.pewresearch.org/hispanic/wp-content/uploads/sites/5/2020/08/PHGMD_2020.08.11_Latinx_FINAL.pdf

Pickett, J. T., Chiricos, T., Golden, K. M., & Gertz, M. (2012). Reconsidering the relationship between neighborhood racial composition and Whites' perceptions of victimization risk: Do racial stereotypes matter? *Criminology, 50*(1), 145–186. https://doi.org/10.1111/j.1745-9125.2011.00255.x

Sadler, M. S., Correll, J., Park, B., & Judd, C. M. (2012). The world is not black and white: Racial bias in the decision to shoot in a multiethnic context. *Journal of Social Issues, 68*(2), 286–313. https://doi.org/10.1111/j.1540-4560.2012.01749.x

Semple, K. (2020, August 6). After a lull, the number of migrants trying to enter the U.S. has soared. *The New York Times.* https://www.nytimes.com/2020/08/06/world/americas/mexico-immigration-usa.html

Simon, G. E. (2003). Social and economic burden of mood disorders. *Biological Psychiatry, 54*(3), 208–215. https://doi.org/10.1016/S0006-3223(03)00420-7

Smith, E. R., & Mackie, D. M. (2016). Group-level emotions. *Current Opinion in Psychology, 11*, 15–19. https://doi.org/10.1016/j.copsyc.2016.04.005

Speight, S. L. (2007). Internalized racism: One more piece of the puzzle. *The Counseling Psychologist, 35*(1), 126–134. https://doi.org/10.1177/0011000006295119

Steele, C. M., & Aronson, J. (1995). Stereotype threat and the intellectual test performance of African Americans. *Journal of Personality and Social Psychology, 69*(5), 797–811. https://doi.org/10.1037/0022-3514.69.5.797

Sue, D. W., Capodilupo, C. M., Torino, G. C., Bucceri, J. M., Holder, A. M. B., Nadal, K. L., & Esquilin, M. (2007). Racial microaggressions in everyday life: Implications for clinical practice. *American Psychologist, 62*(4), 271–286. https://doi.org/10.1037/0003-066X.62.4.271

Sue, D. W., & Sue, D. (2013). *Counseling the culturally diverse: Theory and practice.* John Wiley & Sons.

Toomey, R. B., Ryan, C., Diaz, R. M., Card, N. A., & Russell, S. T. (2010). Gender-nonconforming lesbian, gay, bisexual, and transgender youth: School victimization and young adult psychosocial adjustment. *Developmental Psychology, 46*(6), 1580–1589. https://doi.org/10.1037/a0020705

Tull, E. S., Sheu, Y. T., Butler, C., & Cornelious, K. (2005). Relationships between perceived stress, coping behavior and cortisol secretion in women with high and low levels of internalized racism. *Journal of the National Medical Association, 97*(2), 206–212.

U.S. Department of Labor. (2019). *Labor force statistics from the Current Population Survey.* https://data.bls.gov/cps

Waters, E., Doyle., J., Wolfe, R., Wright, M., Wake, M., & Salmon, L. (2000). Influence of parental gender and self-reported health and illness on parent-reported child health. *Pediatrics, 106*(6), 1422–1428. https://doi.org/10.1542/peds.106.6.1422

Western, B., & Lopoo, L. (2004). *Incarceration, marriage, and family life.* Department of Sociology, Princeton University.

White, M., & Epston, D. (1990). *Narrative means to therapeutic ends.* WW Norton.

Wingo, E., Ingraham, N., & Roberts, S. C. M. (2018). Reproductive health care priorities and barriers to effective care for LGBTQ people assigned female at birth: A qualitative study. *Women's Health Issues, 28*(4), 350–357. https://doi.org/10.1016/j.whi.2018.03.002

Wisconsin v. Mitchell, 508 U.S. 47 (1993).

Wong-Padoongpatt, G., Zane, N., Okazaki, S., & Saw, A. (2017). Decreases in implicit self-esteem explain the racial impact of microaggressions among Asian Americans. *Journal of Counseling Psychology, 64*(5), 574–583. https://doi.org/10.1037/cou0000217

4

COUPLE INSTABILITY

A Focus on Fragile Families, Stepfamilies, Families With a Child on the Autism Spectrum, and Multiracial Families

RESEARCH: FRANCESCA ADLER-BAEDER AND KIM D. GREGSON
CLINICAL APPLICATIONS: C. WAYNE JONES, PATRICIA L. PAPERNOW, SCOTT BROWNING, KELLEY KENNEY, AND MARK KENNEY

RESEARCH: FRANCESCA ADLER-BAEDER AND KIM D. GREGSON

Research on couple instability, particularly earlier work, was built either implicitly or explicitly on family development assumptions of "normative" relationship progression (Sprenkle & Piercy, 1992), and little attention was given to context and characteristics of couples (Karney & Bradbury, 2020). As research on couple instability progressed to match the diversity of couples' demographics and contexts, specialized information has emerged that serves to inform clinical practice and intervention. This chapter provides research information and clinical guidelines for work with several specific types of families in which couples may face a number of challenges that threaten stability: fragile family couples (a term used to describe low-income, non-married partners expecting a child or having a child under age 3), couples with a child on the autism spectrum, stepfamily couples, and multiracial couples. The bulk of research on each of these couple types has focused on cisgender, different-gender couples, and thus the literature review and clinical guidelines are limited to those partnerships.

https://doi.org/10.1037/0000280-004
Treating Contemporary Families: Toward a More Inclusive Clinical Practice, S. Browning and B. van Eeden-Moorefield (Editors)

Note that *stability* is often measured in research as married–divorced or together–separated. As such, research consistently demonstrates that stability and couple relationship quality are related but not always highly correlated (Karney & Bradbury, 2020). Individuals may stay in relationships due to constraints that exist in some commitments, such as religious beliefs discouraging or disallowing separation, economic limitations and employability of each partner, or safety concerns that serve as barriers to separation (Stanley et al., 2010). We assume a primary goal of therapy is enhancing partners' sense of stability and relationship quality rather than solely focusing on keeping couples together. As such, we include in our research summary an emphasis on predictors of couple relationship quality in each of the family types rather than focusing only on predictors of relationship stability. Further, we use a risk and resilience perspective that assumes couples face risk to their stability in varying degrees over time and protective factors serve as intervention targets to promote resilience in the face of those risks (Falconier et al., 2016). This approach undergirds a prevention science approach to research-informed practice (Wandersman et al., 2008).

Across the specific areas of research on the four types of couples, we find some common themes among families (see Table 4.1). Successfully addressing these challenges can lead to greater couple satisfaction and stability. We summarize the research on ways in which each of these manifests within the different couple contexts and present unique factors for each couple type evident in the research that also may be considered in intervention strategies. For each of the four types of couples, we also present a clinical case with an intervention focus that is informed by the research. Psychoeducation, an important component of many couple therapists, plays a particularly critical role in the interventions described.

Research Evidence on Fragile Families

Research on fragile families emphasizes their demographic makeup and the ideal timing for intervention. The Fragile Families and Child Wellbeing Study followed 3,712 children born to unmarried parents over 5 years and found the couples to be primarily in their 20s, low-income/education, and racial/ethnic minorities (Black or Hispanic; Carlson & Högnäs, 2011; McLanahan & Beck, 2010). Further, researchers identify a "magic moment" (McLanahan et al., 2010) for intervention as the prenatal and early postnatal period, when couples reevaluate their relationship investments (e.g., emotional attachment, finances, living arrangements; Carlson & Högnäs, 2011; McHale & Rotman, 2007). By the child's first birthday a large portion of the couples were no longer together (McLanahan et al., 2010).

TABLE 4.1. Couple Instability

Evidence-based area of clinical focus	Type of factor	Appropriateness for use across families	Selected references indicating evidence base
Supportive communication	General	All[a]	Tach & Edin, 2013
Shared responsibility and teamwork	General	All	Sim, Cordier, et al., 2019; Sim, Fristedt, et al., 2019
Social networks/external support	General	All	Sim et al., 2016
Economic stability and financial resources	General	All	Carlson et al., 2004
Family complexity	Unique	Fragile, stepfamilies	Raley & Sweeney, 2020
Asymmetrical attachment	Unique	Fragile, autism spectrum, stepfamilies	Sim, Fristedt, et al., 2019
Aggression/violence	Unique	Fragile, multiracial	Fusco, 2010
Prioritizing couple relationships	Unique	Stepfamilies, autism spectrum, multiracial	Isacco et al., 2010
Coparenting and maternal gate-keeping	Unique	Fragile, stepfamilies	Carlson & Högnäs, 2011
Substance use	Unique	Fragile	Carlson & Högnäs, 2011
Cognitive appraisals	Unique	Autism spectrum	García-López et al., 2016
Racism and racial identity	Unique	Multiracial	Afful et al., 2015; Killian, 2001
Parent role clarity	Unique	Stepfamilies	Ganong & Coleman, 2017

[a]All = This general factor should work with most of the general population.

Studies indicate negative communication patterns are prevalent in the often-ambiguous relationships of fragile families. In qualitative studies with fragile families, tense/conflictual communication was prevalent (Waller, 2008) and cited as a primary reason for dissolution (Reed, 2009). In contrast, **supportive communication** (e.g., expressing love/encouragement, compromise, loyalty, infrequent criticism) between unmarried parents was associated with more **cooperative coparenting** (Carlson & Högnäs, 2011) and greater couple stability (Carlson et al., 2004; Tach & Edin, 2013). As unmarried parents attempt to manage the stress related to communicating, coparenting, uncertainty in relationship status, and economic vulnerabilities (Jamison et al., 2017; McLanahan & Beck, 2010; Seltzer, 2000), mental health challenges are prominent and influence coparenting (Carlson & Högnäs, 2011), as well as couple relationship quality (Isacco et al., 2010). Relatedly, fathers' drug or alcohol problems in fragile families were associated with more disengagement and less couple stability (Carlson et al., 2004).

In addition, the normative strain of raising young children may be exacerbated by fragile families' commitment ambiguity and complications involved in coparenting (Laxman et al., 2013). There is some indication that Black partners may be at a slight advantage because nonresident coparenting is more normative in the Black community (Carlson et al., 2004); mothers reported that nonresident Black fathers (compared with White or Hispanic) were more supportive coparents (Ellerbe et al., 2018). To manage the strains of new parenting, limited resources, and complex relationships, partners' emotional and instrumental support and shared family responsibilities are essential. Broadly, research finds that cohabiting partners, compared with married couples, have more egalitarian beliefs (Seltzer, 2000); however, in these often ambiguous, complex families, arguments over household and childcare tasks are common (Waller, 2008). Thus, collaboration is a crucial skill for family stability and is linked with more frequent, engaged father involvement in fragile families (Waller, 2012).

Importantly, the complex system of relational and parenting challenges faced by fragile families is embedded in strained economic conditions and is of primary concern. Within the couple, resource-sharing decisions are often contentious and deter couple commitment and stability (Gibson-Davis et al., 2005; Tach & Edin, 2013). In contrast, economic supports and advancement for men in fragile families promotes stability and commitment to long-term relationships and marriage (Carlson et al., 2004). Accordingly, fragile families researchers suggest that family resource management is a pertinent intervention target, promoting resiliency as well as effective coparenting (Jamison et al., 2017). Accompanying their financial challenges, fragile families often experience limited external support and even criticism from family and friends. They face a lack of practical support as well as societal and legal challenges (e.g., custody, access to health insurance, hospital visitation) because their family structure is often not formally recognized by the state (Carlson & Högnäs, 2011; Seltzer, 2000).

Several more unique challenges for fragile families emerge as well. Often these couples have a complex family structure due to multiple partner fertility (MPF)—that is, having child(ren) from prior partner(s)—with more than half (59%) of fragile families reporting MPF, compared with 21% of married couples (Carlson & Furstenberg, 2006). Prior children (and partners) can overextend couples' resources. Women with MPF status in the Fragile Families study reported decreases over time in access to money, housing, and child support

(Harknett & Knab, 2007). For the couple relationship, MPF has deleterious effects on coparenting (Carlson & Högnäs, 2011) and couple commitment due to jealousy, mistrust, or sexual infidelity related to previous partners (e.g., Reed, 2009). However, fathers' job status, supportive coparenting, and family engagement serve as protective factors for these MPF couples, promoting their couple stability (Petren et al., 2018).

Also prominent in the research on fragile families is the practice of maternal **gate-keeping** (e.g., criticism, control of family tasks, rules, and time with child), which presents barriers to father involvement in the child's life (Hohmann-Marriott, 2009). This practice is related to **family complexity**, commitment uncertainty, and issues with child support. When "gate-opening" (e.g., encouragement, facilitation) is evident, fathers are more engaged with children (Fagan & Cherson, 2017) and related couple closeness and stability are higher (Hohmann-Marriott, 2009; Olsavsky et al., 2019). Accumulated research suggests that father involvement and couple closeness and stability have bidirectional associations (e.g., McClain, 2011; McClain & Brown, 2017; McLanahan & Beck, 2010; Sobolewski & King, 2005).

Further, research suggests that fragile families, due to their multilayered challenges, are susceptible to unhealthy and abusive relationships (Reed, 2009; Waller & Swisher, 2006), and thus interventions generally promoting commitment and stability may be unwise. The relationship volatility and mental health and substance use issues that often characterize these abusive partnerships (Carlson & Högnäs, 2011) can override constraints that economic conditions and shared parenting may impose, leading to higher rates of relationship dissolution that are in the best interests of the partner and child(ren) (Carlson et al., 2004; Waller & Swisher, 2006). In qualitative interviews with unmarried parents, mothers recounted that partner physical abuse and concomitant drug use were primary reasons they ended the relationship (Waller & Swisher, 2006).

Research Evidence on Families With a Child on the Autism Spectrum

A small but growing body of research on couples with a child with an autism spectrum disorder (ASD) indicates higher divorce rates from early childhood through adulthood, compared with non-ASD families (i.e., divorce rates were 23.5% for couples with an autistic child and 13.8% for a matched set of couples without an autistic child; Hartley et al., 2010). Further, wives report declining marital satisfaction as the ASD child ages (Hartley et al., 2012). As with other couple types, ineffective communication patterns, conflict, and negative affect can be heightened in ASD families (Hartley et al., 2016, 2019). This may be due in part to the greater likelihood that a parent of an autistic child has characteristics associated with "broad autism phenotype" (e.g., aloofness, rigidity, utilitarian language; Hurley et al., 2007). Compared with control couples, 178 couples with an autistic child reported more intense, frequent couple problems, and they were observed to be less engaged and cooperative during conflict (Hartley et al., 2017). Negative affect and poor communication are exacerbated when ASD families have fewer economic resources (Hartley et al., 2016). It is likely that the enhanced financial burden of resources necessary to support the ASD child's needs contributes to the economic strain already experienced by lower resource families. With higher stress (Brobst et al., 2009) and lower relationship satisfaction (Sim et al., 2016) than parents of non-ASD children, developing coping skills is critical. Optimism, benefit finding, positive **cognitive appraisals**, support, and partner support have been found to be particularly beneficial for couples' relationship satisfaction, intimacy, and stability in ASD families (e.g., Ekas et al., 2015; García-López et al., 2016).

Unmanaged stress is linked with other characteristics and conditions common in ASD families. Schnabel and colleagues (2020) reviewed 31 studies and found disproportionately high mental health problems, with 33% and 31% of parents reporting anxiety and depressive disorders, respectively. Further, Sim and colleagues' (2016) meta-analysis of seven studies linked mental health problems with lower relationship satisfaction among these couples. Stress in ASD families is typically centered on challenges with children. Behaviors viewed as disruptive and problematic are exhibited frequently among ASD children (Brobst et al., 2009) and are consistently linked with lower relationship satisfaction and stability (Sim et al., 2016). Negative (or positive) parent–child interactions are often paralleled by couple interactions. A recent study found parents' criticism of their ASD child was associated with more severe criticism of their partners, whereas parental warmth was mirrored with greater couple warmth (Hickey et al., 2019). The considerable demands of parenting an ASD child may help to explain why couples cited shared responsibilities, teamwork, and agreement on beliefs as foundational for their relationship satisfaction (Sim, Fristedt, et al., 2019). Considering the layers of challenge, external support is critical. Indeed, Sim et al.'s (2016) meta-analysis linked social support with higher relationship satisfaction. A unique element in ASD families related to couple instability is **asymmetrical attachment** (i.e., when one partner feels closer to the ASD child or "more burdened" by childcare needs; Hartley et al., 2018). The more peripheral parent may feel as if they are an outsider, while the central parent may resent role and task inequities (Sim, Fristedt, et al., 2019). Tension and instability in the couple relationship can be further aggravated by other incongruous relationships, such as when parents have additional older children and when parents have multiple children with special needs (Hartley et al., 2016).

Research Evidence on Stepfamilies

Couples with children from prior partnerships comprise a significant proportion of families (Smock & Schwartz, 2020), particularly among lower resource families and some minoritized groups (Raley & Sweeney, 2020). Research indicates that healthy, open communication patterns are crucial for managing the complexity inherent in this family structure and for promoting relational stability (Ganong & Coleman, 2017; Raley & Sweeney, 2020). "Step-couples" face an array of potential sources of conflict (e.g., cross-household relationships, changing roles and rules in the family, prior partner involvement, allocation of resources), and thus partners' unity and alliance may protect them from dissolution (Stephenson & DeLongis, 2019). Specifically, communication tone is important; confrontational or withdrawn responses to family stress were linked with negative mood among step-couples (King & DeLongis, 2013) and tension with stepchildren (DeLongis & Preece, 2003), whereas empathic responses reduced subsequent marital tension (O'Brien et al., 2009). Accompanying communication difficulties, mental health problems are prevalent in these complex families, with stepmothers, in particular, reporting higher stress and related depression than biological mothers (Shapiro & Stewart, 2011). A recent report demonstrated that stress in step-couple relationships was linked with dissolution over a 20-year period and partners' depression mediated this link (DeLongis & Zwicker, 2017). That is, stress is associated with increased partner depression, which, in turn, presents a risk for relationship dissolution.

Further, stepfamilies most frequently cite raising children as their principal stressor (in contrast, one study found that first families primarily worried about finances; Stanley et al., 2002), and problems with children are associated with longitudinal increases in step-couple conflict (Jenkins et al., 2005). Conflict typically centers on resource distribution, discipline, and rule setting for biological versus stepchildren (Ganong & Coleman, 2017). The stepmother–child dyad can be particularly tricky (DeLongis & Zwicker, 2017); stepmothers report higher parenting stress and negative child esteem than biological mothers (Shapiro & Stewart, 2011), and this negativity is associated with marital instability (Knox & Zusman, 2001). With the normative challenges of combining families, research indicates that it is particularly important for step-couples to successfully navigate sharing responsibilities and roles because couples in stepfamilies report more egalitarian gender role beliefs compared with their first marriages (Lucier-Greer et al., 2012). Further, role clarity is linked with stepmothers' lower stress, marital satisfaction, and overall stepfamily adjustment (Ganong & Coleman, 2017).

Along with familial stressors related to partner dynamics and parenting, economic hardships put stepfamilies at higher risk for dissolution (Schramm & Adler-Baeder, 2012). Men often have added financial obligations to first families, and remarried wives report economic strain and resentment of their husbands' financial support to his prior family, which is accordingly linked with lower marital quality and instability. Stepfamilies can also feel lacking in external support compared with their experiences in their first families. This may take the form of family and friends' disapproval, negative cultural stereotypes (e.g., stepfamilies as conflictual, detrimental for children), and legal constraints (e.g., underrecognition of stepparent–child relationship, school systems' barriers to stepparent involvement; Ganong & Coleman, 2017). Inadequate family and friend support is associated with wives' lower marital happiness (Knox & Zusman, 2001), and stepmothers with biological children may be uniquely at risk, with smaller support networks and more household and childcare responsibilities.

There are a few additional intervention targets unique to step-couples and derived from research, which are notable. One relates to the degree of **family complexity**, which matters; those stepfamilies with enhanced complexity, including prior children from both partners or multiple previous partners, have greater declines in relationship satisfaction and couple stability over time (Slattery et al., 2011). With ambiguity and tension in family relationships, researchers note family formation processes can take multiple years and may result in varying levels of connectedness between stepfamily members and not a true "blending" (Ganong & Coleman, 2017; Stewart, 2010). Having more realistic expectations can increase couple satisfaction and family success (Adler-Baeder & Higginbotham, 2020; Slattery et al., 2011). In contrast, step-couples who held unrealistic expectations of instant cohesiveness and parent–child adjustment are at risk for lower marital quality and stability (Hetherington & Kelly, 2002; Visher et al., 2003). Another strain on the family formation process may come from step-couples' jealousy or fears related to former partners (Knox & Zusman, 2001) and time and energy spent on parent–child relationships. Because poor stepparent–stepchild relationships are linked with lower couple quality, research provides some indication that building strengths in the step-couple relationship while also working to improve each (step)parent–child relationship can enhance couple satisfaction and stability (e.g., Slattery et al., 2011).

Research Evidence on Multiracial Families

In studies of multiracial couples, most research focuses on Black–White, cisgender heterosexual partnerships. Although comparisons of stability with same-race couples typically indicate greater risk of instability over time, the specific combination matters. Black–White partnerships with a Black woman and White partner are more stable over time compared with same-race couples (Bratter & King, 2008). A meta-analysis of 108 studies provides valuable information on predictors of instability in multiracial couples (Toosi et al., 2012). Findings reveal that negative communication patterns (e.g., lower positive affect, disengaged behaviors, lack of warmth, less effective problem-solving) are more common in multiracial couples than same-race dyads, albeit with small effect sizes. Notably, females in multiracial partnerships may experience acute stress, with lower initial relationship quality (Brown et al., 2019), greater socioeconomic disadvantages (White women only; Bratter & Eschbach, 2006), more severe mental health problems (White women only), and increased prevalence of intimate partner violence (compared with same-race couples; Fusco, 2010). Studies suggest that women's stress in multi-racial couples is strongly related to challenges with children and caregiving (Fu et al., 2001) and incongruent gender role beliefs. The more egalitarian role beliefs of multiracial-coupled women, compared with their partners, and unmet expectations for shared responsibilities and perceived unfairness in financial, parenting, or household duties are linked with poorer marital quality for both men and women (Forry et al., 2007).

Specific to multiracial couples, risks to couple instability are heightened in the context of the stigmatization (e.g., cultural assumptions that same-race unions are happier and more successful) as well as legal and social rejection (Head, 2019). These negative cultural and societal stigmas often spark extended family and friends' disapproval and persistent opposition to their union (Killian, 2001). Greater support from family and friends for their multiracial union is associated with wives' marital happiness (Fu et al., 2001), whereas family and friends' criticism of their multiracial relationship intensifies partners' depression and anxiety symptoms and overall health (Rosenthal et al., 2019). Importantly, evidence also indicates that partners' support can serve a protective function, attenuating the link between family disapproval and depression.

As multiracial couples attempt to establish their own couple ecosystem in the context of potential negative stigmas, racism, and inadequate support from family and friends (Killian, 2001), they also undergo a complex personal process of **racial identity** reclassification, in which White partners may be seen as "less White" and Black partners as "less Black" (Afful et al., 2015). This reclassification process may be more keenly felt for Black partners, who also report stronger links between their racial identity and couple satisfaction than their White counterparts (Killian, 2001). Black racial identity has profound meaning and benefits, including better self-esteem, physical and mental health, and protection against discrimination (Rowley et al., 1998; Sellers & Shelton, 2003; Thompson Sanders et al., 2012). Thus, multiracial coupling may cause Black partners to lose some of the protective factors they held when their racial affiliation was stronger (Afful et al., 2015). Benefits are both individual and relational. Those with stronger Black racial identity report more love and less relationship ambivalence, whereas those who identify more with White culture have greater ambivalence (Leslie & Letiecq, 2004). In contrast, White partners tend to be much less aware of their racial identity and may not be as attuned or sensitive to a racial identity reclassification process. However, if their racial identity includes a superior or racist perspective, the relationship suffers. White partners who hold a superiority view of White culture express less love to their Black partners.

In conjunction with this racial identity reclassification process on the individual level, multiracial couples also have to navigate their cultural and racial differences as a couple. Research provides useful information for intervention. Communicating about and supporting their partners' cultural values bolstered multiracial couples' relationship quality, and this link was stronger than among same-race couples (Reiter & Gee, 2008). Further, a study of multiracial couples enriches our understanding of varying dyadic strategies (Seshadri & Knudson-Martin, 2013). Couples fell into four categories describing how they combined their disparate cultures: (a) integrated (i.e., combine and celebrate both partners' cultures); (b) coexisting (i.e., retain separate cultures but respect each other's differences); (c) singularly assimilated (i.e., allow one partner's culture to dominate, while the other partner seems to convert); and (d) unresolved (i.e., ignore conflicts and tension around culture; Seshadri & Knudson-Martin, 2013). The researchers suggest that identifying these structures is useful for providing a framework to help couples manage their relationships. They also suggest that unresolved couples are more likely to seek therapy. Among all types, couples emphasize finding shared goals, appreciating each culture's peculiarities, expressing insecurities, finding outside support, and underscoring their "we-ness" to family and friends as useful communication and coping strategies.

CLINICAL APPLICATIONS: C. WAYNE JONES, PATRICIA L. PAPERNOW, SCOTT BROWNING, KELLEY KENNEY, AND MARK KENNEY

Clinical Expertise and Interpretation of Evidence: An Overview

Almost all couples periodically face challenges that can threaten the quality of their relationship, regardless of how strong their bond and love for one another are. However, there are couples in certain contexts who face greater stressors and challenges on a more regular basis, leaving them at particularly high risk for becoming destabilized as a couple. As introduced by Adler-Baeder and Gregson in the previous section, these contexts, often tied to social identity locations, include fragile families, families with a child on the autism spectrum (FotS), stepfamilies, and multiracial families. There are unique but predictable stressors and challenges facing couples in each of these four circumstances, many of which interfere with the couples' ability to coparent successfully. These include the challenge of clarifying parental roles (stepfamilies), negotiating **family complexity** (stepfamilies and fragile families), maintaining balance among parent–child attachments (fragile families, FotS, and stepfamilies), and addressing racism and **racial identity** (multiracial couples). See Table 4.1 for a list of challenges and stressors identified in the research literature also discussed in this chapter.

It is critical for therapists to help couples living in these families to recognize typical interactional patterns that undermine the stability of their relationship, identify the characteristic and unique stressors tied to their interactional patterns, and then design interventions that help them come together to navigate their stressors more adaptively. Clinicians are far more likely to be effective in these treatment tasks when they are grounded in empirical knowledge of predictable stressors and they have evidence-based guidance about how to best meet the challenges associated with each couple's unique context. In addition, couples are far more likely to restabilize their relationships when they can recognize and effectively address their very specific stressors and challenges. When this is not understood, partners remain vulnerable to their maladaptive patterns, resulting in conflict and emotional distance and further straining their emotional bonds with one another. Couples with children may decide to preserve the family unit and live for years with chronic unhappiness and instability in their marriage. Others eventually dissolve their relationship. Each of these outcomes is fraught with potentially significant negative impacts for all members of the family and their community.

This section of the chapter translates the research described by Adler-Baeder and Gregson into clinical practice. Rather than describing entire treatment models or approaches, focus is given to a few specific common challenges identified in the research that are likely encountered by each of the four types of couples. One goal for the therapist is to describe how the unique stressors and challenges for each of these couples are represented in the presentation of problems in common clinical practice. Couples do not typically enter treatment naming the specific underlying contextual or systemic issues creating their conflicts. Rather, they tend to be narrowly focused on the content of their current conflicts. Research-informed clinicians can begin treatment with these couples by using research findings to quickly identify underlying contextual or systemic issues and then refocusing the treatment on meaningful processes. Across all four types of couple contexts discussed in this chapter, the children are often a major focus of the couple's presenting concerns. In fragile families, the child is typically the identified patient. In multicultural families, stepfamilies, and FotS, the child may be the identified patient but also just as likely not to be involved in the treatment at all, serving primarily as a major source of interparental conflict. The extent to which a child is included in the treatment is determined by whether the couple locates the source of their problems as in the child or in the couple relationship.

In each of the following subsections—written by clinical experts Wayne Jones (fragile families), Scott Browning (families on the spectrum), Patricia Papernow (stepfamilies), and Kelley and Mark Kenney (multiracial families)—a clinical case is described in detail as well as an intervention focus that is informed by Adler-Baeder and Gregson's research review. Psychoeducation, an important component of many couple therapies, plays a particularly critical role in the interventions described by the clinical experts in three of the four cases presented. Psychoeducation rests on the notion that knowledge can be a powerful antidote to the negative maladaptive processes set in motion when couples face unexpected challenges in their relationship. There is of great value to clinicians knowing the research about the specific types of predictable challenges couples may encounter—factors that increase risks to the couple as well as those that protect them. Included in couple psychoeducation is information about what to expect, what they can do about it, and how they can improve their relationship in the face of the challenges they are facing. When couples are provided this information, it can normalize the stress and help partners frame the causes of their suffering less personally. For many couples, it can be empowering and facilitate openness to deeper clinical interventions.

All clinicians associated with the cases described in the next section understand, however, that it is not enough to simply educate couples about their situations. Another common practice with respect to intervention across the four cases is the clinicians' efforts to facilitate more supportive, direct conversation between spouses about the challenges they are facing. This focus addresses the problem of ineffective and unsupportive communication, a major risk factor identified by Adler-Baeder and Gregson in all four types of couple contexts. One way to view research-informed intervention is that it operates to reduce known risk factors associated with a particular couple context while strengthening known protective factors that can promote the couple's resilience.

Clinical Expertise and Interpretation of Evidence: Fragile Families

Adler-Baeder and Gregson's review highlights two intertwined relational, interactional processes that are particularly important for clinicians to consider as a focus of intervention with couples in fragile families. The first relates to difficulties in collaboration and coparenting among couples in fragile families. Several studies describe a pattern of frequent arguments over household and parenting tasks (Laxman et al., 2013). The clinical implication is that this arena of family life must be given central focus in treatment. Second, interventions must also encourage collaboration, a protective factor. Waller (2012), for example, found that when parents in fragile families collaborated on household and parenting tasks and the father was more engaged with the family, the couple was more stable.

Of course, for couples to collaborate and address the challenges related to household tasks and parenting, they must be able to communicate effectively. Adler-Baeder and Gregson identified multiple studies (e.g., Waller, 2008) that suggest the communication style used during the arguments is a major problem for couples in fragile families. These styles are marked by negative, ineffective communication patterns that leave each member of the couple feeling aggrieved, overwhelmed, and alone. Without effective intervention, these patterns can have damaging effects on children and erode the quality and stability of the couple relationship. Carlson and Högnäs's (2011) study suggests a treatment direction for mitigating these risk factors. For example, they found that **supportive communication** (e.g., expression of love and encouragement, compromise, loyalty, infrequent criticism) was associated with more cooperative **coparenting**.

Clinical Experience: Observations of Common Interactional Patterns

To fully appreciate the complex roots of their problems with coparenting collaboration and communication, it is important to understand how couples in fragile families form. Typically, these couples have not known one another long before they move in together, bringing multiple children with them from previous relationships. The sense of urgency for moving in together is often a combination of hope, survival, and the promise of sharing very limited resources. Fragile families often struggle with communicating, planning, and problem-solving. As such, the couple relationship often begins and ends in chaos. There is little discussion or planning for how they will approach parenting tasks. Everything is ambiguous, including the level of commitment the couple has with one another. A disorganized approach to parenting combined with weak and insecure attachments between caregivers and children living in the household results in increased child behavioral issues and mental health crises. All of this sets the couple up to become overwhelmed, easily disappointed, and frustrated with one another.

When there is perceived inequity and conflict about who is responsible for what task, couples in fragile families often tend toward a communication style that involves rapid symmetrical escalation. That is, both members of the couple may become emotionally dysregulated, with interactions devolving into arguing, yelling, and at times violence. Many times, children are triangulated into these conflicts. Some couples in fragile families tend toward an interactional pattern wherein one member of the couple disengages entirely from parenting while the other member does everything. Given the absence of a tradition that places a value on talking things out, these conflicts do not resolve but continue to build upon one another, creating significant negativity in the relationship and further undermining the couple's fragile bond.

Case Context: Characteristics, Culture, and Preferences

Joe and Alisha have lived together for 2 years. They met in a drug and alcohol treatment program, having known one another only 4 months when they moved in together. He has two children from two previous partners. Stan, who is now 10, lived with Joe and Alisha during the first 4 months of their relationship. However, fighting between Alisha and Stan resulted in Joe sending Stan back to his mother. Joe and his son's mother have a contentious, volatile relationship. Joe distanced himself from his son after he left Joe and Alisha's home, only seeing him a few times over the next 18 months. Alisha has a 3-year-old child from a previous partner who lives with her and Joe full time. After Stan left the household, Joe and Alisha maintained fixed roles and enjoyed relative stability, even though they rarely talked about expectations, disappointments, division of labor, parenting, or the family's future. This is because Alisha preferred to do most of the parenting of her young son, deciding everything, giving little indication that she was disappointed with Joe's peripheral, disengaged role.

Two recent changes triggered intense conflict in this couple. First, Alisha is pregnant. Second, Stan's mother kicked him out of her home, so he is again living with Joe and Alisha. Joe remains disengaged from parenting, even with his own son, who has significant behavioral problems. Alisha now feels overwhelmed and angry that she is doing all the parenting, and she shows it. She does not tell Joe this directly but instead rages at his son Stan. Stan feels abandoned by his father and resentful of what he feels is Alisha's mistreatment of him. The negative interactional pattern could be summarized as follows: The more Joe distances from parenting Stan and the more Alisha tries to control Stan, the more explosive and aggressive Stan becomes with Alisha. The more alone and ineffective Alisha feels with Stan, the more she distances herself from Joe, and the more Joe becomes angry. Because they do not have any established practice of talking through problems in a collaborative manner, their conflicts over family responsibilities cannot be resolved, and their relationship becomes increasingly unstable, with a threat of dissolution of the couple and ejection of Stan from the home.

Clinical Decisions: Intervention Implementation
This couple entered treatment the way most fragile families do: through the child. Stan was identified by the school as showing signs of serious emotional and behavioral problems. The family was subsequently referred to an intensive, in-home program in which treatment was driven by ecosystemic structural family therapy (ESFT; Jones, 2019). The primary intervention in this family relates to the interactional, relational patterns documented in Adler-Baeder and Gregson's research review: negative, ineffective communication patterns. The next most helpful intervention pushes the couple to collaborate as a coparenting team (Laxman et al., 2013). The intervention used to address these research-based interactional, relational problems is facilitated "enactment," a typical ESFT intervention. Enactments require therapists to conduct sessions in a way that facilitates in vivo experiences of more functional communication and collaboration as a coparenting team. It is a "learn by doing" approach. In essence, the therapy is helping the couple to do things better.

The in-home team joined with Joe, Alisha, and Stan, validated their shared emotional experience, and engaged them in a collaborative assessment of how their family works. These facilitated conversations resulted in a mutually derived detailed description of the family's core negative interactional cycle related to parenting. The therapists worked to gain Joe and Alisha's buy-in to the following treatment frame: "To strengthen your family's ability to handle the stress you are facing, particularly with respect to parenting Stan, you need to come together and work as a coparenting team." This could be termed "psychoeducation light" in that this statement informs the couple about one of the more potent protective factors against instability identified in the research on fragile families (Waller, 2012).

The therapists spent half the sessions meeting with Joe and Alisha separately as a couple or parenting subsystem, helping the couple talk directly to one another and to "do" collaboration, while interrupting and redirecting them back to the problem-solving task at hand when one would attack or disengage. Also, in these couple sessions, the therapists helped Joe and Alisha develop and agree on expectations for Stan, as well as decide who was going to take care of the issues he was facing at school. Joe decided he would like to have a closer relationship with his son and agreed to be the one primarily responsible for managing him. Alisha indicated that she wanted them to be more prepared for the arrival of the new baby and convinced Joe to agree to weekly "executive" family planning meetings where they could anticipate potential problems and hash out solutions before they occur.

Stepfamilies

Unlike couples in fragile families, here we focus on couples in married stepfamilies who have a formal commitment to one another. Couples in these stepfamilies are at an especially high risk for instability, particularly within the first 5 years. Many of the complex intense dynamics that contribute to step-couple instability also play out in conflicts over children, which, as Adler-Baeder and Gregson's research section highlights, are a major stressor for step-couples. These struggles are often exacerbated by other areas of difficulty, including unrealistic expectations of instant cohesiveness, step-parents disciplining children too early in the relationship, and lack of clarity about the stepparent role (see Table 4.1).

Clinical Experience: Observations of Common Interactional Patterns

For couples forming a stepfamily, their wishes for "blending" are instead all too often met with experiences of constant tensions centering on children. While couples in first-time families have more time to form a secure bond and develop some mutual understandings, stepfamilies are quite different. Children enter first-time families hardwired for attachment to both parents. In first-time families, shared family habits and values build over time. In stepfamilies, however, established secure attachment bonds and mutual understandings about "how we do things" lie in the parent–child relationship, not in the step-couple. As a result, in stepfamilies where children are present, parents may feel engaged, needed, visible, and cared about, whereas stepparents feel excluded, left out, and invisible. On an often-daily basis stepparents are "stuck outsiders," sitting on the sidelines of parent–child relationships. Parents are "stuck insiders," much closer to everyone (children, new partner, and ex-spouse) but often feeling torn between the evolving families differing needs. Unrealistic expectations of instant "blending" and immediate, loving stepparent–stepchild relationships add to the pain.

Many step-couples continue straining to "blend" but find themselves increasingly tense and anxious with each other and feeling that they are failing at "being a family." Stepparents complain or withdraw. Parents get defensive and critical. Both feel more and more isolated and miserable. Parents may attempt to maintain their family by either prioritizing the couple to the detriment of their child(ren) or by focusing on the parent–child relationship to the detriment of their partners. Some step-couples may move too quickly toward unified family rules and rituals, which can intensify problems and conflicts. Constant misunderstandings spiral into blame and judgement or shame and withdrawal. Children become ever more "resistant." Parents feel even more torn; stepparents feel even more rejected.

Differences over children also play out in struggles over discipline. Stepparents everywhere seem to want more limits and boundaries with their stepchildren. Parents are focused more on providing love and understanding for their kids. For many reasons, what stepparents see as "manipulative," "lazy," or "bad behavior," parents see as "sad," "struggling," or "typical kid behavior." When this goes poorly, stepparents become increasingly desperate and critical. Parents become ever more protective and permissive. Couples find themselves stuck in repeating cycles of painful polarization. Additionally, stepparents often move too quickly into a disciplinary role—or worse, fall into authoritarian (cold and hard) parenting, which, the research tells us, is almost always toxic to stepparent–stepchild relationships.

Case Context: Characteristics, Culture, and Preferences
Amanda and Rob have been together for a year. Rob is 42. He had been divorced for 2 years when he met Amanda. Rob has two adolescents, Max (11) and Maria (13), from his previous marriage. Amanda is 37 and divorced but never had children. "When your kids are here, it's like I'm leftover hamburger," says Amanda disconsolately. Rob bristles, "What's your problem? They're my kids!" He continues, "We've been together for a year and we still aren't acting like a family." Amanda shoots back, "Well if your kids treated me better, maybe we'd have a better time together." Rob retorts, "Maybe if you weren't so hard on them, they'd be nicer to you." Through

clenched teeth Amanda says, "*You* never discipline them. Someone has to." Like many step-couples, Amanda and Rob are struggling over their very different experience of Rob's kids. Their misery is compounded by their expectation of immediate blending, their lack of information about key differences between parenting and stepparenting, and Amanda's expectation that she should discipline her stepchildren. Their inability to communicate effectively about these challenges is only deepening these painful divisions.

Clinical Decisions: Intervention Implementation

Adler-Baeder and Gregson detailed the ways in which psychoeducation can help set realistic expectations and increase **role clarity**. They also described the importance of strong communication skills and solid empathic connection in step-couples. These are key areas for clinical intervention. Like many step-couples, Rob and Amanda have come to their stepfamily with a first-time family vision. A further complication is that rather than becoming a team to face their challenges, poor communication skills contribute to intensifying tensions. Clinical work will need to include both psychoeducation about what is typical, what works, and what does not for children in stepfamilies, as well as helping this couple to forge better interpersonal skills.

We begin with psychoeducation. As with many step-couples, the longing for immediate "blending" is exacerbating Rob and Amanda's distress. This is often a very good place to begin: "That word 'blended' didn't set you up for this, huh!" "It turns out that becoming a stepfamily is not fast food! It's a very slow cooker!" Often, naming and normalizing the recurring stuck insider–outsider positions that result from a step-couple's different relationships with the parent's children is also profoundly helpful in lifting shame and blame and lowering stress and conflict: "This is not happening because you don't love each other. It is happening because you live in a stepfamily. A stepfamily makes one of you, the stepparent, a stuck outsider. It makes the other, the parent, a stuck insider."

It is helpful to step-couples to learn that they can lower stress by practicing "*both/and* rather than *either/or*" (Papernow, 2013, p. 56, italics in original). In other words, all the subsystems need to be satisfied (e.g., the couple, the parent–child, the stepparent–stepchild). Rob and Amanda are encouraged to do some fun things as a family. Equally important, they are urged to carve out regular, reliable alone time for both the couple and the parent–child relationships. For the couple, a few private moments before they get up or go to bed and special date nights can provide time when Rob can focus on Amanda without feeling torn. Feeling seen and cared about enables Amanda to turn away more easily when Rob needs time with his kids. Likewise, one-to-one parent–child time gives Maria and Max the secure attachment they need with their dad, without competing with Amanda, making it a little easier for them to "share" when she is present.

Much of Rob and Amanda's stress centers on differences over discipline. Again, it is extremely helpful to normalize this: "It turns out that stepparents everywhere want more limits, and parents everywhere want more understanding for their kids." It is also vital to share the research that stepfamilies work best when parents retain limit-setting with their own children while stepparents concentrate on slowly building "connection not correction" (Papernow, 2018, p. 13). Amanda is encouraged to leave the disciplining to Rob and begin slowly getting to know her stepchildren by spending time alone with each of them doing something fun.

Not surprisingly, strong communication skills are key. Like many stepcouples, Amanda and Rob often need help to access their curiosity. They are encouraged to refrain from a focus on what each does not like and instead shift the focus to being curious about the other. Slowly, as Amanda and Rob begin to shift from fighting over these differences to summoning enough calm, mutual respect, and curiosity, they begin to become a collaborative team. Often, stepparents can help parents to demand more of their kids, and parents can help stepparents be more understanding of children's needs and wishes. When differences are unresolved, however, a helpful guideline is that until or unless stepchildren have formed a trusting caring relationship with their stepparent, stepparents have *input* and parents have *final say* with their own kids.

Amanda and Rob also need to learn how to reach for each other at moments of difference, rather than attacking or withdrawing. Over and over, Amanda is helped to translate her attack into "I think you're missing Rob. Can you tell him?" With some help, Amanda finds a softer voice: "It's so hard, Rob. It's like I'm invisible." Rob starts to defend himself, "But . . ." Rob then needs help to empathize rather than defend. "Rob, I know you love this woman. Can you take a breath? Can you start by telling Amanda what you DO understand?" Rob sputters a bit. "She feels left out," he says, looking at the floor. "Great! You've got it! Now can you land that on Amanda's heart?" Amanda begins to soften some. Now it is Rob's turn to add a sentence or two: "Just the nub of what you really want Amanda to get." He says, haltingly, "I feel so torn. I try to take care of my kids and you're unhappy. I go to be with you and my kids are unhappy." Amanda starts with "But . . ." Now she is encouraged to take a breath and "find what you DO understand." Going back and forth, very slowly, Amanda and Rob start to feel cared about and connected to each other. As their understanding grows, so does their empathy for each other's quite different experience of their family.

With more realistic expectations and better interpersonal skills, differences over kids become less a signal for alarm and more just "part of being a stepfamily." Rob and Amanda begin to function more and more as a team. They begin to experience closeness and stability that come not from feeling the same way about Rob's kids but from taking a breath at tough moments and finding their empathy for each other's very different positions.

Clinical Expertise and Interpretation of Evidence: Families on the Spectrum

As Adler-Baeder and Gregson indicated, the general stress level for couples in FotS is higher than those with neurotypical children. This stress can significantly influence parental coordination, parental mental health, and relationship satisfaction. It would be impossible to speak of the difficulties experienced in isolation because all psychological factors are to some extent interconnected. However, one area highlighted in Adler-Baeder and Gregson's research section is uniquely important in understanding a common couples' problem. That is *asymmetrical attachment*. This pattern is problematic because it moves the couple away from one another: As one parent begins to become enmeshed with the child, the other parent begins to feel as an outsider (Sim, Fristedt, et al., 2019).

Clinical Experience: Observations of Common Interactional Patterns

What this interpersonal problem looks like in practice may vary, but commonly it involves one parent becoming distant from their child on the spectrum. That parent may feel inadequate or so saddened by the dashed dream of a neurotypical child that they slip into increasing avoidance of their child. It is not unusual for this to occur, often only lasting for a short while. Occasionally, however, an escalating process of complementarity occurs in which one parent becomes completely enmeshed with the child while the other parent moves to the outside world, away from the coparent and the needy child. The enmeshed parent is often spending most of each day researching autism, talking to other parents, and arranging appointments and treatment protocols while the other parent becomes increasingly involved in work or other pursuits outside the family. This common pattern demonstrates "systemic compensation," which occurs when each person in a system moves toward an ever-more-extreme position due to the functioning of the other. For example, when one member of a couple becomes depressed, the other member may pick up the slack and begin to overfunction, thus compensating for the dyadic change. In FotS, the totally involved parent is often balanced with the uninvolved parent. It is critical for clinicians to see this as a systemic function, not as a problem that requires assigning blame. For the following intervention to work, one or both members of the couple must learn to view the entire situation from this very different "systemic" perspective.

Case Context: Characteristics, Culture, and Preferences

Karen and Peter recognized that something about Jason's development was off by his second birthday. Karen immersed herself online to learn more about autism. Jason's upsetting behaviors and frequent doctor's appointments led Karen to leave her job as a software engineer. Peter continued to go to work, becoming gradually more and more consumed by the demands of his job. As Karen became increasingly concerned about Jason's possible autism, Peter seemed numb to this possibility. He also felt strongly that putting his job in jeopardy would not serve the family. Eventually, the developmental pediatrician that Karen consulted confirmed that on multiple screening tests, Jason appeared to meet criteria that suggested a diagnosis of ASD, although it still needed further confirmation. The asymmetrical relationship between Karen and Peter had begun quite innocently. However, as Karen became immersed in understanding autism, and Jason in particular, Peter began to feel more useless at home and mainly felt confident at work. Moving to extreme positions also took a toll on the romantic relationship between Peter and Karen.

By the time that Karen and Peter sought therapy, the couple had become extremely distant. Karen was spending more than 14 hours each day assisting the applied behavioral analysis counselor working with Jason, going online to research other treatments, and actively participating in an online parent support group. Meanwhile, Peter was spending close to the same number of hours per day at work, simply because he found being home so stressful and debilitating to his self-confidence. Karen was disappointed in Peter, and Peter found engaging with Jason frustrating, depressing, and confusing. Note that although this case example identifies the male member of a heterosexual couple as the person who has become disengaged, the pattern of asymmetrical parent–child attachment is not exclusively linked to one gender or to heterosexual couples, and thus an adaptation of this intervention is useful across coparenting couple populations.

Clinical Decisions: Intervention Implementation

The intervention cited here is supported by both the author's clinical expertise and empirical evidence. Research clearly states that **asymmetrical attachment** leads to couple instability and undermines effective parenting. The therapy uses a subsystem emphasis. A six-session treatment sequence follows an initial assessment. This intervention does not commence until an official diagnosis of autism or similar developmental delay condition is made, the family has expressed an interest in treatment, and some external support (such as actively involved grandparents) exists for the family. The initial session takes place with the couple. The intake examines the various ways in which the family has been struggling, with the therapist listening for interpersonal problems that are common to FotS. Certainly, the individual treatment regime, dedicated to developmental issues of the child diagnosed with autism, is essential. The therapist assures the couple that the treatment would examine all issues identified through the intake but that treatment would begin with specific attention to the negative cycle driving the two parents further and further apart so that they were no longer functioning as a team.

The first step is to ascertain that both members of the couple wish to be a unified team, both as coparents and romantic partners. Before the overall couple issues are addressed as part of treatment, obtaining this basic level of commitment is very useful. The second step in the intervention is to identify additional support for the family. This support may be offered by an extended family member, a friend, or a professional. The thinking is that because the system is under pressure, the destructive pattern is best shifted when there is a potential source of temporary relief for the couple, particularly from parenting. This creates some necessary space for the couples to successfully engage in treatment. Once this couple identifies someone who could tend to some of Karen's care-taking responsibilities, that person is contacted, and their willingness confirmed. Next, Karen's accomplishments, regarding caring for Jason, are celebrated. After this occurs (in this case, Peter has no problem acknowledging Karen's work), Karen is encouraged to take some time for herself (which she defines). Peter's efforts at keeping his family financially stable are also recognized and celebrated. Peter's hope to be connected to his wife and son is encouraged and supported.

The specific issue for this couple relates to one parent being enmeshed with the child, while the other partner has become distant. This is identified to the couple as an area of focus that is supported both in the research literature and in clinical expert practice. The systemic nature of this dynamic is explained to the couple. For example, the therapist says,

> The situation occurring between you two is not uncommon in families with a child on the spectrum. Both of you moved to address the stress stemming from Jason's diagnosis, but the movement you made pushed you away from each other, thus weakening the family. Neither of you is at fault, but you must become a team again for the sake of the family, your relationship, and Jason.

Following this frame of the problem, a dramatic shift in the conversations occurs in sessions. Peter and Karen are helped to understand what occurred between them in systemic terms. Rather than either person being entirely right or wrong, the growing distance that occurred between them is framed as a typical pattern, one which the research literature clearly delineates as a normative risk for FotS. They begin to understand that systemic pressures have pushed them in opposite directions. As Karen became more knowledgeable about autism and more connected with Jason, Peter felt increasingly disconnected from both his wife and son. For Peter, work was where he felt most capable, thus he moved in that direction. Karen had become the expert, the only person to really understand Jason; Peter had withdrawn to his own area of competence and had started to see Karen as obsessed. For each person, the extreme position had become terribly lonely. In treatment, Karen and Peter begin to understand that their pattern of compensation would simply intensify unless corrected.

The next step is a session with Peter alone, wherein he is provided psychoeducational guidance on how to begin developing a deeper bond with Jason. The interactional methods of engagement established by Steven Gutstein (2009) informed the coaching provided to Peter. These approaches are highly interactional and are focused more on relationship building than simply behavior change. The therapist informs Peter, "You will learn how to connect with Jason, at a basic level. This is not about you teaching him; it is about you both feeling some relationship." The next session is one in which the disengaged parent and child, Peter and Jason, come in alone, and the whole session involves coaching Peter to relax and "get to know" his son.

In the next, and final, session of this intervention, the couple is brought in together, and the therapist facilitates a discussion with the goal of establishing a more equal coparenting arrangement. Certainly, the hours dedicated to Jason will remain unequal because, in this case, Peter is the only parent working outside the home. However, Karen and Peter begin to understand that this inequality does not need to continue in asymmetrical positions that lead to a destructive pattern. Peter becomes increasingly involved, interested, and connected (and is working to gain connection) with Jason. Karen begins to feel Peter's "return" to the family, while also resuming or developing interests outside of Jason's treatment. In addition, the couple searches for a method to begin a dating life, even in a restricted, but regular, arrangement.

Clinical Expertise and Interpretation of Evidence: Multiracial Families

As Adler-Bader and Gregson's research section on multiracial families indicates, one factor that leaves these couples at risk for instability is how they navigate their racial and cultural worldview background differences (Reiter & Gee, 2008; Seshadri & Knudson-Martin, 2013). Although this may be specific to all multiracial families, the dynamics and manifestations around these differences may be more heightened in multiracial families involving Black–White partners, which is the focus here.

Clinical Experience: Observations of Common Interactional Patterns

One partner or the other, or both partners, in a multiracial couple may be totally unaware of, avoid, or ignore the concept of cultural worldview background, its impact, and influence in shaping who they are and how they view the world. They may not acknowledge that cultural worldview background differences exist between them. Furthermore, cultural norms manifest in values and beliefs about finances, expressions of emotion, gender role beliefs and expectations, parenting, and importance of family. As such, and as suggested by the research described by Adler-Baeder and Gregson in the first part of this chapter, cultural norms inform communication patterns and styles and can have a profound impact on partners' interactions.

Multiracial partners also have different experiences related to their **racial identity** development and racial socialization. According to the research, this too may affect the relationship in terms of whether or how each partner understands the other's lived experiences. This can be further exacerbated by lack of communication. Multiracial couples may view the issues and concerns that arise as endemic of an individual partner's flaws or shortcomings and either take things personally or become defensive as a way of dealing with situations or with each other. An understanding of the significance of racial and cultural worldview background differences, especially those related to communication styles and patterns, is important and can play a critical role in marital and family functioning, well-being, and success.

Case Context: Characteristics, Culture, and Preferences

Chuck is a 48-year-old White man of German and Irish heritage. He has been looking to advance as a technical engineer and has been offered an opportunity to do so in Seattle, Washington. Pamela is a 47-year-old Black woman and is an attorney for a small family law practice in Baltimore. The couple has a 12-year-old son, Troy. The family currently lives in the Washington, DC, metropolitan area near where they both grew up. The couple has been in counseling because of stress and disagreements that have surfaced related to their various roles and responsibilities, as well as issues related to Troy's schooling and educational and extracurricular involvements. Chuck's eagerness to accept a new job offer and quickly move the family across the country has added to their conflicts. Pamela is about to become a partner at the law firm where she works. Although the scheduling of Troy's activities has been a source of stress for the couple and the family, he is in a diverse school environment where he is happy and experiencing success. Pam is opposed to the idea of moving to the West Coast, where the family knows no one, except for Chuck's brother, with whom they are not close.

Pamela yells, "You just don't get it, Chuck. Moving Troy all the way across country, to a place with little or no diversity, at his age, and where we have no family—no community, scares me!" "He's been doing well in school and has a great group of friends!" And "What about me? I don't know anybody out there—you're moving us away from my family, from my roots! What about my career? I'm about to become partner! There aren't a lot of Black folks out there!" Chuck retorts, "Here we go again with the, I don't understand the Black thing!" "Troy's going to be fine." "I'm trying to think of our future, and this opportunity will be good for all of us." "You're a good attorney, you'll find something out there."

It is clear at this point during the session that Chuck and Pamela have not discussed their racial and cultural worldview background differences as a multiracial couple. The conflict and tension that exist around the move to Seattle, Washington, relates to the lack of, or poor, communication between them about the importance of their racial and cultural identities in the context of their family.

Clinical Decisions: Intervention Implementation

As highlighted by Adler-Bader and Gregson in their research review, a psychoeducational approach can be used with "unresolved couples" such as Chuck and Pamela. Ibrahim and Schroeder (1990) provided a useful psychoeducational model for working with multiracial couples to help them understand and appreciate their racial and cultural worldview background differences, identify shared goals as a couple and family, and help them improve the overall effectiveness of their communication. To address the obvious racial and cultural worldview differences illustrated in this case, the clinician must raise questions during the session about each of their backgrounds and upbringing. The clinician must also ask, "How did the two of you make decisions about your own family, with regard to roles and responsibilities, career, parenting, family, and community and geographic location?" Again, this line of questioning opens the door for partners to engage one another in dialogue that allows for what may be new understanding of each other's values and beliefs from a cultural worldview context and enhance their ability to empathize with each other.

The clinician may also ask questions related to racial identity development and racial socialization:

> I'm wondering, Pamela and Chuck, about your conversations about race and racism, your individual experiences, the implications for your family, and the importance for your family of living in a racially diverse environment, and what these discussions have been like for you both.

The clinician is assessing the extent to which the couple has talked about race and racism in general, in the context of their family and in the context of their family's living environment. It is also important to explore the extent to which the couple has engaged in dialogue about the implications of their discussions of race and racism for their son and for how they raise their son. Providing the space and time for the partners to talk about their conversations about race and racism may provide an opportunity for new understandings of each other's, and their son's, contexts and experiences. Regarding Chuck's reaction to Pamela, it may present an opportunity for him to empathize with his partner.

Conclusion

Many couples experiencing instability are overwhelmed by the content of their arguments and caught in unproductive debates. The clinician can assist the couple to see that the unique structure of their family (e.g., being in a stepfamily) produces stressors that are misunderstood and misidentified. A skilled therapist can help the family reframe contention and understand how the pressures of the family structure lead to conflicts. This will allow each member to be less likely to blame the other and recognize that both people in the dyad play a role in the couple's problems. This is not to suggest the content of the fights are not important, but systemic dynamics need equal attention and, if done correctly, can create moments of connection and closeness otherwise lost.

REFERENCES

Adler-Baeder, F., & Higginbotham, B. (2020). Efforts to design, implement, and evaluate community-based education for stepfamilies: Current knowledge and future directions. *Family Relations*, *69*, 559–576. https://doi.org/10.1111/fare.12427

Afful, S. E., Wohlford, C., & Stoelting, S. M. (2015). Beyond "difference": Examining the process and flexibility of racial identity in interracial marriages. *Journal of Social Issues*, *71*(4), 659–674. https://doi.org/10.1111/josi.12142

Bratter, J. L., & Eschbach, K. (2006). What about the couple? Interracial marriage and psychological distress. *Social Science Research*, *35*(4), 1025–1047. https://doi.org/10.1016/j.ssresearch.2005.09.001

Bratter, J. L., & King, R. B. (2008). "But will it last?": Marital instability among interracial and same-race couples. *Family Relations, 57*(2), 160–171. https://doi.org/10.1111/j.1741-3729.2008.00491.x

Brobst, J. B., Clopton, J. R., & Hendrick, S. S. (2009). Parenting children with autism spectrum disorders: The couple's relationship. *Focus on Autism and Other Developmental Disabilities, 24*(1), 38–49. https://doi.org/10.1177/1088357608323699

Brown, C. C., Williams, Z., & Durtschi, J. A. (2019). Trajectories of interracial heterosexual couples: A longitudinal analysis of relationship quality and separation. *Journal of Marital and Family Therapy, 45*(4), 650–667. https://doi.org/10.1111/jmft.12363

Carlson, M., McLanahan, S., & England, P. (2004). Union formation in fragile families. *Demography, 41*(2), 237–261. https://doi.org/10.1353/dem.2004.0012

Carlson, M. J., & Furstenberg, F. F., Jr. (2006). The prevalence and correlates of multipartnered fertility among urban US parents. *Journal of Marriage and the Family, 68*(3), 718–732. https://doi.org/10.1111/j.1741-3737.2006.00285.x

Carlson, M. J., & Högnäs, R. S. (2011). Coparenting in fragile families: Understanding how parents work together after a nonmarital birth. In J. P. McHale & K. M. Lindahl (Eds.), *Coparenting: A conceptual and clinical examination of family systems* (pp. 81–103). American Psychological Association. https://doi.org/10.1037/12328-004

DeLongis, A., & Preece, M. (2003). Emotional and relational consequences of coping in stepfamilies. *Marriage & Family Review, 34*(1–2), 115–138. https://doi.org/10.1300/J002v34n01_06

DeLongis, A., & Zwicker, A. (2017). Marital satisfaction and divorce in couples in stepfamilies. *Current Opinion in Psychology, 13*, 158–161. https://doi.org/10.1016/j.copsyc.2016.11.003

Ekas, N. V., Timmons, L., Pruitt, M., Ghilain, C., & Alessandri, M. (2015). The power of positivity: Predictors of relationship satisfaction for parents of children with autism spectrum disorder. *Journal of Autism and Developmental Disorders, 45*(7), 1997–2007. https://doi.org/10.1007/s10803-015-2362-4

Ellerbe, C. Z., Jones, J. B., & Carlson, M. J. (2018). Race/ethnic differences in nonresident fathers' involvement after a nonmarital birth. *Social Science Quarterly, 99*(3), 1158–1182. https://doi.org/10.1111/ssqu.12482

Fagan, J., & Cherson, M. (2017). Maternal gatekeeping: The associations among facilitation, encouragement, and low-income fathers' engagement with young children. *Journal of Family Issues, 38*(5), 633–653. https://doi.org/10.1177/0192513X15578007

Falconier, M. K., Randall, A. K., & Bodenmann, G. (2016). *Couples coping with stress: A cross-cultural perspective.* Routledge. https://doi.org/10.4324/9781315644394

Forry, N. D., Leslie, L. A., & Letiecq, B. L. (2007). Marital quality in interracial relationships: The role of sex role ideology and perceived fairness. *Journal of Family Issues, 28*(12), 1538–1552. https://doi.org/10.1177/0192513X07304466

Fu, X., Tora, J., & Kendall, H. (2001). Marital happiness and inter-racial marriage: A study in a multi ethnic community in Hawaii. *Journal of Comparative Family Studies, 32*(1), 47–60. https://doi.org. https://doi.org/10.3138/jcfs.32.1.47

Fusco, R. A. (2010). Intimate partner violence in interracial couples: A comparison to white and ethnic minority monoracial couples. *Journal of Interpersonal Violence, 25*(10), 1785–1800. https://doi.org/10.1177/0886260509354510

Ganong, L., & Coleman, M. (2017). *Stepfamily relationships: Development, dynamics, and interventions* (2nd ed.). Springer. https://doi.org/10.1007/978-1-4899-7702-1

García-López, C., Sarriá, E., Pozo, P., & Recio, P. (2016). Supportive dyadic coping and psychological adaptation in couples parenting children with autism spectrum disorder: The role of relationship satisfaction. *Journal of Autism and Developmental Disorders, 46*(11), 3434–3447. https://doi.org/10.1007/s10803-016-2883-5

Gibson-Davis, C. M., Edin, K., & McLanahan, S. (2005). High hopes but even higher expectations: The retreat from marriage among low-income couples. *Journal of Marriage and the Family, 67*(5), 1301–1312. https://doi.org/10.1111/j.1741-3737.2005.00218.x

Gutstein, S. E. (2009). Empowering families through relationship development intervention: An important part of the biopsychosocial management of autism spectrum disorders. *Annals of Clinical Psychiatry, 21*(3), 174–182.

Harknett, K., & Knab, J. (2007). More kin, less support: Multipartnered fertility and perceived support among mothers. *Journal of Marriage and the Family, 69*(1), 237–253. https://doi.org/10.1111/j.1741-3737.2006.00356.x

Hartley, S. L., Barker, E. T., Baker, J. K., Seltzer, M. M., & Greenberg, J. S. (2012). Marital satisfaction and life circumstances of grown children with autism across 7 years. *Journal of Family Psychology, 26*(5), 688–697. https://doi.org/10.1037/a0029354

Hartley, S. L., Barker, E. T., Seltzer, M. M., Floyd, F., Greenberg, J., Orsmond, G., & Bolt, D. (2010). The relative risk and timing of divorce in families of children with an autism spectrum disorder. *Journal of Family Psychology, 24*(4), 449–457. https://doi.org/10.1037/a0019847

Hartley, S. L., Hickey, E. J., DaWalt, L., & Rodriguez, G. (2019). Broader autism phenotype and couple interactions in parents of children with autism. *Autism: An International Journal of Research and Practise, 23*(8), 2068–2079. https://doi.org/10.1177/1362361319841312

Hartley, S. L., Papp, L. M., Blumenstock, S. M., Floyd, F., & Goetz, G. L. (2016). The effect of daily challenges in children with autism on parents' couple problem-solving interactions. *Journal of Family Psychology, 30*(6), 732–742. https://doi.org/10.1037/fam0000219

Hartley, S. L., Papp, L. M., & Bolt, D. (2018). Spillover of marital interactions and parenting stress in families of children with autism spectrum disorder. *Journal of Clinical Child and Adolescent Psychology, 47*(Suppl. 1), S88–S99. https://doi.org/10.1080/15374416.2016.1152552

Hartley, S. L., Papp, L. M., Mihaila, I., Bussanich, P. M., Goetz, G., & Hickey, E. J. (2017). Couple conflict in parents of children with versus without autism: Self-reported and observed findings. *Journal of Child and Family Studies, 26*(8), 2152–2165. https://doi.org/10.1007/s10826-017-0737-1

Head, T. (2019). *Interracial marriage laws history & timeline.* https://www.thoughtco.com/interracial-marriage-laws-721611

Hetherington, E. M., & Kelly, J. (2002). *For better or for worse: Divorce reconsidered.* W. W. Norton & Co.

Hickey, E. J., Nix, R. L., & Hartley, S. L. (2019). Family emotional climate and children with autism spectrum disorder. *Journal of Autism and Developmental Disorders, 49*(8), 3244–3256. https://doi.org/10.1007/s10803-019-04037-6

Hohmann-Marriott, B. E. (2009). Father involvement ideals and the union transitions of unmarried parents. *Journal of Family Issues, 30*(7), 898–920. https://doi.org/10.1177/0192513X08327885

Hurley, R. S. E., Losh, M., Parlier, M., Reznick, J. S., & Piven, J. (2007). The Broad Autism Phenotype Questionnaire. *Journal of Autism Developmental Disorders, 37*(9), 1679–1690. https://doi.org/10.1007/s10803-006-0299-3

Ibrahim, F. A., & Schroeder, D. G. (1990). Cross-cultural couples counseling: A developmental, psychoeducational intervention. *Journal of Comparative Family Studies, 21*(2), 193–205. https://doi.org/10.3138/jcfs.21.2.193

Isacco, A., Garfield, C. F., & Rogers, T. E. (2010). Correlates of coparental support among married and nonmarried fathers. *Psychology of Men & Masculinity, 11*(4), 262–278. https://doi.org/10.1037/a0020686

Jamison, T. P., Ganong, L., & Proulx, C. M. (2017). Unmarried coparenting in the context of poverty: Understanding the relationship between stress, family resource management, and resilience. *Journal of Family and Economic Issues, 38*(3), 439–452. https://doi.org/10.1007/s10834-016-9518-z

Jenkins, J., Simpson, A., Dunn, J., Rasbash, J., & O'Connor, T. G. (2005). Mutual influence of marital conflict and children's behavior problems: Shared and non-shared family risks. *Child Development, 76*(1), 24–39. https://doi.org/10.1111/j.1467-8624.2005.00827.x

Jones, C. W. (2019). *Setting the stage for change: An eco-systemic approach to in-home family-based treatment* (2nd ed.). Center for Family Based Training.

Karney, B. R., & Bradbury, T. N. (2020). Research on marital satisfaction and stability in the 2010s: Challenging conventional wisdom. *Journal of Marriage and the Family, 82*(1), 100–116. https://doi.org/10.1111/jomf.12635

Killian, K. D. (2001). Reconstituting racial histories and identities: The narratives of interracial couples. *Journal of Marital and Family Therapy, 27*(1), 27–42. https://doi.org/10.1111/j.1752-0606.2001.tb01137.x

King, D. B., & DeLongis, A. (2013). Dyadic coping with stepfamily conflict: Demand and withdraw responses between husbands and wives. *Journal of Social and Personal Relationships, 30*(2), 198–206. https://doi.org/10.1177/0265407512454524

Knox, D., & Zusman, M. E. (2001). Marrying a man with "baggage": Implications for second wives. *Journal of Divorce & Remarriage, 35*(3–4), 67–79. https://doi.org/10.1300/J087v35n03_04

Laxman, D. J., Jessee, A., Mangelsdorf, S. C., Rossmiller-Giesing, W., Brown, G. L., & Schoppe-Sullivan, S. J. (2013). Stability and antecedents of coparenting quality: The role of parent personality and child temperament. *Infant Behavior and Development, 36*(2), 210–222. https://doi.org/10.1016/j.infbeh.2013.01.001

Leslie, L. A., & Letiecq, B. L. (2004). Marital quality of African American and White partners in interracial couples. *Personal Relationships, 11*(4), 559–574. https://doi.org/10.1111/j.1475-6811.2004.00098.x

Lucier-Greer, M., Ketring, S. A., Adler, B. F., & Smith, T. (2012). Malleability of gender role attitudes and gendered messages in couple and relationship education. *Family and Consumer Sciences Research Journal, 41*(1), 4–17. https://doi.org/10.1111/j.1552-3934.2012.02125.x

McClain, L., & Brown, S. L. (2017). The roles of fathers' involvement and coparenting in relationship quality among cohabiting and married parents. *Sex Roles, 76*(5–6), 334–345. https://doi.org/10.1007/s11199-016-0612-3

McClain, L. R. (2011). Better parents, more stable partners: Union transitions among cohabiting parents. *Journal of Marriage and the Family, 73*(5), 889–901. https://doi.org/10.1111/j.1741-3737.2011.00859.x

McHale, J. P., & Rotman, T. (2007). Is seeing believing? Expectant parents' outlooks on coparenting and later coparenting solidarity. *Infant Behavior and Development, 30*(1), 63–81. https://doi.org/10.1016/j.infbeh.2006.11.007

McLanahan, S., & Beck, A. N. (2010). Parental relationships in fragile families. *The Future of Children, 20*(2), 17–37. https://doi.org/10.1353/foc.2010.0007

McLanahan, S., Garfinkel, I., Mincy, R. B., & Donahue, E. (2010). Introducing the issue. *The Future of Children, 20*(2), 3–16. https://doi.org/10.1353/foc.2010.0005

O'Brien, T. B., DeLongis, A., Pomaki, G., Puterman, E., & Zwicker, A. (2009). Couples coping with stress: The role of empathic responding. *European Psychologist, 14*(1), 18–28. https://doi.org/10.1027/1016-9040.14.1.18

Olsavsky, A. L., Yan, J., Schoppe, S. S. J., & Kamp Dush, C. M. (2019). New fathers' perceptions of dyadic adjustment: The roles of maternal gatekeeping and coparenting closeness. *Family Process.* https://doi.org/10.1111/famp.12451

Papernow, P. L. (2013). *Surviving and thriving in stepfamily relationships: What works and what doesn't.* Routledge. https://doi.org/10.4324/9780203813645

Papernow, P. L. (2018). Clinical guidelines for working with stepfamilies: What family, couple, individual, and child therapists need to know. *Family Process, 57*(1), 25–51. https://doi.org/10.1111/famp.12321

Petren, R. E., Garneau-Rosner, C. L., & Yildirim, E. D. (2018). Union stability among mothers and stepfathers: Contributions of stepfathers and biological fathers. *Journal of Family Psychology, 32*(8), 1142–1151. https://doi.org/10.1037/fam0000482

Raley, R. K., & Sweeney, M. M. (2020). Divorce, repartnering, and stepfamilies: A decade in review. *Journal of Marriage and the Family, 82*(1), 81–99. https://doi.org/10.1111/jomf.12651

Reed, J. (2009). Anatomy of the breakup: How and why do unmarried couples with children break up. In P. England & K. Edin (Eds.), *Unmarried couples with children* (pp. 133–156). Russell Sage Foundation.

Reiter, M. J., & Gee, C. B. (2008). Open communication and partner support in intercultural and interfaith romantic relationships: A relational maintenance approach. *Journal of Social and Personal Relationships, 25*(4), 539–559. https://doi.org/10.1177/0265407508090872

Rosenthal, L., Deosaran, A., Young, D. L., & Starks, T. J. (2019). Relationship stigma and well-being among adults in interracial and same-sex relationships. *Journal of Social & Personal Relationships, 36*(11–12), 3408–3428. https://doi.org/10.1177/0265407518822785

Rowley, S. J., Sellers, R. M., Chavous, T. M., & Smith, M. A. (1998). The relationship between racial identity and self-esteem in African American college and high school students. *Journal of Personality and Social Psychology, 74*(3), 715–724. https://doi.org/10.1037/0022-3514.74.3.715

Schnabel, A., Youssef, G. J., Hallford, D. J., Hartley, E. J., McGillivray, J. A., Stewart, M., Forbes, D., & Austin, D. W. (2020). Psychopathology in parents of children with autism spectrum disorder: A systematic review and meta-analysis of prevalence. *Autism: An International Journal of Research and Practise, 24*(1), 26–40. https://doi.org/10.1177/1362361319844636

Schramm, D. G., & Adler-Baeder, F. (2012). Marital quality for men and women in stepfamilies: Examining the role of economic pressure, common stressors, and stepfamily-specific stressors. *Journal of Family Issues, 33*(10), 1373–1397. https://doi.org/10.1177/0192513X11428126

Sellers, R. M., & Shelton, J. N. (2003). The role of racial identity in perceived racial discrimination. *Journal of Personality and Social Psychology, 84*(5), 1079–1092. https://doi.org/10.1037/0022-3514.84.5.1079

Seltzer, J. A. (2000). Families formed outside of marriage. *Journal of Marriage and the Family, 62*(4), 1247–1268. https://doi.org/10.1111/j.1741-3737.2000.01247.x

Seshadri, G., & Knudson-Martin, C. (2013). How couples manage interracial and intercultural differences: Implications for clinical practice. *Journal of Marital and Family Therapy, 39*(1), 43–58. https://doi.org/10.1111/j.1752-0606.2011.00262.x

Shapiro, D. N., & Stewart, A. J. (2011). Parenting stress, perceived child regard, and depressive symptoms among stepmothers and biological mothers. *Family Relations, 60*(5), 533–544. https://doi.org/10.1111/j.1741-3729.2011.00665.x

Sim, A., Cordier, R., Vaz, S., & Falkmer, T. (2016). Relationship satisfaction in couples raising a child with autism spectrum disorder: A systematic review of the literature. *Research in Autism Spectrum Disorders, 31*, 30–52. https://doi.org/10.1016/j.rasd.2016.07.004

Sim, A., Cordier, R., Vaz, S., & Falkmer, T. (2019). "We are in this together": Experiences of relationship satisfaction in couples raising a child with autism spectrum disorder. *Research in Autism Spectrum Disorders, 58*, 39–51. https://doi.org/10.1016/j.rasd.2018.11.011

Sim, A., Fristedt, S., Cordier, R., Vaz, S., Kuzminski, R., & Falkmer, T. (2019). Viewpoints on what is important to maintain relationship satisfaction in couples raising a child with autism spectrum disorder. *Research in Autism Spectrum Disorders, 65*, 1–13. https://doi.org/10.1016/j.rasd.2019.04.008

Slattery, M. E., Bruce, V., Halford, W. K., & Nicholson, J. M. (2011). Predicting married and cohabiting couples' futures from their descriptions of stepfamily life. *Journal of Family Psychology, 25*(4), 560–569. https://doi.org/10.1037/a0024538

Smock, P. J., & Schwartz, C. R. (2020). The demography of families: A review of patterns and change. *Journal of Marriage and the Family, 82*(1), 9–34. https://doi.org/10.1111/jomf.12612

Sobolewski, J. M., & King, V. (2005). The importance of the coparental relationship for nonresident fathers' ties to children. *Journal of Marriage and the Family, 67*(5), 1196–1212. https://doi.org/10.1111/j.1741-3737.2005.00210.x

Sprenkle, D. H., & Piercy, F. P. (1992). A family therapy informed view of the current state of the family in the United States. *Family Relations, 41*(4), 404–408. https://doi.org/10.2307/585582

Stanley, S. M., Markman, H. J., & Whitton, S. W. (2002). Communication, conflict, and commitment: Insights on the foundations of relationship success from a national survey. *Family Process, 41*(4), 659–675. https://doi.org/10.1111/j.1545-5300.2002.00659.x

Stanley, S. M., Rhoades, G. K., & Whitton, S. W. (2010). Commitment: Functions, formation, and the securing of romantic attachment. *Journal of Family Theory & Review, 2*(4), 243–257. https://doi.org/10.1111/j.1756-2589.2010.00060.x

Stephenson, E., & DeLongis, A. (2019). A 20-year prospective study of marital separation and divorce in stepfamilies: Appraisals of family stress as predictors. *Journal of Social and Personal Relationships, 36*(6), 1600–1618. https://doi.org/10.1177/0265407518768445

Stewart, S. D. (2010). The characteristics and well-being of adopted stepchildren. *Family Relations, 59*(5), 558–571. https://doi.org/10.1111/j.1741-3729.2010.00623.x

Tach, L., & Edin, K. (2013). The compositional and institutional sources of union dissolution for married and unmarried parents in the United States. *Demography, 50*(5), 1789–1818. https://doi.org/10.1007/s13524-013-0203-7

Thompson Sanders, V. L., Clark, E. M., & Purnell, J. Q. (2012). The role of African American racial identification in health behavior. In J. M. Sullivan & A. M. Esmail (Eds.), *African American identity: Racial and cultural dimensions of the Black experience* (pp. 189–220). Lexington Books/Rowman & Littlefield.

Toosi, N. R., Babbitt, L. G., Ambady, N., & Sommers, S. R. (2012). Dyadic interracial interactions: A meta-analysis. *Psychological Bulletin, 138*(1), 1–27. https://doi.org/10.1037/a0025767

Visher, E. B., Visher, J. S., & Pasley, K. (2003). Remarriage families and stepparenting. In F. Walsh (Ed.), *Normal family processes: Growing diversity and complexity* (3rd ed., pp. 153–175). Guilford Press. https://doi.org/10.4324/9780203428436_chapter_6

Waller, M. R. (2008). How do disadvantaged parents view tensions in their relationships? Insights for relationship longevity among at-risk couples. *Family Relations, 57*(2), 128–143. https://doi.org/10.1111/j.1741-3729.2008.00489.x

Waller, M. R. (2012). Cooperation, conflict, or disengagement? Coparenting styles and father involvement in fragile families. *Family Process, 51*(3), 325–342. https://doi.org/10.1111/j.1545-5300.2012.01403.x

Waller, M. R., & Swisher, R. (2006). Fathers' risk factors in fragile families: Implications for "healthy" relationships and father involvement. *Social Problems, 53*(3), 392–420. https://doi.org/10.1525/sp.2006.53.3.392

Wandersman, A., Duffy, J., Flaspohler, P., Noonan, R., Lubell, K., Stillman, L., Blachman, M., Dunville, R., & Saul, J. (2008). Bridging the gap between prevention research and practice: The interactive systems framework for dissemination and implementation. *American Journal of Community Psychology, 41*(3–4), 171–181. https://doi.org/10.1007/s10464-008-9174-z

5 INTIMATE PARTNER VIOLENCE

A Focus on Queer Families, Families and Substance Use, and Military Couples

RESEARCH: AUTUMN M. BERMEA
CLINICAL APPLICATIONS: PETER FRAENKEL, KRISTEN BENSON, CAMILLE ST. JAMES, AND MATTHEW BOWEN

RESEARCH: AUTUMN M. BERMEA

Intimate partner violence (IPV) is multifaceted and encompasses a number of acts and experiences between romantic or sexual partners (Breiding et al., 2015). Throughout this chapter, we use the term *partner* or *partners* when referencing IPV to be inclusive of multiple relationship types. Generally, IPV refers to psychological, physical, and sexual violence as well as stalking. Psychological violence includes verbal abuse (e.g., name-calling, belittling), systematic isolation, economic control, making threats, and playing mind games (e.g., gaslighting). Physical violence can include hitting, slapping, hair pulling, and punching, as well as more severe tactics such as hitting a partner hard enough to leave a mark, choking, slamming a partner against something hard, or throwing objects. Stalking includes repeated and unwanted contact—in person, through the mail, or electronically (e.g., over the phone, text messages, social media). It can be directed toward the victim but might also include their loved ones, such as friends, family members, and pets. Stalking can also escalate into physical violence.

https://doi.org/10.1037/0000280-005
Treating Contemporary Families: Toward a More Inclusive Clinical Practice, S. Browning and B. van Eeden-Moorefield (Editors)

Forms of IPV have been categorized into a typology that highlights distinct patterns and suggests unique correlates. Three of the most common forms of intimate partner **violence types** are situational couple violence, coercive controlling violence, and violent resistance (Kelly & Johnson, 2008). *Situational couple violence* is when violence is perpetrated by both partners and often in the context of an argument or conflict escalation. This form of IPV is often what is captured on national or population-based surveys, lending support to the idea of *gender symmetry*, or that both men and women perpetrate IPV at relatively equal rates. The second category is *coercive controlling violence*, which is when one partner attempts to gain control in the relationship through tactics including isolation, fear, and the limiting of resources (e.g., financial control). In this case, physical violence is only one aspect of the abuse. In coercive controlling relationships, only one partner, commonly conceptualized as a cisgender man toward a cisgender woman in a different-gender relationship, perpetrates abuse toward the other. Oftentimes, this form of IPV is captured in locations where survivors receive services, such as hospitals, shelters, and within legal systems, such as in police interactions and the courts. Finally, *violent resistance* is when one partner is violent toward the other in self-defense or in defense of another, typically a child. Violent resistance can occur either during a violent event or before it, in anticipation of violence (Kelly & Johnson, 2008).

This chapter discusses the experiences of IPV in three unique contexts: queer relationships, military families, and substance use disorders (see Table 5.1). We first present some of the research evidence and follow with an overview of some of the major treatment considerations. Finally, we present a clinical case with an intervention focus that is informed by the research for each family type.

Research Evidence on Queer Families

Queer individuals, used here as an inclusive signifier for those who identify within the LGBTQ+ community, are disproportionately more likely to experience IPV than those who are both cisgender and heterosexual (Walters et al., 2013). This means that those who are a sexual minority (e.g., lesbian, gay, bisexual) report IPV more frequently than those who are not, as do people who are a gender minority (e.g., transgender), regardless of their sexual identity, compared with those who are cisgender. These trends should be viewed in light of processes influenced by larger structural contexts related to discrimination (i.e., **minority stress**), discussed subsequently. Here, I review three unique components of IPV in queer relationships: queer-related tactics, minority stress, and **barriers to leaving**.

TABLE 5.1. Intimate Partner Violence

Evidence-based area of clinical focus	Type of factor	Appropriateness for use across families	Selected references indicating evidence base
Violence dynamics	General	All[a]	Breiding et al., 2015
Violence types	General	All[a]	Kelly & Johnson, 2008
Queer-specific tactics	Unique	Queer couples	Cook-Daniels, 2015; Dyar et al., 2021
Minority stress	Unique	Queer couples	Edwards & Sylaska, 2013; McKenry et al., 2006
Barriers to leaving	Unique	Queer couples	Hardesty et al., 2011; Jordan et al., 2020
Instability	Unique	Military families	Jennings-Kelsall, 2012
The Combat Effect	Unique	Military families	Sullivan & Elbogen, 2014; Webermann et al., 2020
Insularity	Unique	Military families	Lutgendorf et al., 2012
Blaming the victim	Unique	Substance use disorders	Yamawaki et al., 2012
Trust within the family system	Unique	Substance use disorders	Kilroy et al., 2014
Contextual influences on help-seeking	Unique	Substance use disorders	Gezinski et al., 2019; McCann & Lubman, 2018

[a]The general factor could work for other family types included in this chapter but needs a small adaptation to ensure cultural relevance. Information about potential adaptations is included in the text.

Tactics

In addition to experiencing IPV more often, **queer survivors** report distinct forms of violence. The tactics documented most often include threatening to disclose the survivor's sexual identity without their consent ("out" them), questioning their sexual identity, attempting to isolate them from other members of the queer community, telling a person to present as heterosexual or, conversely, forcing them into unwanted public displays of affection, and using slurs related to their identity (Dyar et al., 2021). Although many of these tactics can be applied across different groups, there are also certain tactics that survivors experience that are unique to their sexual identities. For example, those who perpetuate IPV against bisexual survivors might force their bisexual partner into unwanted sexual acts by justifying it with the idea that bisexuals are promiscuous (Head & Milton, 2014). Similarly, among transgender and gender nonbinary (TGNB) survivors, perpetrators sometimes purposefully misgender them, tell them they are unlovable because they are TGNB, forbid or withhold access to gender-confirming resources (e.g., hormones, chest binders, gender-aligned clothing, surgery), or forcibly touch them in areas that cause gender dysphoria (e.g., genitals; Cook-Daniels, 2015).

Minority Stress
The role of minority stress has been increasingly recognized as related to violence perpetration in queer relationships (Edwards & Sylaska, 2013). *Minority stress* is the psychological effects of cultural prejudice against queer individuals, including discrimination, rejection, and hostility (Meyer, 2003). Some researchers have theorized that this is because those who experience minority stressors might use substances to cope, which, in turn, might lower inhibitions and exacerbate violence (Shorey et al., 2019). However, this perspective does not consider issues related to power and control. Perpetrators who feel as though their power has been taken away through experiences of discrimination might turn to violence in an intimate relationship to regain power (McKenry et al., 2006).

Barriers to Leaving
Queer survivors often face **barriers to leaving** abusive relationships that cisgender and heterosexual survivors do not. Broadly, there are limited IPV-related services that queer survivors view as welcoming and affirming, and therefore, they might feel their options are limited in accessing formal supports (Jordan et al., 2020). A queer survivor might be further hesitant to reach out to formal resources out of fear that it will stigmatize queer relationships as being dysfunctional or unhealthy (Hassouneh & Glass, 2008; Turell & Herrmann, 2008). Queer survivors might also be hesitant to reach out to police due to the minimization of queer IPV (Hardesty et al., 2011). These feelings might also be further exacerbated for groups who are marginalized within the queer community, such as bisexuals (Head & Milton, 2014) and those who identify as TGNB (Tesch & Bekerian, 2015). TGNB people are disproportionately more likely to be the victims of police violence, and thus they might be reluctant to report violence for their own safety (Jordan et al., 2020). In addition to formal supports, a lack of social supports, either real or perceived, can make it difficult for queer survivors to leave a violent partnership. In some cases, a perpetrator might limit their connections with other members of the queer community or, alternatively, share a similar social circle, making it difficult for others to believe that the perpetrator could be abusive (Turell & Herrmann, 2008). In the case of same-gender relationships, a perpetrator might also tell the survivor that a partner of the

same gender cannot be abusive (Hassouneh & Glass, 2008). These barriers to informal and formal resources often make it difficult for a queer survivor to leave a violent relationship.

Research Evidence on Military Families

Military families are another group with unique considerations to their experiences of family violence. Here we review factors (i.e., locational instability of military families that can cause stress, trauma of **the combat effect**, **insularity** of the military community) that are distinct to military families and can make it difficult for survivors to seek help. The majority of partner violence in the military appears to be perpetrated by men toward a female survivor (Lutgendorf et al., 2012). This is critical because the vast majority of active-duty military personnel are men and most of them are married to civilian spouses (Council of Economic Advisors, 2018).

Instability

Relocation has been identified as a primary stressor in the lives of most military families (Burrell et al., 2006). Military families relocate frequently, can rarely refuse to do so, and may be given little advance notice of an impending move (Dimiceli et al., 2010). Greatly compounding the issue of constant, and often abrupt, relocation is the deployment of the enlisted partner for lengthy and undetermined time periods. Extended deployments cause cumulative, long-lasting strain on enlisted individuals who do not see their children or partners for many months (O'Neal et al., 2019). Within the larger framework of lack of control imbued by military life, research with spouses/partners identified six stressors: (a) stuck in a state of flux, (b) going through changes, (c) relational uncertainty, (d) loneliness, (e) alienation, and (f) anxiety related to deployment (Jennings-Kelsall et al., 2012). The confluence of these stressors holds the potential for these families to experience IPV. These stressors are also often worsened in the presence of the combat effect.

The Combat Effect

The **combat effect** is a form of posttraumatic stress disorder (PTSD) that is specific to those who have served in combat. Past trauma has been linked to violence perpetration in civilian populations (Webermann et al., 2020), which can be amplified for military personnel given the correlation between combat experience and family violence (Sullivan & Elbogen, 2014). This might be because those who experience such trauma are at an increased risk of hyperarousal as well as being quick to anger. Further, those who exhibit trauma might turn to substances to cope, which has also been linked to violence perpetration (Martin et al., 2010).

Insularity

Although the preceding stressors might be predictive of family violence, the **insularity** of the military community can sometimes be a **barrier to ending the abuse**. As a largely self-contained institution and culture, the military exerts control over the lives of service members, which presents unique challenges for identifying and resolving domestic violence. The military largely comprises several autonomous cities that function differently from their civilian counterparts, and many other military personnel are stationed overseas, where adherence to norms and legal procedures differ. In 2006, the Department of Defense removed its requirement for mandatory reporting of suspected domestic violence against adults.

Contrasting with the civilian realm, significant decision-making power can be delegated to a service member's unit commander in response to a domestic violence incident on military bases. Among civilian recourses, boundaries exist with an individual's employer and the medical and legal systems, whereas this is not the case within the military. The Department of Defense established the Family Advocacy Program (FAP) in 1992, which does not include the right of confidentiality under military law. Any evidence gathered during investigations may be used in military justice proceedings, which has led to a decrease in reports of family violence compared with victimization in civilian families (Lutgendorf et al., 2012). Rather than representing a decrease in family violence among military families, this discrepancy indicates that family members are less likely to seek help. Further, in the case of female military personnel, female family violence survivors' experiences of victimization might also be linked to trauma from sexual assault experienced in the military during service (Portnoy et al., 2020). Victims also often hesitate to report abuse due to its potential impact on their partners' careers. Reliance on an abuser can also be a reason that a survivor is reluctant, or might find it difficult, to leave the relationship. Given the distinct context of military families, it is therefore important to consider the unique circumstances and challenges they face in IPV and help-seeking.

Research Evidence on Substance Use Disorders in Families

As previously noted, substance abuse often plays a role in family violence, both within the broader population and within distinct communities, such as queer and military families. This section highlights three important factors when considering family violence in the context of a substance use disorder: **blaming the victim**, **trust within the family system**, and the contextual factors that influence the survivors' experiences of violence and **help-seeking**.

Blaming the Victim

Although substance abuse has been established as a factor in perpetrating family violence, it also plays a role in victimization (Cafferky et al., 2018). Survivors' substance use disorder can create obstacles to receiving necessary help. Additionally, survivors with substance use disorders are vulnerable to "victim blaming," whereby the culpability of violence is turned toward the person who has been harmed (Yamawaki et al., 2012). Victims of violence may be subjected to blame if they are intoxicated, especially in cases of sexual assault (Sims et al., 2007). Although victims are unable to consent to sexual acts when intoxicated, they will sometimes be told they should not have placed themselves in a dangerous or vulnerable situation. Victim blaming can retraumatize survivors and negatively affect functioning.

Trust Within the Family System

Experiences of family violence toward members with substance use disorder can also lead to mistrust within the family system. For example, if a survivor previously lied about substance abuse, family members might be reluctant to believe the survivor's reports of violence. Such outcomes allow the violence to continue and can be detrimental to their recovery, if survivors continue to abuse substances as a means of coping with the trauma (Hawn et al., 2020). If and when family members, such as older parents, eventually uncover the truth about the violence after previously denying survivors' disclosures, feelings of self-blame among those family members may occur (Kilroy et al., 2014). Such dynamics can adversely affect family functioning. Notably, **contextual factors** are also important to consider among families contending with violence and substance use disorders.

Contextual Influences on Help-Seeking

Contextual factors unique to families of survivors with substance use disorder can include judgment, which can be a source of shame for family members (McCann & Lubman, 2018). As such, family members may be less inclined to discuss factors related to substance abuse, which largely mirrors the often-taboo subject of family violence (Murray et al., 2018). Although this may be the case in most cultures, an intersectional approach reveals a more nuanced perspective (Barrios et al., 2020) of families operating in very different types of contexts. For example, in some patriarchal religious communities, family violence can be condoned when female submission to a male partner is encouraged and divorce is discouraged (Gezinski et al., 2019), yet substance use, either recreational or disordered, is immoral. As such, family members may not acknowledge the violence or the substance use. Other contexts, such as those of survivors from minoritized racial populations, may result in detracting survivors from seeking help due to fear of further potential persecution by the police and legal systems (Barrios et al., 2020). These dynamics highlight the need to understand substance abuse in the context of family violence, as well as other contextual considerations.

CLINICAL APPLICATIONS: PETER FRAENKEL, KRISTEN BENSON, CAMILLE ST. JAMES, AND MATTHEW BOWEN

Due to the complexity of treatment of IPV, this clinical section uses a slightly different format than other chapters to clarify the specific factors that need to be understood in pursuing clinical work with this population. We begin with an overview of the history and range of interventions used for couples engaged in IPV and in which both partners are heterosexual and cisgender. We discuss the controversy about whether it is safe and appropriate to conduct conjoint couple therapy for IPV. Next, we briefly describe the integrative feminist–systemic–psychodynamic theory developed by Goldner et al. (1990; Goldner, 2004) that delineates the multiple levels of influence that result in IPV among couples in which both partners are heterosexual and cisgender. In what follows, we briefly summarize two additional behaviorally oriented, empirically supported approaches to treatment shown to be effective, both independently and in a meta-analysis (Karakurt et al., 2016). In the last part of this chapter, we describe several issues (see Table 5.1) and clinical interventions for three specific populations, with each section written by experts in these areas: queer couples, families in which a member has a substance use disorder or addiction, and military couples.

Clinical Expertise and Interpretation of Evidence: An Overview

Beginning in the 1970s, approaches for addressing IPV often highlighted societally reinforced patriarchal power differences between heterosexual cisgender men and women (Hare-Mustin, 1978), which remain intervention options today (Walker, 2017). These include women escaping the violence by temporarily living (often with children) in a shelter and getting support to end the relationship and attain legal protections such as restraining orders. They also include support groups for survivors, as well as for batterers (Babcock et al., 2004; Pence & Paymar, 1993). These group interventions include a culturally sensitive approach that acknowledges intersectional stressors for men of color who batter women and for women victimized by men (Almeida & Durkin, 1999). Larger scale interventions aim to affect structural systems and include social and political movements that result in legal and other policy changes to attain equal rights and protections for women, more stringent laws punishing men for IPV, and the challenging of the patriarchal cultural narrative of men's assumed greater entitlement to power (Hare-Mustin, 1978; Walker, 2017). Other necessary larger systems and cultural transformations pertain to reducing IPV in LGBTQ+ couples and providing safety when IPV occurs. These include decreasing the stigma of non–cisgender and heteronormative identities and relationships more generally vis-à-vis the broader society—a stigma that is often internalized and causes a range of negative psychological effects, including reluctance to seek therapeutic and protective services (Carvalho et al., 2011; Jordan et al., 2020). Before continuing, we would like to note the language used to refer to persons who are the targets of IPV. Although much clinical and popular literature has substituted the term *survivor* for the earlier term *victim* so as not to further stigmatize or add to a sense of powerlessness for women who have experienced IPV, the research literature generally uses the term *victim*. This is probably because at the time the studies were conducted, women were still in these violent relationships; they had not left the abusers and their "survival" of the violence is not solely in the past but also in the present. Therefore, we use the term *victim* in this section.

The "cycle of violence" described in the first edition of Walker's (2017) classic book remains useful for many cases. Originally described in reference to couples in which both partners are heterosexual and cisgender, the cycle of violence is a pattern in which a male partner becomes challenged and frustrated and engages in physical violence and other forms of abuse. Such forms include emotional, sexual, and economic threats; intimidating gestures and looks; and controlling the woman's relationship to time in general as well as where she goes outside the home and when she returns. This is followed by feelings of remorse and apology, and the victim's acceptance of declarations that this will not happen again, after which the couple reconnects.

In considering the current taxonomy of violent couples described in the research (Johnson, 2008), this pattern may pertain mostly to "coercive controlling violence" in which a man perpetrates abuse against a woman to achieve domination. In situational violence where both partners engage in violence, it may be one or both partners who seek forgiveness for their behavior, but in either case, the couple reunites. The main point for the clinician to bear in mind is that these couples typically stay together despite repeated violent episodes and the urgings of others to separate. It is the nature of this powerful connection that must be explored and addressed so that partners can make choices either to change their attitudes and behaviors or separate without fear of further violence or other consequences, such as loss of economic support, housing, threats against the children or other family members, or destructive sharing of information about the partner with family, friends, or workplace colleagues (Walker, 2017).

Controversy About Conjoint Couple Therapy

Notably, there has long been a fair amount of controversy, particularly among many feminist thinkers, about whether it is appropriate to conduct couple therapy for IPV (Bograd, 1984; see reviews of the debate by Maharaj, 2017; Walker, 2017). However, a strong clinical/conceptual and empirical case has been made for couple therapy over individual treatment and for gender-specific group treatment, as well as no treatment (usually with recommendations by shelter staff or others for the battered woman to leave the man) for couples who engage in situational violence and want to try to stay together. There are also support groups focused on cognitive-behavioral and feminist principles and practices for male batterers that typically address anger management, communication and appropriate assertiveness skills, critique of patriarchal beliefs that assign greater power to men than women, and heighten awareness of the negative effects on the victims of violence and their children. Such groups have been found to yield mixed results at best, with some research indicating high dropout rates, peer-influenced normalization of violence (Babcock et al., 2004; Stover et al., 2009), and no difference in recidivism rates for men who attended groups over those who were simply arrested (Babcock et al., 2004). The popular and often mandated community-based "Duluth model" (Pence & Paymar, 1993) used with male perpetrators is based on a feminist analysis of patriarchy and introduces men to the Power and Control Wheel to heighten their awareness of the many ways that men abuse socially sanctioned power. However, this model has not been shown to reduce recidivism of violence either (Stover et al., 2009).

In contrast, a meta-analysis of six well-controlled studies showed couple therapy to be more effective than alternative treatments or no treatment (Karakurt et al., 2016). The approaches described in this chapter integrate feminist concerns about women's safety with the reality that many women maintain or return to abusive relationships despite counseling to leave (Goldner at al., 1990; Stith et al., 2011). All include feminist-based psychoeducation or consciousness-raising about violence and its larger societal determinants that are delivered either conjointly or in gender-specific groups occurring before the conjoint couple work. In contrast to approaches that counsel women to leave abusive relationships irrespective of the level of violence, these approaches recognize that in many cases of situational violence, the violence is bidirectional and can be initiated by the woman as well as by the man (Straus, 2011) and that couples in which there has been IPV often seek couple therapy. As such, rejecting victims' requests on ideological grounds raises other ethical concerns about denial of treatment. As Fals-Stewart and Clinton-Sherrod (2009) noted, "to select intervention approaches in developing treatment plans that the preponderance of research reveals is not as effective as couples therapy raises its own set of ethical concerns" (p. 262).

Integrative Systemic-Feminist Theory and Practice in IPV: The Ackerman Institute

In the late 1980s into the early 1990s, building on the feminist movement in family therapy (Goldner, 1985; Hare-Mustin, 1978), Goldner and colleagues (1990) at the Ackerman Institute for the Family developed an integrative feminist/systemic approach to working with couples in which there had been violence. This approach also included a psychoanalytic perspective on internalized representations of intimate relationships derived from family-of-origin and attachment theory, as well as social learning theory's perspective on how gendered relational beliefs and behaviors are learned and reinforced. Although never assessed as to its effectiveness through empirical study, it remains the most theoretically nuanced and integrative systemic analysis of the many factors that converge in acts of intimate violence, at least for couples in which both partners are heterosexual and cisgender. We describe it here to complement the more straightforward behavioral and solution-focused approaches that have garnered the most empirical support (Fals-Stewart & Clinton-Sherrod, 2009; Stith et al., 2011).

Goldner et al. (1990) found that working with IPV required a significant reconceptualization of basic systems theory, especially around the fundamental notions of circular causality and the function of the symptom–homeostasis. Whereas systems theory traditionally held that all participants in a relational problem contributed equally (and therefore with equal power) to the maintenance of the problem in a repeated circular, reciprocal fashion, Goldner and colleagues (1990) held that this construction implicitly suggested that women have equal power in perpetuating men's violent behavior, a notion that went against feminism's emphasis on the social-structural privileging of men's power over women. Likewise, the general notion that problems or symptoms serve the function of maintaining or stabilizing a family system whose equilibrium or homeostasis is disrupted—for instance, when a woman stated her displeasure with a man's behavior or other conditions of their lives together—was rightly deemed seriously problematic by feminists (Bograd, 1984) because it ignored the manner in which coercion, threat, and violence represented a one-way, or linear, attempt by a male partner to exert control and silence a woman's objections.

Holding the "double vision" (Goldner et al., 1990, p. 344) of feminism and systems theory led to an approach to treatment that simultaneously addresses the broader social narrative that affirms men's power over and violence toward women, while also addressing the circular, reciprocal interactions between men and women that precede a man perpetrating violence. This approach acknowledges the distress experienced by the man before his violent behavior, which is cast as an explanation, not an excuse. However, abusers needed to take full responsibility for the choice to engage in violence and were encouraged to reflect on other, nonviolent ways in which they could respond to perceived provocation. Both partners were engaged in changing their interactional cycle and in understanding how their respective behaviors triggered family-of-origin–based attachment insecurity and other vulnerabilities.

The Ackerman approach also sought to help couples separate from the simplistic script of "perpetrator and victim" by separating the man's tendency toward violence from his broader personhood. Doing so appeals to the latter to enact change in beliefs and behavioral responses and also empowers the woman to view herself not only as a victim but as a person. Men's violence was often conceptualized as instrumental—a means of dominating and silencing the female partner—yet experienced by many men as spontaneous and impulsive. This belief on the part of male perpetrators that their violence is due to "loss of control" results in shame and remorse, expressions of which reengage the female partner to maintain the relationship.

Central to this approach is an analysis of how persons become gendered in early childhood and how this socialization affects men's and women's orientation to their own and other's emotions and their relational exchanges. Drawing on gender studies in anthropology, developmental psychology, and psychoanalysis, girls are understood to develop gender identity through identification with the mother, still the primary parent despite an increase in men's involvement in parenting over the past few decades (Fraenkel & Capstick, 2012), whereas boys develop an identity that is centered on being *different* from the mother. Thus, to be a man is largely defined as being not like a woman. Given that women are socialized to accept and even highlight their emotional vulnerability and their greater role in preserving connection, men's sense of masculinity requires them to reject vulnerable feelings and to rely on women to maintain a positive emotional quality to the relationship and repair ruptures when these occur.

Goldner et al. (1990) found that in couples in which there has been violence, the violence is often preceded by events that leave the man feeling hurt, criticized, weak, disempowered, dependent, and afraid of abandonment. Goldner's (2004) later writing incorporates research by Dutton (1998) indicating that abusive men often suffer from an extreme version of insecure attachment, as well as experiences of shame and humiliation at the hands of their fathers, which later provide the intrapsychic fuel for self-protective rage. When combined with rigid gender norms about avoiding vulnerability or expressing needs for connection, this insecure attachment leads men to engage in controlling behavior to ensure that their dependency needs are met.

These vulnerable feelings—largely disavowed consciously and seen by the man as "caused" by the woman—are viewed as feminine and therefore as subverting the man's sense of gender identity. As such, he attempts to reassert his masculinity by engaging in expressions of dominance, including violence. This in turn pushes the woman, who may have been attempting to assert herself and equalize power, back into a subordinate role and elicits her feminine socialization, especially qualities of empathy and acts of emotional protection, so as to repair the relationship. Based on her relationship with her often similarly subjugated mother, the woman's gender socialization leads her to preserve connection despite conflict, suppress her own voice, needs, and autonomy, accept a lack of empathy from her partner, and privilege the needs of others. Further, doing so can contribute to her difficulty in leaving a violent relationship.

Goldner et al.'s (1990) formulation of the psychological precursors to violence also includes a detailed description of the loyalty binds and confusing identifications both men and women in these relationships experienced in their families of origin. (Please note that this brief summary does not do justice to the theory's thoughtful description of these complex, gendered loyalty binds and how they are activated in IPV. Interested readers should consult the original articles.) They found that men often had fathers who were violent, who did not establish a warm bond with their sons, and who insisted on and modeled hypermasculine behavior—being "tough" and not experiencing or expressing vulnerable feelings. As adults, because they still longed to experience connection and vulnerability, these men were found to rely on their female partners to demonstrate these needs and feelings for them—an extreme version of gender-based emotional polarization described by Fraenkel (2019) and observed in other high-conflict "last-chance couples." At moments when it was no longer possible to deny these feelings as their own, these men felt feminized and therefore challenged in their identification with their fathers. They then sought to reassert their sense of masculinity and connection with their internalized fathers by reasserting control over their female partners through violence and intimidation.

As a result of these complex gender beliefs, emotion-regulatory processes, and family-of-origin factors that get activated within seconds during conflict with their female partner, therapy with violent men requires repeatedly and slowly "deconstructing the violent moment" (Goldner et al., 1990, p. 353). Doing so enables both unpacking of the internal sources of violence and modeling for the client a slowed-down way of thinking about himself in relation to his partner. Slowing down their experiences and reflections in these violence-prone moments allows all of the current triggers and relational meanings, as well as the internalized scripts from families of origin, to be identified, understood, and modulated, making it possible for men to choose to respond nonviolently.

Another important attribute of Goldner et al.'s (1990) approach to therapy is that it creates a safe space in which to reveal the complex bond or "alliance" between partners and thereby allows both partners, especially the woman, to evaluate her choices more clearly. Often, women feel they know the secret vulnerable part of their abusive partners, often revealed in the apologetic, remorseful denouement of a violent episode, and feel compelled to stand by their abusers, even if sacrificing their own well-being. In particular, therapy needs to honor women's caregiving tendencies as a general strength, while also reevaluating it in the context of IPV and made conditional on loving and equitable treatment. Therapy also needs to highlight positive aspects of the relationship that exist in parallel to the violence, while inviting thinking about whether the relationship can continue without violence so that mutual, healthy caregiving becomes possible. Goldner et al. (1990) wrote, "In our view, it is only when both partners become committed to transcending the rigid categories of gender difference and can begin to tolerate their disowned similarities, that real change is possible" (p. 349).

Obviously, given the centrality of traditional feminist analysis of male–female identity and relationships, the Goldner et al. (1990) approach to IPV does not immediately transfer to queer couples but could be adapted with a broader view of the development of sexual orientation and gender identity and the family-of-origin dynamics surrounding those identities.

Empirically Supported Conjoint Couple Therapy for IPV

This section briefly summarizes two empirically supported approaches to couple therapy with IPV followed by specific interventions for the family types included in this chapter. Most existing models have been tested with couples in which partners are heterosexual and cisgender. To date, no controlled studies have examined couple treatment of IPV in queer couples. However, it is likely that most of the interventions tested thus far would apply for such couples, with necessary additions that address the unique dynamics, sources of heteronormative societal oppression, and internalized stigma experienced by queer persons and couples (Carvalho et al., 2011).

Domestic Violence–Focused Couple Therapy

Stith and colleagues (2004, 2011) developed and empirically tested domestic violence–focused couple therapy. The approach combines psychoeducation, a feminist orientation, and solution-focused therapy, as well as contributions from narrative, Bowen intergenerational, and cognitive-behavioral theories and practices. The treatment begins with careful screening of each partner in confidential individual meetings to determine whether conjoint treatment is appropriate for the couple. The Revised Conflict Tactics Scale (Straus et al., 1996) is used to determine the **severity of the violence** and the degree of similarity in partners' respective reports of severity. Couples in which partners' reports of violence severity are discrepant are not accepted for treatment. Neither are couples in which partners do not feel they could speak openly about their conflicts, fear experiencing retribution after sessions for revealing violent episodes, or in which one partner feels coerced by the other to enter therapy. However, couples are more likely to be accepted when the violence has been more severe, but the perpetrator acknowledges and takes responsibility for it and is motivated for treatment.

The therapy begins with 6 weeks of separate groups for men and women. These groups center on psychoeducation about IPV, help partners become more comfortable with being in treatment, prepare them emotionally for the couple work, afford an opportunity for ongoing evaluation of appropriateness for conjoint work, and foster (especially for perpetrators of abuse) greater acknowledgment of responsibility for the violence. Following these groups, conjoint therapy (either with individual couples or in a group format) is conducted by two therapists and teaches mindfulness skills to reduce physiological/emotional arousal. Referred to as the "time-out" practice, it guides how to avoid escalations, engages couples in broader safety planning, and invites couples to answer and refine the solution-focused Miracle Question. Subsequent sessions center on asking couples about instances of conflict or violence but focus more on exceptions to the problem, using agency questions (the classic Kim Soo Berg question, "How did you do that?" when couples avoided an escalation or got along well) and scaling questions (tracking improvement or regression on a Likert-type scale) to highlight progress in avoiding violence and engaging in positive interactions. In the final (sixth) session, partners are once again interviewed individually to confidentially assess their sense of progress. Last, the cotherapists provide a joint statement to the couple to encourage their continued progress.

Six months after treatment, couples who completed the multicouple treatment reported significant changes in relationship satisfaction, attitudes about wife beating, and relational aggression. At the 2-year follow-up, men in both treatment conditions were less likely to recidivate than men in the no-treatment comparison group. Stith et al. (2004) also noted that compared with outcome data from male batterer programs, recidivism rates were much lower for couples who had received conjoint treatment in either format. They also argued that because both men and women who received the treatment had more negative attitudes about wife beating before treatment, this demonstrates the viability of couple therapy for violence and should assuage concerns that couple therapy (at least with those couples who meet criteria for treatment) creates increased risk of violence against women.

General Couple Therapy for IPV With a Substance-Abusing Partner

Building on earlier studies that demonstrated the effectiveness of behavioral couples therapy (BCT) in reducing IPV in couples with an alcoholic male partner, Fals-Stewart and Clinton-Sherrod (2009) conducted an intervention study with a large sample of couples in which there had been IPV and the male partner was in outpatient substance abuse treatment ($n = 207$ couples). This study did not screen out couples in which there had been more severe forms of IPV. Couples were randomly assigned to two possible groups. One group attended 12 weekly sessions of BCT paired with 20 sessions of standard 12-Step–based individual treatment for the substance-abusing male. Another group entailed 32 weeks of individual behavior therapy (IBT) for the substance-abusing partner, also based on the 12-Step approach.

Results indicated that overall, men who received BCT engaged in significantly less male-to-female violence posttreatment over the 12-month follow-up period compared with men who received only individual substance abuse treatment. Importantly, there was no difference in IPV rates on days when the men had not used substances among men in both the BCT and IBT groups; both treatments reduced incidence of violence on days when the substance-abusing partner abstained. The main difference observed between the treatments centered on frequency of violence on days when the men relapsed: Men who participated in BCT were significantly less likely to initiate violence when using substances compared with men who received IBT.

Clinical Expertise and Interpretation of Evidence: Queer Couples

Treatment protocols for therapy with queer and trans couples are emerging. Historically, IPV has maintained a heteronormative bias that assumes perpetrators are cisgender men and victims are cisgender women (Cannon & Buttell, 2015). Given that couple therapy for IPV was initially somewhat controversial (see the earlier review by Fraenkel), treatment typically followed gender-specific tracks where men completed psychoeducational groups and women received victim support services (McCollum & Stith, 2011). Although rates of IPV among same-gender couples are similar to or even higher than rates of IPV in couples in which partners are heterosexual and cisgender, heteronormative approaches to treatment rooted in gender assumptions are not helpful to queer couples (Subirana-Malaret et al., 2019); therapy must center on gender identity and sexual orientation. Couples may not define themselves as violent or report violence during a clinical intake, and queer couples may be less forthcoming about violence. As noted in the research review, some couples may feel pressure to legitimize their relationships as "healthy" given **minority stress** and heteronormative assumptions (Bornstein et al., 2006). Heterosexual clinicians must be aware of their own heterosexual assumptions to provide inclusive services to queer clients (McGeorge & Carlson, 2011). Awareness of heterosexism and heteronormative influences are critical to understanding the systemic process that marginalizes queer people (McGeorge & Carlson, 2011), as sexual minority stressors both contribute to IPV and also create **barriers to treatment** and services (Carvalho et al., 2011).

Clinical Experience: Observations of Common Interactional Patterns

The nature of violence and the willingness to discuss IPV vary in queer relationships, requiring therapists to establish a queer inclusive and nonjudgmental environment. Clinicians should first meet with the couple in a conjoint therapy session and assess their relationship history and strengths (Linville et al., 2012). Throughout the initial conversation, the therapist should pay attention to intersectionality and how those combined locations play into their issues around violence. The therapist can ask follow-up questions about each partner's unique experiences regarding how their identities relate to IPV and assess social and family supports.

Next, the therapist should individually interview each partner to assess the type of IPV that has occurred to determine the nature of the IPV in the couple. If the couple experienced situational violence, conjoint therapy may be applicable; in cases where intimate terrorism or coercive controlling violence is present, conjoint therapy is not appropriate (McCollum & Stith, 2011). Situational violence occurs when a specific situation escalates and, unlike intimate terrorism, does not involve ongoing pervasive fear and control of one partner over the other, such as threats to out a closeted partner or restrict access to gender-confirming resources (Woulfe & Goodman, 2021). The therapist may use an IPV assessment instrument if language on the measure is suitable for use with queer and nonbinary clients (e.g., Dyar et al., 2021). The therapist should inquire about how out, or public, partners are about their sexual orientation and gender identity and if their partner ever threatens to "out" them to force them to comply (e.g., a queer person who is not out at work and may face discrimination). For couples who experience situational couple violence and express an interest to stop using violence, conjoint couple therapy may continue.

Case Context: Characteristics, Culture, and Preferences
Angel (age 34, White, cisgender, queer) and Tai (age 37, Latinx, nonbinary, queer) are an out queer couple who have been partnered for 7 years. They are active in their local queer community, and enjoy socializing with friends, but recently have noticed that friends increasingly decline invitations to spend time with them. They recognize that "things get out of hand" on occasion and want to communicate better. The couple agrees that they get along well for the most part, yet when they are frustrated with one another, arguments quickly escalate to yelling and throwing whatever items are within reach. Angel will "get in Tai's face" and push them when she feels they won't listen to her. Tai gets defensive and will shove Angel to get their away. Angel has hit Tai on the arms and left bruises on a few occasions when she was attempting to get their attention. They sought couple therapy after a recent incident involving law enforcement. A neighbor overheard an argument and called the police, who came to Angel and Tai's home. The officer referred to Tai as "sir," although they clarified their gender as nonbinary. Tai disclosed that they did not want police involvement because they feared being placed in the men's jail based on the gender marker in their driver's license. Angel believed the police officer seemed to assume that Tai was to blame even

though Angel was yelling and had hit Tai. When she attempted to explain, the officer threatened to arrest both of them.

Clinical Decisions: Intervention Implementation

The intervention is guided by research on conjoint couple therapy for IPV (Stith et al., 2011) and by research and recommendations specific to queer populations (Carvalho et al., 2011; Linville et al., 2012). The first session included Angel and Tai, with the goals of establishing rapport, getting to know the couple's history and current primary concerns, and what has kept them together despite conflict and other challenges. The therapist determined how willing the couple was to talk during the conjoint session about their relationship and their experiences of violence. Angel and Tai indicated that they had engaged in low-level bidirectional partner violence and want to stop using violence in their relationship. Angel expressed her embarrassment after the incident involving police and her fear that her behavior could have resulted in a high-risk situation for Tai if they had been arrested. The therapist asked further questions about what risk and safety mean for Angel as a cisgender White woman and how Tai experiences risk and safety as a nonbinary Latinx person. Angel acknowledged that while she tends to initiate escalation of violence in their relationship conflicts, Tai is more likely to face dangerous consequences. In contrast to these violent episodes, the couple reported that for the most part, they have fun together, share similar values, and want to stay together.

The therapist then met individually with each partner to (a) further explore Angel's and Tai's concerns in the relationship, (b) assess if either of them are using substances, and (c) further assess IPV by asking questions about their sense of safety in the relationship and specific behaviors during conflict. The therapist normalized IPV assessment by directly and matter-of-factly asking questions such as the following: Have you ever pushed your partner? Does your partner ever hit you? How often does this happen? Are you committed to finding ways to resolve conflict that do not involve physical and hurtful verbal altercations? What do you do to resolve conflicts in your relationship? To assess issues specific to this couple's queer relationship, the therapist asked Angel and Tai to each complete the Revised Conflict Tactics Scale (CTS2; Straus & Douglas, 2004), which helps to identify familiar behaviors on the Gay, Lesbian, Bisexual, and Trans Power and Control Wheel (Texas Council on Family Violence, 1995). Additionally, the therapist asked Tai to point out relevant issues listed on the Trans-Specific Power and Control Tactics handout (FORGE, 2013). The therapist compared responses on the CTS2 to detect similarities and discrepancies, as well as the concerns specific to sexual orientation and gender identity, and concluded that Angel and Tai are not fearful of one another and have a desire to resolve conflicts.

Angel revealed that she often initiates pushing, hitting, or throwing objects during an argument, and Tai becomes physical to push her away, but has never hit her. Angel stated that she would be comfortable talking about these incidences and her feelings with Tai in the room. Tai disclosed they are sometimes concerned that neighbors hear their arguments, which draws attention to them. Tai does not hide being nonbinary, yet they prefer not to draw attention to themself to "avoid trouble." They do not believe that Angel intentionally wants to endanger them. The therapist asked Tai if they ever discuss how they navigate cisnormative spaces, and Tai agreed this would be an important conversation to have with Angel in a future session. Individual assessments indicated that both partners minimally use substances socially, and neither appeared to experience addiction or substance abuse issues. Both stated that they would like to engage in couple therapy and are open to challenging conversations. As such, the therapist recommended conjoint couple therapy and scheduled their next appointment with the understanding that assessment is a process rather than an event and will occur throughout therapy (McCollum & Stith, 2011).

Ongoing couple therapy is guided by a relational approach and requires that the therapist be skilled in deescalation. In this case, the therapist was informed by narrative therapy (White, 2007), which allows for a curious stance to explore the meaning Angel and Tai make of their relationship within a critical cultural context (Tilsen, 2013). The therapist asked Angel and Tai deconstructing questions, which included: "What are the unspoken rules within your relationship? Who enforces the rules and what are the penalties for breaking them?" Angel responded that she would never strike Tai with a closed fist or hit near their head and that she believed Tai would end the relationship if she crossed that line. Tai stated that it is OK to be physical to defend themself when Angel was aggressive, but they did not initiate violent behaviors. The therapist then asked follow-up questions regarding where they learned these rules and "Do you think the rules about your relationship are the same as other couples given your social location as a queer couple of different ethnicities? How are they the same or different? Are you OK with this?"

Angel and Tai came to realize that the violence in their relationship was less likely to be taken seriously by their cisgender, heterosexual friends and family because of social assumptions about gender and violence, as Angel is a cis woman and Tai is nonbinary who was assigned male at birth. They went on to talk about how these rules invalidate Tai's gender identity and hold Angel less accountable for her behaviors. They agreed that this was problematic and wanted to work together against these social inequities and to take more stands for justice.

When the couple returned for a fourth session, they reported a unique outcome: They had gotten into a conflict a few days earlier, were able to take a time-out and come back to talk about the problem without it escalating. As couple therapy continued, the therapist asked inoculation questions about unique outcomes: "What do you know now that you think 'injustice' would want you to forget during a fight?" and a reauthoring question: "What skills and knowledge did you have to be able to stop that fight from escalating?" The therapist asked additional consultative questions, such as, "What advice do you have for other queer interracial couples whose fights sometimes become violent?" Therapy encouraged Angel and Tai to better understand the meaning they made about IPV in their relationship, how it connects to larger social contexts, and how they prefer to be as a couple.

Clinical Expertise and Interpretation of Evidence: IPV in Military Couples

Military families are unique with regard to factors that influence them (see the research section by Bermea) and are a relatively understudied population (Palmer, 2008). The incidence of domestic violence within the military is consistently much higher than for civilian families. Rates in the civilian population are reported to have declined significantly over a 20-year period to 3.6 per 1,000 people age 12 or older; during this same period, rates within the military were found to range between 18.6 and as high as 25 per 1,000 personnel (Hourani et al., 2017).

Clinical Experience: Observations of Common Interactional Patterns

Within the clearly defined hierarchy of a given military base, intervention for IPV begins with a complaint typically fielded by a supervisory non-commissioned officer and then brought to the attention of the commander. After consultation with the Law Center, the appropriate course of action is determined at numerous levels (involving military lawyers, family support program staff, and, finally, the defendant's immediate commander) and is influenced by the nature of the evidence and relational circumstances. Once the couple involved expresses a willingness to engage in therapy, the parties are referred to treatment. A common systemic pattern has been found in which the soldier becomes overwhelmed emotionally, leaving the spouse to try to interpret whether the outburst is related to PTSD or issues in the relationship.

Case Context: Characteristics, Culture, and Preferences

As a 21-year-old infantry platoon commander in the Marine Corps, Jeremy embarked on the first of two 7-month deployments to Iraq. It was during a period of heavy fighting, and he was repeatedly engaged in significant combat. He was awarded for very high valor for action in his second tour. This resulted in what he experienced as overwhelming adulation and attention. He chose a job as drill instructor as his stateside career track. Several months postdeployment, he was plagued by continuous nightmares of deceased comrades and was coping through heavy alcohol abuse. He was readily found unfit to function in the demanding role of drill instructor and transferred to part-time duty on a landscape crew. Referred for evaluation, he was diagnosed with PTSD and prescribed psychotropic and pain medication. Jeremy would have been discharged as a result of the diagnosis if not for his decoration.

He rejected group therapy. The psychotropics caused lethargy, and he was chronically sleep deprived. Married to his high school sweetheart, 20-year-old Becky, just before his first deployment, she was quickly overwhelmed by the severe downward spiral in Jeremy upon his return. She was employed on base as a cosmetologist. Since returning stateside, Jeremy had become disengaged and withdrawn overall. At the onset of violence, he was secluded in the spare room on the computer when Becky went in to ask if he needed anything. In despair due to his lack of response, she took him firmly by the shoulder. He reacted by backhanding her in the head. She was dazed by the blow and fled to the bedroom. Jeremy remained on the computer for several more hours, drinking beer before falling asleep on the couch.

They did not discuss the incident, but Becky had confided in her sister across the country. Because of Jeremy's high profile and the lack of confidentiality, the sisters agreed that reporting or calling for professional help on base was out of the question. For the next several weeks, they maintained their routine, which for Jeremy was either his part-time work or being isolated in their apartment. At night she watched television while he passed the evening almost exclusively playing video games predicated on the Iraq war. Sex had entailed only several perfunctory episodes in over 2 months, and their original plan to get pregnant when he returned from war was forsaken. Becky was enormously disappointed in this, and she had also largely withdrawn from her network of several friends on base because they were in relationships and Jeremy had ceased socializing. When one of those friends probed her, she glossed over the issues and felt more compelled to withdraw for fear she might end up confiding about the violence.

Two weeks after the initial incident a second one occurred. On that occasion, Jeremy impulsively flung her across the small kitchen after she bumped into him as they prepared dinner. She bounced off the wall and fell to the floor. Cursing, he started to help her up, but she scrambled away and ran into the bedroom and locked the door. When she refused to open it, Jeremy kicked it in. Rather than advancing on her, he abruptly retreated to his computer room and drank the night away. Becky left a message at work that she had to fly home on account of a sudden death, called her sister to say she was coming home to get away from Jeremy, and left the next morning for the airport while Jeremy slept on the couch.

Both families supported Becky, and all agreed that she and Jeremy needed to receive psychological treatment as a condition of Becky returning home. Becky and Jeremy talked for hours each of the 5 days she was gone. That process, and the loss of her physical presence, was literally a sobering experience for Jeremy. Becky advocated that they go into therapy as a couple (a tack suggested to her by her former high school guidance counselor, whom she had consulted for lack of any mental health contacts), which resonated with Jeremy and to which he committed. The key feature of their plan was to seek treatment outside the VA hospital to conceal the domestic violence from the Marine Corps. As such, they would pay privately versus using military benefits. Becky connected with a male clinical social worker who was a noncombatant Marine Corps veteran. He specialized in domestic violence wherein he facilitated a male batterers group as jail diversion for first-time offenders.

Clinical Decisions: Intervention Implementation

The extended intake session established that the process would entail a starting structure of six weekly sessions. Each session would be attended as a couple, but Jeremy readily acknowledged that he was the problem focus and was highly motivated to regain his former self. It was understood that Becky's role was as a supportive participant who wanted to have no further fear of being battered and to save her marriage. That she grew up close to a cousin and uncle with alcoholism contributed helpful background for that essential component of the treatment approach. Jeremy affirmed that keeping his marriage and getting back on track to become parents were paramount goals.

Among the presenting problems, it was emphasized that, first and foremost, the goal was to stop the violence. As noted in the research section by Bermea in this chapter, Sullivan and Elbogen (2014) established that the hyperarousal common to PTSD is a major factor in the instigation and perpetuation of IPV. The two violent incidents were carefully reviewed; highlighting how Jeremy's PTSD led him instinctively to lash out after Becky inadvertently and without notice violated his physical space. It was helpful for both of them to understand that the violence was not a reflection of Jeremy being hateful toward Becky or a flaw in their relationship, but rather solely a function of a primitive reflex in service of self-preservation classic to combat engendered PTSD. Concrete approaches to avoid such moments were discussed, and for self-educational purposes, several related web links about PTSD were provided for the couple to review between sessions. The second session initially reviewed the readings, which both members of the couple reported found useful. Moreover, they had discussed the material at length during the week. They reported sleeping together every night in the interim, breaking Jeremy's pattern of staying up late and sleeping on the couch. Satisfying sexual relations occurred on two occasions. They reported feeling reconnected as a couple now, joined in understanding and commitment to overcoming the consequences of combat trauma on Jeremy and their marriage.

As a next step, the highlights of a U.S. Department of Defense report was presented, which strongly recommended the development of effective violence risk reduction interventions in military populations postdeployment. This entailed identifying protective factors that have proven to decrease the risk of violence. Additionally, this model establishes the domains of basic functioning and well-being, which helped the couple identify and process how Jeremy's war trauma had caused regression in basic functioning, which also affected their relationship. Much of this work is also geared to help educate both members of the couple about the effects of war on the ability to trust, share, and feel safe. Helping the couple to experiment with ways to reconnect and establish safety was highly effective in stabilizing the couple. For example, in one intervention, the therapist asked Jeremy, "How can Becky believe that you love her when the violence occurs?" Jeremy stared down and said, "I never stop loving her, it just is not me when I am triggered." The therapist then turned to both said, "So the key will be that we need to learn the triggers so that we can assist Jeremy to not get lost."

Alcohol was isolated as the priority domain to address for Jeremy's self-care and the couple's well-being. This problem focus was particularly addressed in terms of its extremely well-established correlation with IPV. Despite his new understandings about PTSD, Jeremy felt guilty and apologetic for aggressing against Becky and had a strong sense of shame. Indeed, the two battering episodes served to highly motivate him to gain control of his alcohol abuse. Thus, the treatment process at this phase isolated a two-factor basis for the violence as (a) PTSD creating a brittle trigger and (b) the alcohol disinhibiting that trigger. Because the latter could be much more readily intervened with than the former, eliminating alcohol abuse was prioritized through a collaboratively drafted contract.

Furthermore, to enhance Jeremy's well-being by critically burning energy for both physical and emotional benefit, an exercise schedule that included Becky was also drafted. By virtue of Jeremy's Marine Corps training, and the couple both having an athletic background, this initiative was very much embraced as a means for returning to healthy activities together, reminiscent of the time the couple shared before Jeremy's deployments. This return to exercising together, along with Jeremy's motivation to regain his recently disciplined, responsible, and high-functioning self, combined optimally to help the couple invest in, and adhere to, the treatment protocol. With the violence and alcohol abuse contained and the couple reunited as a positively functioning unit, the treatment could then progress to individual work with Jeremy to address the PTSD.

Clinical Expertise and Interpretation of Evidence: IPV and Families in Which a Member Has a Substance Use Disorder

As highlighted in Bermea's research section of this chapter, an overarching culture of secrecy is pervasive among families in which a member struggles with addiction and substances, making IPV more likely to occur and less likely to be reported. Hawn et al. (2020) reported that the fear of not being believed can lead to additional substance abuse and concomitant exposure to IPV. The combined issue of substance abuse and sexual violence (a form of interpersonal violence) is complex and influenced by individual and systemic factors. Treatment must involve both individual and family therapy, particularly when an adolescent is involved (Baldwin et al., 2012). Ideally, the addicted individual receives specific support for their substance abuse via inpatient or outpatient services. Family therapy focuses on interactional patterns and emotional themes associated with the presenting issues such as disconnection, shame, guilt, splitting, and enmeshment. Further, family therapy is generally organized into three phases: assessment, structural changes (including subsystem work), and reinforcement of new patterns. In addition, ongoing support via Al-Anon, Alateen, Alcoholics Anonymous, Narcotics Anonymous, and other support groups is recommended. Psychoeducation related to trauma is provided and covers the importance of safety within the therapy space, particularly when working with adolescents (Greenwald, 2005), the psychological effects of trauma, and the role of families in the process of recovering from trauma (Figley & Figley, 2009). Psychoeducation about addiction is provided if necessary and situates addiction as a disease rather than as an individual moral failing.

Clinical Experience: Observations of Common Interactional Patterns
The secrecy and disconnection that often accompany addiction make psychoeducation highly relevant in these cases. Members of these families often report having limited connection to their extended families and friendship/community circles, and live with an assumption that they would not be believed, even if they were to report what was occurring. Psychoeducation about trauma should cover the importance of safety within the therapy space, particularly when working with adolescents, and about the psychological effects of trauma and the role of families in the process of recovering from trauma. In cases of addiction and sexual trauma, it is important to encourage structural and interactional changes that create resilient and supportive relationships throughout the system so that the victim feels safe and empowered. Research has shown that the most powerful variable predicting a child, teen, or young adult victim's recovery from sexual trauma is that the victim receives clear emotional support and protection from nonoffending family members (see review by Sheinberg & Fraenkel, 2001). It is crucial to consider cultural factors and values, and this is especially true with families of faith, as the following case vignette illustrates.

Case Context: Characteristics, Culture, and Preferences
Kimberly has just completed inpatient treatment for substance abuse at a facility specializing in co-occurring disorders. She is 16 years old and has been drinking alcohol and smoking marijuana for 2 years. In that time period, Kimberly's grades declined, her friend group changed, and she became sexually active with several partners. Her parents felt that her current boyfriend was a bad influence and were concerned that he was abusing her. Just before entering treatment, Kimberly ran away from home with a known drug dealer who reportedly raped her and left her in a car. She was able to call a friend, who contacted Kimberly's parents. Understandably upset by the situation, her parents insisted on treatment.

Kimberly comes from a suburban, White middle-class family. Her parents are married and financially stable. Kimberly has an older brother, Mike, who is a good student and athlete. Kimberly's mother, Joanne, is a teacher in the local school system and active in the family's church and community. Her father, Marcus, is in sales and coaches her brother's travel soccer team. Joanne and Marcus have quite different reactions to their daughter's sexual behavior and drug addiction, causing strain in the marriage. Joanne feels the family needs to do more to support Kimberly and is worried about what others in their social network think about what happened, particularly colleagues at work and church. Marcus is concerned about how Kimberly's issues affect his reputation and repeatedly blames her for being intoxicated and putting herself in the position to be abused.

While in treatment, Kimberly received support for her substance use disorders and psychoeducation regarding trauma. In addition, the family participated in psychoeducational workshops and family sessions, which focused on her substance use and highlighted some of the dysfunctional relational patterns within the family. As part of Kimberly's aftercare treatment plan, the family committed to engage in family therapy.

Clinical Decisions: Intervention Implementation

The work with this family was informed by both feminist and structural family therapy (SFT) approaches to family therapy. A feminist perspective recognizes the influence of socialization and stereotyped gender roles that contribute to women engaging in self-blame and feeling powerless to defend themselves and the normalization of aggressive male behavior. In addition, a feminist perspective empowered Kimberly to make relational choices that kept her comfortable and safe and offered a pathway to rebalance the power dynamics within the family. This allowed for greater collaboration and mutual support among the members (Hare-Mustin, 1978). A structural family therapy perspective focuses on interactional patterns and allows change to occur while recognizing strongly held values related to individual or collective identity (Micucci, 2009). In addition, a structural approach invites all family members to be part of the solution by emphasizing the symptomatic cycle and circular transactions in the family that fuel the presenting issue. By combining these theories, personal and collective issues of shame and disconnection are addressed and replaced with connection and resiliency by realigning power dynamics and interrupting the symptomatic cycle.

A critical part of the initial assessment is to create a detailed genogram to highlight the nature of relationships within the family and, importantly, the influence of broader cultural factors such as the family's faith and their roles within the community. This provides a context to explore the family's values and the gender stereotypes that influence how they interact around a family member's substance abuse and experience of sexual violence.

A critical intervention early in treatment with Kimberly and her parents helped the family see how the parents' sense of shame and disconnection contributed to Kimberly's negative sense of self, which led her to engage in the types of negative behaviors that aroused her own and her parents' feelings of shame in a repeating cycle. Understanding this symptomatic cycle fueled by shame led to a realignment between Joanne and Marcus and provided Kimberly the space to be empowered and gain the therapeutic support needed to feel connected to her parents.

Aware of the family's commitment to community and faith, as identified through the assessment genogram, the therapist asked about the strain between the family and their faith community. All reported feeling shame and disconnection. As was noted earlier, Marcus focused on how Kimberly's behavior reflected on him as a coach. Joanne was worried about what friends at church and school thought about Kimberly's behavior. Both reported feeling disconnected now from these community supports. Kimberly stated her parents' shame and her own feelings about the rape made her feel "like crap about myself," which led to isolating herself from them and an increase in risky behavior and substance use. The therapist pointed out the symptomatic cycle of shame fueling negative behaviors and disconnection, disempowering all involved.

Marcus challenged the therapist's suggestion that he was disempowering Kimberley, or contributed to her risky behavior, restating his belief that she would not have been raped had she been sober. The intervention offered to the family was as follows:

> Feeling shame sets up a vicious cycle. Although it is natural to think that feeling shame will help one avoid bad behavior, ironically, it often has the opposite effect. Filled with shame, people begin to feel they deserve to be hurt. Kimberly needs to feel that you see her as worthwhile.

Using the SFT technique of *enactments*—creating novel healthier interpersonal interactions during the session—the therapist directed Marcus to ask Kimberly how his statements affected her. In response, Kimberly described feeling blamed and alone, which made her want to "act out." Furthering the enactment, and to help Kimberly feel empowered and shift out of the victim role, the therapist encouraged her to express her needs to her parents. She stated she did not feel safe to do so.

To further build alignment between Joanne and Marcus, the therapist encouraged them to consider their daughter's sense of safety and how safety and care are values reflected in their faith and community commitments. They both quickly affirmed their commitment to keeping Kimberly safe. The therapist emphasized their alignment and acknowledged how their shared values guide the family, including their attitudes about sex, gender roles, and substance use. In an effort to reduce the extreme power discrepancy between father and daughter, Kimberly was again encouraged to express her needs, and Marcus was guided to simply listen and validate her experience. When he did so, Kimberly visibly brightened and said she felt safer, less ashamed, and more connected to him as a result. When asked to reflect on this session, all involved noted the importance of discussing their faith and connection to their community. By leveraging the family's faith and values, Kimberly's symptomatic cycle of addiction and sexual behavior fueled by shame was disrupted, and the connections within the family and to the community were strengthened. The family was able to address all three key elements of trauma recovery: safety, connection, and a model for well-managed emotional expression. In addition, these same elements contribute to Kimberly's sobriety, empowerment, and overall well-being.

Conclusion

This chapter briefly summarized couple and family therapy approaches to working with interpersonal violence with couples in which partners are heterosexual and cisgender, queer couples, military couples, and families in which a young person with substance abuse issues has experienced IPV. In studies of couples in which partners are heterosexual and cisgender and in which IPV occurs, couple therapy approaches to IPV have begun to demonstrate effectiveness in treating at least those couples that fit the category of situational, lower intensity/frequency, and more bidirectional violence. At least one study (Fals-Stewart & Clinton-Sherrod, 2009) demonstrated that couple therapy can be effective with couples in which the violence has been perpetrated by the male against the female in a unidirectional fashion, even when the male has a history of substance abuse.

REFERENCES

Almeida, R. V., & Durkin, T. (1999). The cultural context model: Therapy for couples with domestic violence. *Journal of Marital and Family Therapy*, *25*(3), 313–324. https://doi.org/10.1111/j.1752-0606.1999.tb00250.x

Babcock, J. C., Green, C. E., & Robie, C. (2004). Does batterers' treatment work? A meta-analytic review of domestic violence treatment. *Clinical Psychology Review*, *23*(8), 1023–1053. https://doi.org/10.1016/j.cpr.2002.07.001

Baldwin, S. A., Christian, S., Berkeljon, A., & Shadish, W. R. (2012). The effects of family therapies for adolescent delinquency and substance abuse: A meta-analysis. *Journal of Marital and Family Therapy*, *38*(1), 281–304. https://doi.org/10.1111/j.1752-0606.2011.00248.x

Barrios, V. R., Khaw, L. B. L., Bermea, A., & Hardesty, J. L. (2020). Future directions in intimate partner violence research: An intersectionality framework for analyzing women's processes of leaving abusive relationships. *Journal of Interpersonal Violence*. Advance online publication. https://doi.org/10.1177/0886260519900939

Bograd, M. (1984). Family systems approaches to wife battering: A feminist critique. *The American Journal of Orthopsychiatry*, *54*(4), 558–568. https://doi.org/10.1111/j.1939-0025.1984.tb01526.x

Bornstein, D. R., Fawcett, J., Sullivan, M., Senturia, K. D., & Shiu-Thornton, S. (2006). Understanding the experiences of lesbian, bisexual and trans survivors of domestic violence: A qualitative study. *Journal of Homosexuality, 51*(1), 159–181. https://doi.org/10.1300/J082v51n01_08

Breiding, M. J., Basile, K. C., Smith, S. G., Black, M. C., & Mahendra, R. (2015). *Intimate partner violence surveillance uniform definitions and recommended data elements.* National Center for Injury Prevention and Control, Division of Violence Prevention. https://www.cdc.gov/violenceprevention/pdf/ipv/intimatepartnerviolence.pdf

Burrell, L. M., Adams, G. A., Durand, D. B., & Castro, C. A. (2006). The impact of military lifestyle demands on well-being, army, and family outcomes. *Armed Forces and Society, 33*(1), 43–58. https://doi.org/10.1177/0002764206288804

Cafferky, B. M., Mendez, M., Anderson, J. R., & Stith, S. M. (2018). Substance use and intimate partner violence: A meta-analytic review. *Psychology of Violence, 8*(1), 110–131. https://doi.org/10.1037/vio0000074

Cannon, C., & Buttell, F. (2015). Illusion of inclusion: The failure of the gender paradigm to account for intimate partner violence in LGBT relationships. *Partner Abuse, 6*(1), 65–77. https://doi.org/10.1891/1946-6560.6.1.65

Carvalho, A. F., Lewis, R. J., Derlega, V. J., Winstead, B. A., & Viggiano, C. (2011). Internalized sexual minority stressors and same-sex intimate partner violence. *Journal of Family Violence, 26*(7), 501–509. https://doi.org/10.1007/s10896-011-9384-2

Cook-Daniels, L. (2015). Intimate partner violence in transgender couples: "Power and control" in a specific cultural context. *Partner Abuse, 6*(1), 126–139. https://doi.org/10.1891/1946-6560.6.1.126

Council of Economic Advisors. (2018). *Military spouses in the labor market.* The Council of Economic Advisers. https://trumpwhitehouse.archives.gov/wp-content/uploads/2018/05/Military-Spouses-in-the-Labor-Market.pdf

Dimiceli, E., Steinhardt, M., & Smith, S. (2010). Stressful experiences, coping strategies, and predictors of health-related outcomes among wives of deployed military servicemen. *Armed Forces and Society, 36*(2), 351–373. https://doi.org/10.1177/0095327X08324765

Dutton, D. (1998). *The abusive personality: Violence and control in intimate relationships.* Guilford Press.

Dyar, C., Messinger, A. M., Newcomb, M. E., Byck, G. R., Dunlap, P., & Whitton, S. W. (2021). Development and initial validation of three culturally sensitive measures for intimate partner violence for sexual and gender minority populations. *Journal of Interpersonal Violence, 36*(15–16), NP8824–NP8851. https://doi.org/10.1177/0886260519846856

Edwards, K. M., & Sylaska, K. M. (2013). The perpetration of intimate partner violence among LGBTQ college youth: The role of minority stress. *Journal of Youth and Adolescence, 42*(11), 1721–1731. https://doi.org/10.1007/s10964-012-9880-6

Fals-Stewart, W., & Clinton-Sherrod, M. (2009). Treating intimate partner violence among substance-abusing dyads: The effect of couples therapy. *Professional Psychology, Research and Practice, 40*(3), 257–263. https://doi.org/10.1037/a0012708

Figley, C. R., & Figley, K. R. (2009). Stemming the tide of trauma systemically: The role of family therapy. *Australian and New Zealand Journal of Family Therapy, 30*(3), 173–183. https://doi.org/10.1375/anft.30.3.173

FORGE. (2013). *Trans-specific power and control tactics*. http://www.ncdsv.org/images/FORGE_Trans-specificPowerAndControlTactics_updated_2013.pdf

Fraenkel, P. (2019). Love in action: An integrative approach to last chance couple therapy. *Family Process*, *58*(3), 569–594. https://doi.org/10.1111/famp.12474

Fraenkel, P., & Capstick, C. (2012). Contemporary two-parent families: Navigating work and family challenges. In F. Walsh (Ed.), *Normal family processes* (4th ed., pp. 78–101). The Guilford Press.

Gezinski, L. B., Gonzalez-Pons, K. M., & Rogers, M. M. (2019). "Praying does not stop his fist from hitting my face": Religion and intimate partner violence from the perspectives of survivors and service providers. *Journal of Family Violence*. Advance online publication. https://doi.org/10.1177/0192513X19830140

Goldner, V. (1985). Feminism and family therapy. *Family Process*, *24*(1), 31–47. https://doi.org/10.1111/j.1545-5300.1985.00031.x

Goldner, V. (2004). When love hurts: Treating abusive relationships. *Psychoanalytic Inquiry*, *24*(3), 346–372. https://doi.org/10.1080/07351692409349088

Goldner, V., Penn, P., Sheinberg, M., & Walker, G. (1990). Love and violence: Gender paradoxes in volatile attachments. *Family Process*, *29*(4), 343–364. https://doi.org/10.1111/j.1545-5300.1990.00343.x

Greenwald, R. (2005). *Child trauma handbook: A guide for helping trauma-exposed children and adolescents*. The Haworth Maltreatment and Trauma Press.

Hardesty, J. L., Oswald, R. F., Khaw, L., & Fonseca, C. (2011). Lesbian/bisexual mothers and intimate partner violence: Help seeking in the context of social and legal vulnerability. *Violence Against Women*, *17*(1), 28–46. https://doi.org/10.1177/1077801209347636

Hare-Mustin, R. T. (1978). A feminist approach to family therapy. *Family Process*, *17*(2), 181–194. https://doi.org/10.1111/j.1545-5300.1978.00181.x

Hassouneh, D., & Glass, N. (2008). The influence of gender role stereotyping on women's experiences of female same-sex intimate partner violence. *Violence Against Women*, *14*(3), 310–325. https://doi.org/10.1177/1077801207313734

Hawn, S. E., Bountress, K. E., Sheerin, C. M., Dick, D. M., & Amstadter, A. B. (2020). Trauma-related drinking to cope: A novel approach to the self-medication model. *Psychology of Addictive Behaviors*, *34*(3), 465–476. https://doi.org/10.1037/adb0000552

Head, S., & Milton, M. (2014). Filling the silence: Exploring the bisexual experience of intimate partner abuse. *Journal of Bisexuality*, *14*(2), 277–299. https://doi.org/10.1080/15299716.2014.903218

Hourani, L., Williams, J., Lattimore, P., Trudeau, J., & Van Dorn, R. (2017). Psychological model of military aggressive behavior: Findings from population-based surveys. *Military Psychology*, *29*(5), 381–395. https://doi.org/10.1037/mil0000172

Jennings-Kelsall, V., Aloia, L. S., Soloman, D. H., Marshall, A. D., & Leifker, F. R. (2012). Stressors experienced by women within Marine Corps families: A qualitative study of discourse within an online forum. *Military Psychology*, *24*(4), 363–381. https://doi.org/10.1080/08995605.2012.695255

Johnson, M. P. (2008). *A typology of domestic violence: Intimate terrorism, violent resistance, and situational couple violence*. Northeastern Press.

Jordan, S. P., Mehrotra, G. R., & Fujikawa, K. A. (2020). Mandating inclusion: Critical trans perspectives on domestic and sexual violence advocacy. *Violence Against Women*, *26*(6–7), 531–554. https://doi.org/10.1177/1077801219836728

Karakurt, G., Whiting, K., van Esch, C., Bolen, S. D., & Calabrese, J. R. (2016). Couples therapy for intimate partner violence: A systematic review and meta-analysis. *Journal of Marital and Family Therapy, 42*(4), 567–583. https://doi.org/10.1111/jmft.12178

Kelly, J. B., & Johnson, M. P. (2008). Differentiation among types of intimate partner violence: Research updates and implications for interventions. *Family Court Review, 46*(3), 476–499. https://doi.org/10.1111/j.1744-1617.2008.00215.x

Kilroy, S. J., Egan, J., Maliszewska, A., & Sarma, K. M. (2014). "Systemic trauma": The impact on parents whose children have experienced sexual abuse. *Journal of Child Sexual Abuse, 23*(5), 481–503. https://doi.org/10.1080/10538712.2014.920458

Linville, D., Chronister, K., Marsiglio, M., & Brown, T. B. (2012). Treatment of partner violence in gay and lesbian relationships. In J. J. Bigner & J. L. Wetchler (Eds.), *Handbook of LGBT-affirmative couple and family therapy* (pp. 327–342). Brunner-Routledge.

Lutgendorf, M. A., Snipes, M. A., Rau, T., Busch, J. M., Zelig, C. M., & Magann, E. F. (2012). Reports to the Navy's Family Advocacy Program: Impact of removal of mandatory reporting for domestic violence. *Military Medicine, 177*(6), 702–708. https://doi.org/10.7205/MILMED-D-11-00436

Maharaj, N. (2017). Perspectives on treating couples impacted by intimate partner violence. *Journal of Family Violence, 32*(4), 431–437. https://doi.org/10.1007/s10896-016-9810-6

Martin, S. L., Gibbs, D. A., Johnson, R. E., Sullivan, K., Clinton-Sherrod, M., Walters, J. L. H., & Rentz, E. D. (2010). Substance use by soldiers who abuse their spouses. *Violence Against Women, 16*(11), 1295–1310. https://doi.org/10.1177/1077801210387038

McCann, T. V., & Lubman, D. I. (2018). Stigma experience of families supporting an adult member with substance misuse. *International Journal of Mental Health Nursing, 27*(2), 693–701. https://doi.org/10.1111/inm.12355

McCollum, E. E., & Stith, S. M. (2011). Conjoint couples treatment and intimate partner violence: Best practices. In J. L. Wetchler (Ed.), *Handbook of clinical issues in couple therapy* (pp. 115–128). Routledge.

McGeorge, C., & Carlson, T. S. (2011). Deconstructing heterosexism: Becoming an LGB affirmative heterosexual couple and family therapist. *Journal of Marital and Family Therapy, 37*(1), 14–26. https://doi.org/10.1111/j.1752-0606.2009.00149.x

McKenry, P. C., Serovich, J. M., Mason, T. L., & Mosack, K. (2006). Perpetration of gay and lesbian partner violence. *Journal of Family Violence, 21*(4), 233–243. https://doi.org/10.1007/s10896-006-9020-8

Micucci, J. A. (2009). *The adolescent in family therapy: Harnessing the power of relationships* (2nd ed.). The Guilford Press.

Meyer, I. H. (2003). Prejudice, social stress, and mental health in lesbian, gay, and bisexual populations: Conceptual issues and research evidence. *Psychological Bulletin, 129*(5), 674–697. https://doi.org/10.1037/0033-2909.129.5.674

Murray, C. E., Crowe, A., & Overstreet, N. M. (2018). Sources and components of stigma experiences by survivors of intimate partner violence. *Journal of Interpersonal Violence, 33*(3), 515–536. https://doi.org/10.1177/0886260515609565

O'Neal, W., Greer, M., & Mancini, J. (2019). The role of community context and psychological well-being for physical health: A dyadic study of military couples.

Military Psychology, 31(3), 200–211. https://doi.org/10.1080/08995605.2019. 1579608

Palmer, C. (2008). A theory of risk and resilience factors in military families. *Military Psychology, 20*(3), 205–217. https://doi.org/10.1080/08995600802118858

Pence, E., & Paymar, M. (1993). *Education groups for men who batter: The Duluth model.* Springer. https://doi.org/10.1891/9780826179913

Portnoy, G. A., Relyea, M. R., Street, A. E., Haskell, S. G., & Iverson, K. M. (2020). A longitudinal analysis of women veterans' partner violence perpetration: The roles of interpersonal trauma and posttraumatic stress symptoms. *Journal of Family Violence, 35*(4), 361–372. https://doi.org/10.1007/s10896-019-00061-3

Sheinberg, M., & Fraenkel, P. (2001). *The relational trauma of incest: A family-based approach to treatment.* Guilford Press.

Shorey, R. C., Stuart, G. L., Brem, M. J., & Parrott, D. J. (2019). Advancing an integrated theory of sexual minority alcohol-related intimate partner violence perpetration. *Journal of Family Violence, 34,* 357–364. https://doi.org/10.1007/s10896-018-0031-z

Sims, C. M., Noel, N. E., & Maisto, S. A. (2007). Rape blame as a function of alcohol presence and resistance type. *Addictive Behaviors, 32*(12), 2766–2775. https://doi.org/10.1016/j.addbeh.2007.04.013

Spencer, C. M., Stith, S. M., & Cafferky, B. (2019). Risk markers for physical intimate partner violence victimization: A meta-analysis. *Aggression and Violent Behavior, 44,* 8–17. https://doi.org/10.1016/j.avb.2018.10.009

Stith, S. M., McCollum, E. E., & Rosen, K. H. (2011). *Couples treatment for domestic violence: Finding safe solutions.* American Psychological Association. https://doi.org/10.1037/12329-000

Stith, S. M., Rosen, K. H., McCollum, E. E., & Thomsen, C. J. (2004). Treating intimate partner violence within intact couple relationships: Outcomes of multi-couple versus individual couple therapy. *Journal of Marital and Family Therapy, 30*(3), 305–318. https://doi.org/10.1111/j.1752-0606.2004.tb01242.x

Stover, C. S., Meadows, A. L., & Kaufman, J. (2009). Interventions for intimate partner violence: Review and implications for evidence-based practice. *Professional Psychology, Research and Practice, 40*(3), 223–233. https://doi.org/10.1037/a0012718

Straus, M. A. (2011). Gender symmetry and mutuality in perpetration of clinical-level partner violence: Empirical evidence and implications for prevention and treatment. *Aggression and Violent Behavior, 16*(4), 279–288. https://doi.org/10.1016/j.avb.2011.04.010

Straus, M. A., & Douglas, E. M. (2004). A short form of the Revised Conflict Tactics Scales, and typologies for severity and mutuality. *Violence and Victims, 19*(5), 507–520. https://doi.org/10.1891/vivi.19.5.507.63686

Straus, M. A., Hamby, S. L., Bony-McCoy, S., & Sugarman, D. (1996). The Revised Conflict Tactics Scale (CTS2): Development and preliminary psychometric data. *Journal of Family Issues, 17,* 283–316. https://doi.org/10.1177/019251396017003001

Subirana-Malaret, M., Gahagan, J., Parker, R., & Crowther-Dowey, C. (2019). Intersectionality and sex and gender-based analyses as promising approaches in addressing intimate partner violence treatment programs among LGBT couples: A scoping review. *Cogent Social Sciences, 5*(1), 1644982. https://doi.org/10.1080/23311886.2019.1644982

Sullivan, C. P., & Elbogen, E. B. (2014). PTSD symptoms and family versus stranger violence in Iraq and Afghanistan veterans. *Law and Human Behavior, 38*(1), 1–9. https://doi.org/10.1037/lhb0000035

Tesch, B. P., & Bekerian, D. A. (2015). Hidden in the margins: A qualitative exploration of what professionals in the domestic violence field know about transgender domestic violence. *Journal of Gay and Lesbian Social Services, 27*(4), 391–411. https://doi.org/10.1080/10538720.2015.1087267

Texas Council on Family Violence. (1995). *Gay, Lesbian, Bisexual and Trans power and control wheel*. National Center on Domestic and Sexual Violence. http://www.ncdsv.org/images/TCFV_glbt_wheel.pdf

Tilsen, J. (2013). *Therapeutic conversations with queer youth: Transcending homonormativity and constructing preferred identities*. Jason Aronson, Inc.

Turell, S. C., & Herrmann, M. M. (2008). "Family" support for family violence: Exploring community support systems for lesbian and bisexual women who have experienced abuse. *Journal of Lesbian Studies, 12*(2–3), 211–224. https://doi.org/10.1080/10894160802161372

Walker, L. E. A. (2017). *The battered woman syndrome* (4th ed.). Springer.

Walters, M. L., Chen, J., & Breiding, M. J. (2013). *The National Intimate Partner and Sexual Violence Survey: 2010 findings on victimization by sexual orientation*. https://www.cdc.gov/violenceprevention/pdf/nisvs_sofindings.pdf

Webermann, A. R., Maldonado, A., Singh, R., Torres, S., Bushee, S., & Murphy, C. M. (2020). Centrality of traumatic events and men's intimate partner violence perpetration. *Psychological Trauma: Theory, Research, Practice, and Policy, 12*(2), 200–206. https://doi.org/10.1037/tra0000497

White, M. (2007). *Maps of narrative practice*. W. W. Norton & Co.

Woulfe, J. M., & Goodman, L. A. (2021). Identity abuse as a tactic of violence in LGBTQ communities: Initial validation of the Identity Abuse Measure. *Journal of Interpersonal Violence, 36*(5–6), 2656–2676. https://doi.org/10.1177/0886260518760018

Yamawaki, N., Ochoa-Shipp, M., Pulsipher, C., Harlos, A., & Swindler, S. (2012). Perceptions of domestic violence: The effects of domestic violence myths, victim's relationship with her abuser, and the decision to return to her abuser. *Journal of Interpersonal Violence, 27*(16), 3195–3212. https://doi.org/10.1177/0886260512441253

6

COPARENTING

*A Focus on Divorced Families, Stepfamilies,
Intergenerational Families, and Families
With a Child on the Autism Spectrum*

RESEARCH: TAMARA D. AFIFI, ALISON MAZUR, AND
CHRIS OTMAR
CLINICAL APPLICATIONS: AMY C. WAGNER,
PATRICIA L. PAPERNOW, BINDU METHIKALAM, AND
BRYAN M. PEIGHTAL

RESEARCH: TAMARA D. AFIFI, ALISON MAZUR, AND
CHRIS OTMAR

The family is a complex and dynamic system. When change occurs, such as divorce; the creation of a new stepfamily; or having a child with cognitive, emotional, or physical challenges, that change affects the entire family. Across these transitions, as well as throughout daily life for many types of families, how adults in a family coparent with one another has a profound impact on the entire family's well-being. Coparenting involves efforts by each parent to support the other's parenting practices, the dynamic exchange of beliefs and expectations between the coparents about their caregiving for a child, and family management of roles and rules (Lamela et al., 2016). As Lamela et al. (2016) noted, "successful coparenting is not equivalent to the non-existence of overt and covert coparenting conflict, but also encompasses a proactive and cooperative coparenting alliance and a shared commitment to childrearing" (p. 717). Nevertheless, conflict can

https://doi.org/10.1037/0000280-006
Treating Contemporary Families: Toward a More Inclusive Clinical Practice, S. Browning and B. van Eeden-Moorefield (Editors)

impede coparenting and make successful coparenting difficult to achieve (Amato et al., 2011). This chapter provides a brief overview of the research on coparenting in four areas that are often a common source of stress and conflict in today's families: divorce, stepfamilies, families on the spectrum, and intergenerational families (see Table 6.1).

Coparenting can vary in its effectiveness and the ways it is achieved, which is a reflection of the multitude of family types and the unique challenges they face (see Amato et al., 2011). For example, the research on coparenting after divorce has centered on the impact of interparental conflict on children and on identifying coparenting practices that best support well-being in children after divorce. The research on coparenting in stepfamilies has focused on two areas: coparenting across households (between

TABLE 6.1. Coparenting

Evidence-based area of clinical focus	Type of factor	Appropriateness for use across families	Selected references indicating evidence base
Reduce conflict/ tailoring programs to degree of conflict	Unique	Divorcing, stepfamilies	Backhouse & Graham, 2012
Shifting from romantic partners to coparents	Unique	Divorcing, stepfamilies	Cartwright & Gibson, 2013
Supportive communication	General	All[a]	Afifi et al., 2015
Parent role clarity	General	All[a]	Perry-Fraser & Fraser, 2018
Shared responsibility and teamwork	General	All[a]	Callander & Lindsay, 2018
Setting of predictable schedules, expectations, rules, boundaries across households	Mostly general	Divorcing, stepfamilies, intergenerational	Braithwaite et al., 2003
Social networks/ external support	Mostly general	Stepfamilies, intergenerational, spectrum	Prendeville & Kinsella, 2019
Attunement and respect for cultural sensitivity	General	Relevant to all,[a] particularly for intergenerational families	Wagner & Diamond, 2017a

[a]The general factor could work for other family types included in this unit but needs a small adaptation to ensure cultural relevance. Information about potential adaptations is included in the text.

the step-couple and the children's other parent) and coparenting challenges within the step-couple. Contemporary families, however, face an array of other challenges. With the rise in rates of autism in the United States, coparenting a child on the autism spectrum has become an important area of research across disciplines (Callander & Lindsay, 2018; Hartley et al., 2010). Current research tends to focus on the caregiver burden of the mother when a child is on the spectrum and the impact of this on a marriage, as well as siblings of a child on the spectrum (e.g., Cohrs & Leslie, 2017). Finally, as families become more diverse, they often struggle with intergenerational differences in opinions on how to parent children, particularly if there are generational or intercultural differences. In the pages that follow, we outline the research on coparenting in the aforementioned areas, beginning with the research on coparenting after divorce. We follow that with the presentation of a clinical case for each family type and describe an intervention focus that is informed by the research evidence. Psychoeducation also is included.

Research Evidence on Divorce

Divorce arguably has been one of the most studied topics in the social sciences. This section focuses on postdivorce coparenting practices that research suggests are linked most strongly to various child outcomes, thereby making this focus particularly clinically relevant. To understand coparenting, however, it is important to understand the challenges that divorced families often experience, especially concerning the well-being of children. In the short term, children of divorce may experience greater internalizing (e.g., anxiety, depressive symptoms) and externalizing (e.g., problems in school, aggressive tendencies) problems, fears of abandonment, less contact with one or both parents, and greater economic difficulty compared with children of nondivorced parents (van der Wal et al., 2019). Long-term effects from divorce include a greater likelihood of divorce themselves compared with children of never-divorced parents, fear of commitment, and continued psychological challenges (Amato, 2001). Nevertheless, meta-analyses show that most of the short-term effects of divorce dissipate over time and that there are few statistically significant differences between children of divorced and nondivorced parents if conflict between parents is kept to a minimum, and most long-term effects dissipate if the relationship between parents is amicable (Amato, 2001).

Most important for our purposes, the strongest predictor of children's well-being is not family structure (e.g., single-parent family, divorce, step-family) but the degree of **interparental conflict** and the parents' ability to effectively coparent (Amato, 2001). Part of effective coparenting in divorced families means that parents' decisions about parenting and caretaking put the child's well-being first (Lamela et al., 2016). It also means that they communicate with each other in a respectful and supportive manner while managing their conflict. At a minimum, effective coparenting means that they do not put their child in the middle of their disputes with each other. A wealth of research details the detrimental impact of parental conflict on both divorced and continuously married families (Booth & Amato, 2001; O'Mara & Schrodt, 2017). A key finding in divorce scholarship over the past 2 decades is that parental conflict is as important, if not more important, than divorce in determining child outcomes. In fact, research shows that children with high conflict never-divorced parents tend to have worse mental, relational, and physiological outcomes than children whose parents divorce and maintain a low-conflict relationship (Booth & Amato, 2001). For example, Amato and Afifi (2006) found that when postdivorce interparental conflict remained low, adult children's feelings of being caught between their parents diminished 10 years postdivorce. However, adult children whose parents remained in a high-conflict marriage still felt caught between their parents after 10 years. Conflict can disrupt the effectiveness of coparenting, regardless of whether a divorce is involved. Similarly, in the lab setting, Afifi et al. (2015) asked parents and adolescents from divorced and continuously married families to describe stressful elements related to the parents' relationship. Adolescents and young adults from divorced and continuously married families responded differently when their parents were more communicatively incompetent (e.g., less social support, greater conflict). Adolescents with high-conflict, married parents had the most difficulty recovering physiologically from a stressful parental interaction. At a minimum, effective parenting involves managing the conflict effectively and not involving the children directly in parental disputes. Effective coparenting beyond this, however, includes an active partnership (an aspect of **parental role clarity**) where parents work together to meet their child's social and emotional needs (Fidler & McHale, 2020).

The active partnership between coparents often translates into parenting that is **supportive, cooperative, and involves positive communication** between the parents and with the child (Schrodt & Afifi, 2018). Beckmeyer et al. (2020) operationalized effective coparenting as cooperatively parenting together, supportive and frequent communication, a lack of boundary ambiguity regarding the roles of the parents, and satisfaction with the custody arrangement and child support. They found that effective coparenting was associated with more prosocial behaviors and less internalizing and externalizing behavior problems in adolescents. Schrodt and Afifi (2018) also discovered that coparental communication that is supportive and not antagonistic was positively associated with young adults' mental health, largely through reduction in children's feelings of being caught between their parents. This finding held true for children of divorced and continuously married families and was especially evident in the mother–child relationship. Karberg and Cabrera (2020) also showed that although the impact of parents' divorce on children's aggression was small, it was also mediated by supportive coparenting. Specifically, the more the mother felt that her parenting decisions were supported and respected by the father and the more cooperative their communication with each other, the less aggressive the child was as a result of the divorce. Similarly, Herrero et al. (2020) discovered that positive family communication and coparental communication were associated with better psychological adjustment and fewer economic consequences for children after a divorce. In high-conflict families, however, a lack of parental support hurt children's adjustment. In general, research demonstrates that it is important for parents to be supportive, cooperative, and respectful of each other's parenting and childrearing, as well as positive in their communication with one another.

Research has also focused on evaluating interventions and parenting programs designed to assist parents in creating effective parenting plans, improve parenting skills, and help children navigate the divorce transition (see Fidler & McHale, 2020). Scholars studying educational programs for divorcing parents emphasize the need to tailor the program to the specific relationship between the parents and their degree of conflict (Sandler et al., 2015). Ideally, parents would be able to work together collaboratively and cooperatively to create parenting plans and caregiving decisions that prioritize the emotional and social functioning of child (Becher et al., 2019). Many such programs, such as the New Beginnings Program (Sandler et al., 2015), have been extremely beneficial for parents and children. The New Beginnings Program focuses on authoritative and consistent parenting with children across households, promoting positive family interactions, engaging in active listening with children, and other practical parenting skills. The program also emphasizes the importance of parents practicing the skills they learn with their children throughout the program. The positive effects of the program on parenting lasted 6 years, and positive effects on children (e.g., decreases in internalizing problems and at-risk behaviors, improvements in self-esteem, coping efficacy, educational goals) lasted between 6 and 15 years after participation (Sandler et al., 2015). If collaborative parenting is not possible, however, parents might need to engage in parallel parenting, where they parent separately from one another (Pryor, 2004). Research has also found that improving the coparenting relationship might have indirect effects on children by improving the child's relationship with both parents (Saini, 2019), bringing the child closer emotionally to both parents.

Research Evidence on Stepfamilies

Coparenting becomes increasingly important when new stepfamilies are formed. Not only are the families often managing the emotions of a divorce or death of a parent, but they are combining new families together that already have a preestablished history. Two coparental relationships are particularly important in stepfamilies: (a) the coparental relationship between the step-couple and the parent in the other household and (b) the coparental relationship within the step-couple itself.

One of the primary aspects of a stepfamily that needs to be determined for a stepfamily to function well is the renegotiation of **boundaries** between former spouses. Former spouses need to separate the remaining upset feelings of their marriage enough to forge a long-term, cooperative coparenting relationship for their children. Parents must renegotiate intimacy and power boundaries with one another and reenvision themselves as coparents rather than romantic partners (Cartwright & Gibson, 2013). Doing so will allow them to manage the negative emotions they might feel toward their former spouse. It will also help ease concerns about a new stepparent entering the family. Coparenting in stepfamilies involves negotiating a complex set of issues across households, including a visitation schedule, household rules across the two households, discipline and other parenting practices (between the parents and with the new stepparent), and finances. The former spouses need to formulate a parenting plan that is consistent between households, is authoritative, and allows the child to easily transition from one household to the other (Braithwaite et al., 2003). Some research has shown that mothers are often the "hub" of the coparenting system in stepfamilies. If they feel they can trust the parenting of the father and can cooperatively and actively coparent with each other, they can then allow the stepparent to enter that coparental relationship (Ganong et al., 2015). Having two sets of households can be stressful for children, and effective coparenting between households can help children manage this stress.

The second, essential coparental relationship in stepfamilies is the step-couple, as well as the coparental relationship between the original parent and the stepparent. This coparental relationship can be challenging because although there is guidance for how parents should parent their children, there is less guidance for stepparents. They are often unsure whether and how to parent their stepchildren (Perry-Fraser & Fraser, 2018). Research tends to show that a warm, flexible, and emergent authoritative parenting style tends to be the most effective parenting style for most stepparents (Ganong & Coleman, 2017). The stepparent should also support and reinforce the parenting of the parents, which can be stressful for stepparents as they attempt to determine their disciplinary role in the family (Schrodt & Braithwaite, 2011). The age of the child is also an important factor. If the child is young when the stepfamily forms, it tends to be easier for the parent to assume a firm parenting role. If the child is an adolescent, the stepparent might face greater challenges exerting his or her authority. Regardless of the age of the child, research shows that children benefit from stepparents who reaffirm and provide rationales for the household rules of the family, while simultaneously remaining warm and approachable.

Within both coparental types, loyalty conflicts can emerge that challenge them. When both parent and stepparent have an antagonistic coparental relationship with the other parent, children can feel caught in the middle (e.g., Schrodt, 2015). Another type of loyalty conflict can occur when a parent feels caught between their child and the stepparent (Afifi, 2003). Divorce can lead to power shifts within the family between the custodial parent and the child. The child might assume a more powerful position in the family, often due to emotional parentification where the parent treats the child like a peer and relies on them for emotional support. In addition to forming a close emotional bond with one parent, the child holds a more powerful position in the family in the absence of the other parent, making it difficult for the new stepparent to penetrate that preexisting parent–child bond. **Conflict** likely ensues between the child and stepparent, with the parent being caught in the middle. In addition, stepparents can feel caught between the parent and the child. In general, it is important for the parent and stepparent couple to communicate a unified front to the child, signaling to them that they love each other and are always going to be together (Afifi, 2003). Additionally, children might test the parent–stepparent relationship because they are afraid they might get divorced. Communicating solidarity across all the coparental relationships will help convey a sense of security and trust to the child.

Finally, stepfamilies need to remember that it often takes years for stepfamilies to "feel like a family." Stepparents sometimes fall into a "myth of instant love" where they assume that everyone in their new stepfamily will instantly feel a strong, positive emotional connection. These feelings take time to develop and emerge through committed maintenance of the relationships within the family (Braithwaite et al., 2001).

Research Evidence on Families With a Child on the Autism Spectrum

Families with a child on the autism spectrum also represent an important context for coparenting challenges. Autism spectrum disorder (ASD) is a developmental disability that is characterized by difficulties with social communication, repetitive and restricted behaviors and interests, and emotional and behavioral problems (American Psychiatric Association, 2013). An estimated one in 59 children is identified with ASD in the United States (Centers for Disease Control and Prevention, 2019). Parents of children with ASD are at risk for experiencing a high level of parenting stress and are more prone to psychological disorders such as depression and anxiety (Cohrs & Leslie, 2017). This excess of stress can cause tension and place strain on the family relationships, including both the parent–child and parent–parent relationships. These relational issues include the marginalization of one parent, a loveless relationship for the parents, an expanded critical period of vulnerability for divorce, neglect of the neurotypical children, and **lack of support from the extended family**.

The burden of caretaking for the child with ASD typically falls on mothers (lack of **shared responsibility**), who take on the majority of daily parenting responsibilities in families of children with ASD (Callander & Lindsay, 2018). Mothers of children with ASD also report higher levels of parenting stress than fathers (Foody et al., 2015). Hickey et al. (2019) found that mothers were more likely than fathers to express high criticism of their child with ASD, potentially because they are shouldering more of the parenting stress burden. Additionally, families with children with ASD can experience greater financial, employment, and time-related burdens compared with families with a child with a developmental disability, mental health condition, or a combination of both (Vohra et al., 2014). These burdens can cause parents to cut back on work or stop working to care for their child, and mothers are significantly more likely than fathers to have their work life affected (Gau et al., 2012). These are major areas of **conflict** as well.

This marginalization of the mother can cause stress in the marriage and influence relationship satisfaction. Parents of children with ASD experience lower relationship satisfaction than other parenting couples, although there were no significant differences in levels of perceived spousal support, respect for one's partner, and commitment to the relationship (Harper et al., 2013). However, Brown et al. (2020) found a positive relationship between dyadic coping and marital satisfaction in parents of children with ASD. Parents of children with ASD also report lower levels of marital happiness, family cohesion, and family adaptability compared with parents of children without ASD (Higgins et al., 2005). Gau et al. (2012) found that mothers of children with ASD felt significantly less dyadic satisfaction and affection expression than fathers. In addition, overall parents of children with ASD had significantly less dyadic satisfaction than parents of children without ASD (Gau et al., 2012). Lower levels of marital satisfaction may be expressed through partner criticism, and mothers of children with ASD were found to be more likely than fathers to express high criticism of their partner (Hickey et al., 2019).

Furthermore, marital stress and relational dissatisfaction can ultimately lead to divorce. Approximately 23.5% of parents with children with ASD are divorced compared with 13.8% of parents of children without developmental disabilities (Hartley et al., 2010). Hartley et al. (2010) also found that divorce rates taper off for parents of children without a disability when the child is around 8 years old, whereas the divorce rate for parents of children with ASD does not taper off until the child is 30 years old. This finding suggests that there is an expanded critical period for divorce among parents of children with ASD compared with other parents.

Marital stress can have a negative impact for all family relationships, not just the parents. When marital stress was high in families, neurotypical siblings of children with ASD expressed less satisfaction in their sibling relationships and directed more negative behaviors and fewer positive behaviors toward the sibling with ASD (Rivers & Stoneman, 2003). Siblings of children with autism are often thought of as the "forgotten child" because they receive less attention and time from their parents compared with the child with ASD, which causes the neurotypical sibling to become more independent (Chan & Goh, 2014). However, findings from studies about siblings of children with ASD are inconclusive; some show positive outcomes, whereas others demonstrate negative outcomes or no perceptible difference (Kovshoff et al., 2017). Chan and Goh (2014) found that siblings of children with ASD perceived double-standard parenting and differential treatment of them and their sibling. However, the neurotypical siblings understood this differential treatment and empathized with their parents, made do with their family situation, and some even viewed it in a positive manner (Chan & Goh, 2014).

Social support has been found to reduce stress and depression and improve well-being among parents of children with ASD (Meadan et al., 2010). Grandparents have been found to be a source of support for both the grandchildren with ASD and the parents of the children with ASD because they can provide care for the children and respite for the parents (Prendeville & Kinsella, 2019). However, some extended family members are not as supportive. Altiere and von Kluge (2009) found that some families had significant trouble with their extended family members when they found out their child had ASD. Some family members could not understand the concept of autism or found it embarrassing, which led to estrangement at a time when the family needed social support (Altiere & von Kluge, 2009).

Research Evidence on Intergenerational Families

Intergenerational coparenting has become more prevalent over the past 2 decades as a result of an increasing aging population, such that many more grandparents are available to help with parenting (Chiang & Park, 2015). Additionally, scholars have suggested that the influx of single-parent homes and the growing number of dual-income families have resulted in the need for additional childrearing support (Leonce, 2020). However, the reliance on multiple generations to raise children may have its roots in evolutionary adaptiveness. Indeed, the grandmother hypothesis postulates that females have an extended life expectancy beyond menopause to support younger generations in childrearing, freeing up resources for the parents to grow the family, as well as shift their attention to securing additional resources for the well-being of the familial system (Hawkes & Coxworth, 2013). However, these evolutionary benefits do not eliminate the potential for intergenerational coparenting to lead to interpersonal **conflict**. Intergenerational family turmoil over coparenting can be caused by a wide range of issues. This section reviews two prominent situations likely to spark disagreement: stress and resentment stemming from **role ambiguity** and conflict related to multicultural assimilation.

Although intergenerational coparenting is usually motivated by a grandparent's willingness to help the family unit, an external event often makes intergenerational coparenting necessary in the first place. Custodial grandparenting, wherein grandparents assume the central caregiver role for their grandchildren, is a common type of coparenting. This type of coparenting is often preceded by events such as the adult child's absence due to death, incarceration, financial instability, or abuse of the grandchild (Fruhauf & Hayslip, 2013; Hayslip & Kaminski, 2005). It is therefore not surprising that custodial grandparents experience heightened stress compared with peers who not raising grandchildren. The additional stress from raising children at an older age can lead to a decline in mental and physical health (Hayslip & Kaminski, 2005), financial insecurity (Nelson et al., 2010), and a strained relationship with their adult child (Fruhauf & Hayslip, 2013). Children of custodial grandparents are also at a higher risk of negative outcomes.

Indeed, many of the precursors to having custodial grandparents, such as child neglect, may induce feelings of grief for both the children and their caregivers (Pruchno & McKenney, 2002).

Custodial grandparents report intrafamily strain and an increase in family conflict (Musil et al., 2013; Oburu & Palmérus, 2005). In fact, research on conflict in teenage-mother and grandmother coparents found that grandmothers are at a higher risk for depressive symptoms (Caldwell et al., 1998). Additionally, a wide age gap between the grandmother and mother coparents may increase conflict in the relationship (Hoang et al., 2020). This may be due to grandparents experiencing role conflict while coparenting with their adult child (Landry-Meyer & Newman, 2004). Researchers have theorized that this role conflict stems from dissatisfaction with not being able to assume the traditional grandparent role as they fulfill the role of parent (Backhouse & Graham, 2012). Landry-Meyer and Newman (2004) report that role ambiguity is also common among coparenting grandparents, which may cause conflict within the coparenting relationship, due to the lack of clear societal role for the grandparent. Extending this rationale suggests that grandparents who are expected to coparent may feel resentful about making sacrifices later in life to raise an additional child (Kelley et al., 2013).

With the rise of cultural diversity in the United States and intergenerational and multicultural homes becoming more common, the potential for cultural differences among intergenerational coparents also increases. There is a wealth of literature that points to the positive influences of being raised in a home with diverse cultural practices (Chang et al., 2014; Raval & Walker, 2019). In fact, Li et al. (2018) found that filial piety beliefs moderated the relationship between grandparental involvement and cognitive well-being in a sample of Hong Kong college students. In the United States, intergenerational coparenting tends to be more common among African American families than Western European families due to greater reliance on extended family relationships for support (Jones et al., 2007). Similarly, Hispanic and Latino families have traditionally relied on grandparents to help raise children and are more likely to assist in coparenting children than African American grandparents (Goodman & Silverstein, 2002). East Asian cultures also differ from Western European cultures in their approach to intergenerational ties. One study found that in Indian and Vietnamese families, grandparents and other extended family members do not just look after the children when the parents are away but are considered "cocaregivers" (Hoang et al., 2020).

However, intergenerational multicultural coparenting comes with a unique set of challenges. The acculturation process in the United States for immigrant families can be a tumultuous time and potentially lead to conflict among children, parents, and grandparents. Some studies suggest that the potential for such conflict is heightened due to the challenge of preserving cultural values and norms while simultaneously integrating mainstream culture (Bámaca-Colbert et al., 2019). For example, an adolescent who grows up in the United States might exert more individualistic attitudes, which could clash with the parents' more collectivistic tendencies. Such a clash may be because many immigrants' countries of origin emphasize collective community values in stark contrast with the individualism prevalent in the United States (Höllinger & Haller, 1990). Provided that intergenerational coparenting may cause turmoil that impedes the family system, it is not surprising that studies have reported that such conflicts can negatively affect immigrant caregivers and their children (Conn et al., 2013). Nonetheless, despite the disagreements that culture can spark among intergenerational coparents, the positive benefits of diverse households and multicultural upbringings should not be understated in future research and clinical practice (Chang et al., 2014; Raval & Walker, 2019). In sum, there is a wide array of situations that rely extensively on coparenting, which occurs within and across generations. This complexity can sometimes create conflict and stress, but it also provides opportunities for acceptance, empathy, and personal and relational growth.

CLINICAL APPLICATIONS: AMY C. WAGNER, PATRICIA L. PAPERNOW, BINDU METHIKALAM, AND BRYAN M. PEIGHTAL

Overview of Clinical Expertise and Interpretation of Evidence

As discussed in the previous sections, research indicates that the degree to which adults can communicate and harmoniously cooperate in childrearing is essential to children's well-being (O'Mara & Schrodt, 2017). This is especially true for families that have experienced a high level of stress and transition. When the **coparenting relationship** breaks down, it is not only the coparents who experience stress; the children in these families become especially vulnerable. Although the systemic pressures experienced in the families covered in this section are not all the same, similar complex family dynamics and issues emerge (see Table 6.1).

Regardless of family structure, the **degree of conflict** between adults who are coparenting is a strong predictor of how children function within or across any type of household. Additionally, a wealth of research has long supported the importance of both warm and moderately firm (authoritative) parenting. Successful coparenting is highly dependent on a clear definition of roles and division of parenting labor. This is not dependent on equal division but on mutual respect and satisfaction with the coparenting arrangement. Clinically, the process of helping coparents come to these agreements is often the focus of the therapeutic work. Working together effectively in caretaking is critical. Former spouses do not have to agree on everything, but they must be able to form a partnership. A positive parenting alliance includes the absence of undermining one another in the coparental role as well as shared beliefs concerning childrearing issues and values. Therapy can assist coparents with the process of constructing and maintaining a mutually agreed-on partnership structure and negotiating conflicts.

Family scholars agree that how coparents manage interactions within the larger family system is also essential to children's well-being. With complex family structures, this may involve many other adults in relationship with the children, both within and outside the home. Complicated **kin and social networks** are often challenging to navigate for coparents, as they attempt to balance their needs, their children's needs, and those of others in the family. Therapists can help coparents navigate what may feel like "shark-filled waters" with ex-partners, stepparents, multiple sets of grandparents, or other relatives living in the home. In addition, therapists can help coparents find ways to enlist support from extended family to share the parenting work. In this clinical section, we explore clinical interventions with four specific family types that follow directly from empirically based evidence shown to increase children's well-being.

Clinical Expertise and Interpretation of Evidence: Divorcing Families

Coparenting after divorce is challenging for many parents. The majority of divorces are not based on a mutual decision, and, as such, conflict is inherent. The inability to resolve and reconcile the marital relationship often morphs into the inability to coparent. As Afifi and colleagues discussed in their review, recent research has indicated that **conflict**, not divorce per se, is damaging to children (O'Mara & Schrodt, 2017). As such, parents' ability to coparent harmoniously without interpersonal conflict is the most important factor in determining children's postdivorce functioning (Amato, 2001). The transition from being divorced as partners while remaining cooperative parents occurs over time. Family scholars agree that myriad factors influence the ease and speed of this process. These include each parent's individual experience of the divorce process, their emotional and financial stability and ability to adjust to change, the amount of cooperation and conflict in the parental relationship, religious and cultural variables, and the level of stress caused by the child's behavior problems (Wagner & Diamond, 2017a).

Clinical Experience: Observations of Common Interactional Patterns
As every marriage is different, so too is every divorce, including the unique needs of each individual in the family. However, there are many shared dynamics particular to divorcing families, and effective coping strategies and therapeutic interventions that can positively influence the ability to coparent. The goal of successful coparenting is to assist parents to unite in putting the child needs first. Becoming a healthy binuclear family entails keeping the child out of any conflicts that occur between parents in the divorce process. In addition, a **clear schedule (i.e., expectations and rules)** for visitation and parental agreements around childrearing provides children with a more predictable and stable environment, which reduces conflict.

Parents may seek therapy at many points in the pre- and postdivorce process, which is not a discrete event but a nonlinear process. Clients may enter therapy contemplating divorce (e.g., prefiling or contemplating separation), i n the midst of the divorce (e.g., in unison with attorney negotiations and court proceedings), or postseparation adjustment (e.g., after physical separation; Wagner & Diamond, 2017b). Thus, the therapist may play many roles dependent on client needs, which vary greatly based on where each family member is in the process of change. These roles may include supporting parents as divorce coach, child specialist, mediator, coparenting coordinator, and individual, couple, or family therapist. What makes coparenting especially challenging for divorced parents is the need for them to set aside their emotions or negative feelings about their marital relationship with their former spouse to cooperate with them in continuing to love and parent their children effectively. Divorced parents are often coping with feelings of anger, loss, fear, grief, guilt, and loss of individual and family identity. The therapist's role is to help create harmony and order in a system often filled with conflict and chaos and help parents focus on keeping the child out of their disputes.

Successful coparenting relies on the ability of the former nuclear family to reorganize and adapt to a new binuclear structure, and the therapist can facilitate this transition by helping parents establish **boundaries** and redefine their roles as parents, not partners (Wagner & Diamond, 2017a). By maintaining predictability and order through organized and **clear schedules** and open exchange of information, child care is more consistent. Additionally, supporting consistent parental empathetic **attunement** increases children's ability to emotionally self-regulate and feel secure.

Case Context: Characteristics, Culture, and Preferences

Alexa and Ted decided to divorce after 15 years of marriage. They had attempted couple therapy years before, but Ted was having an extramarital affair that he was unwilling to end. Nearly a year after their parents' separation, the couples' two children, Noah (age 12) and Anabelle (age 9), were struggling. Noah was often defiant, especially with his mother, and Anabelle was frequently tearful at separations from Alexa. Both parents came to therapy with the goal of helping their children to better adjust to living in two households.

Alexa and Ted had ongoing conflict around **parenting schedules** and decision making, as well as differences in responding to both children's behavior. A typical problem sequence involved the process of Ted picking up the kids from Alexa's house during the week for his visitation. Ted often arrived after the agreed-on time, and Alexa would become upset about the delay in the children's dinner hour and the impact on completing homework and bedtime. Noah reacted to the conflict between his parents by resisting Ted's efforts to have him stop playing his video games and get in the car. Anabelle reacted to the tension by crying and protesting leaving the house while clinging to her mother. Both parents felt exhausted by this situation and unable to work together to ensure a smooth transition for the children between households.

Clinical Decisions: Intervention Implementation

The therapist began by meeting with the parents together and each of them alone to better understand each of their narratives about the divorce process and current child-related problems. It was clear that they each were struggling to separate their angry and hurt feelings related to their former marriage and divorce process from their new roles as **cooperative coparents**. In the joint session the couple began to argue: "You are so irresponsible Ted, you always put your work and own needs first!" Alexa exclaimed. Ted countered, "You are so rigid and controlling, you have never understood how hard I have to work!" The therapist intervened by acknowledging and normalizing their angry feelings. She stated, "It's hard for most couples to not fall into an argument as if you are still a married couple. However, what your children need from you right now is to set aside those feelings and work together for their best interests." The therapist shared with them the current research about the impact of ongoing parental conflict on their children's emotional and physical health and the benefits of parental cooperation and **good communication**. Both acknowledged that they often let their own emotions interfere with their ability to be partners in parenting.

Alexa and Ted agreed that they wanted to make their divorce as positive as they could for their children. They talked about how hard it was to cooperate with each other when they were both holding onto the hurt and resentment from their marriage. The therapist stated, "I understand from my meetings with both of you alone that you both still carry a lot of strong feelings about the loss of your relationship, and it has been hard to forgive yourself and one another. I hope over time with therapy I can help you heal those wounds and let go of that pain and anger, so your lives can move forward." Alexa and Ted agreed, and Alexa stated, "I know that the children love Ted and that I shouldn't let my feelings about him as a partner get in the way of his relationship with the kids." Ted replied, "Thank you for saying that, I know I messed up as a husband; I want to do better as a father."

In subsequent sessions, the therapist discussed with Alexa and Ted some ways they could work together to make transitions between households easier for the kids and brainstormed ideas specific to the problematic pickup situation. It was agreed that the children would remain at an aftercare program and Ted would leave work earlier on his parenting days to pick them up directly from school, rather than Alexa's house. Both agreed not to have disagreements in front of the children and to use therapy to discuss any child-related issues that they could not resolve themselves. They decided to use an online communication platform (e.g., Talking Parents, Our Family Wizard) to share information and concerns. In addition, they arranged to have transitions that were consistent and predictable for the children. To address the children's anxiety or defiant behavior during transitions between households, they agreed to try to maintain a sense of calm, positivity, and reassurance. After several weeks of the new plan, both parents reported that both Noah and Anabelle were coping better with transitioning between households.

Clinical Expertise and Interpretation of Evidence: Coparenting Conflict in Stepfamilies

Coparenting between parents and stepparents is fundamentally different from a first-time family and often much more complex than the term *blended family* might imply. Indeed, compared with first-time families, couples in stepfamilies report lower levels of parenting satisfaction (Whitton et al., 2008). Coparenting stressors arise in stepfamilies in two areas that intersect with each other: within the step-couple and across households with the children's other parent.

Clinical Experience: Observations of Common Interactional Patterns

Within the step-couple, differences around parenting are often a primary source of conflict and the most common presenting problem in therapy. Often, stepparents want more limits and **boundaries** with their stepchildren, and parents want their new partner to love their stepchildren. This is understandable because parents have previously established attachment bonds with their children and share a longstanding understanding of "how we do things"; stepparents have neither. Additionally, the entry of a stepparent often creates significant losses and loyalty binds for children. As a result, many stepchildren are often decidedly cool and even rejecting of their stepparents. Although a stepparent may care deeply for a stepchild, the experience of being with a child since birth creates a more expansive love. Hence, a parent and a stepparent frequently experience the same child very differently (Papernow, 2018).

Furthermore, all too often, an ex-partner carries conflict from the previous union into the coparenting relationship. Thus, although keeping a nonresidential parent connected to one's child can be positive, the effect on the step-couple, who are trying to discipline together, can be difficult. These two arenas interact when one feels caught between acceding to a new partner's wishes and keeping the peace with an ex-partner. This may be further exacerbated given that often when an ex-partner recouples, the former partner may become anxious about losing their children and sharing control with an "outsider."

Case Context: Characteristics, Culture, and Preferences

Carla (age 35) and Skip (age 47) came to therapy for help "communicating about the kids." The couple had been together for 18 months, immediately after Skip's divorce. Carla had never been married and had no children, and Skip had two children, Suzie (age 15) and Seth (age 11). In the session Carla immediately stated, "Your kids are slobs. They don't listen to me. And you don't back me up." Skip retorted, "But they're just being kids. Besides, if you were nicer to them, maybe they'd listen to you." Carla and Skip were being torn apart by a toxic combination of normal stepfamily challenges intensified by unrealistic expectations for immediate "blending" and ineffective interpersonal practices (e.g., believing in the "instant family" and forming an immediate dislike of the new steprelation).

Clinical Decisions: Intervention Implementation

To meet this challenge, family scholars recommend that therapists provide evidence-based psychoeducation about parenting, stepparenting, and discipline in stepfamilies (Adler-Baeder & Higginbotham, 2020; Ganong & Coleman, 2017; Papernow, 2018). "I'm betting this is a familiar conversation," the therapist says to Carla and Skip. "Did you know that you're having this conversation because you live in a stepfamily? It turns out, parents and stepparents feel very differently about kids! And kids need both warmth and limits." Indeed, authoritative (warm and moderately firm) parenting is best for kids in many respects and is a key predictor of child well-being in stepfamilies. However, the research is also clear that parents need to retain the disciplinary role (Ganong & Coleman, 2017) until or unless stepparents have formed a trusting, caring relationship.

The therapist explained that research has shown that authoritarian (harsh and demanding) parenting by stepparents is almost always toxic to stepparent–stepchild relationships (Ganong & Coleman, 2017). This was the very style that Carla, like most stepparents, was being pulled toward, especially when she felt unheard and dismissed by Skip.

Over the course of therapy, the therapist began to help Carla ease out of the disciplinary role, encouraging her to concentrate on "connection not correction" and getting to know her stepkids rather than trying to control them. The therapist shared the research that successful stepparents concentrate on "affinity-building behaviors": expressing warmth, caring, and interest, and handling concerns constructively and respectfully. Connection would likely be easier with Seth, who is a younger boy, and harder with Suzie, an early adolescent girl. The therapist encouraged Carla to carve out one-on-one time with each of the kids, doing something fun without their dad. Weaving back into the couple relationship, the therapist helped Skip to empathize with the painful impact of Suzie's rejection on Carla and helped Carla reach for comfort, rather than withdrawing or attacking.

The therapist helped the couple understand that while stepparents have input about kids, parents have the final say about their own children. When this works well, stepparents can help parents to "firm up" and make more demands of their kids, and parents can help stepparents to "soften up." During sessions with the couple, the therapist worked on interpersonal practices that could help Skip and Carla stay connected and caring across their differences. We traced their "Polarization Polka": The harsher Carla was, the more protective Skip became, leaving the children with the worst of both of them: increasingly indulgent parenting from Skip and authoritarian parenting from Carla. The couple began working on making this toxic cycle the enemy rather than each other. They began to catch themselves, take a breath, and begin again. Over time they learned basic skills, such as turning criticisms ("Seth is a slob") into requests ("I'd love it if you'd ask Seth to put his dishes away").

In addition, the therapist helped Skip understand the consequences of his making decisions and plans with his ex-wife without consulting Carla. They agreed on a process in which he and Carla would discuss any requests he received from the children's mother with Carla before agreeing to **schedule changes**. In addition, he agreed to be more mindful of protecting the **boundary** around their couple time by setting limits on the **amount of communication** with his ex-wife when he and Carla were alone together. Over time, gaining clarity on their very different roles in their family and empathizing with each other brought the couple out of their polarized positions and into a more collaborative **coparenting partnership**.

Clinical Expertise and Interpretation of Evidence: Intergenerational Families

In the United States, an estimated 4 million children under age 6 live with parents and grandparents (U.S. Census Bureau, 2011). Although intergenerational families can be a source of support, assisting with the caretaking of children, they face many challenges. As discussed in the research section of this chapter, intergenerational coparents can find it difficult to manage adjustment to coparenting with the additional challenges of role ambiguity and multicultural assimilation (Musil et al., 2013; Oburu & Palmérus, 2005).

Clinical Experience: Observations of Common Interactional Patterns
The three most common systemic challenges within intergenerational families are (a) cultural differences between the parent and the intergenerational family, (b) unresolved issues around power and grief between generations, and (c) a lack of models of how to **appropriately coparent**. Cultural differences are relevant because coparents across generations may have different cultural identities that influence all facets of parenting. Further, in many cultures the extended family is seen to play a significant role in the parenting process. For example, in many Asian or Eastern traditions, aunts, uncles, and grandparents participate in the childrearing process. However, in more Western traditions, the nuclear family structure is more typical. Thus, conflict can occur when the parent is more acculturated than the extended family. Religious differences between generations can also **contribute to conflict**.

Additionally, unresolved issues with power, grief, and resentment can also affect coparenting. External events such as loss, incarceration, financial hardship, or abuse may have been precipitating factors that led to the development of the intergenerational family unit. For example, loss of or abandonment by a parent can influence how much or how little that parent is involved in the coparenting relationship. Additionally, intrafamily strain and conflict between extended family members can affect the coparenting relationship.

Finally, it is important to consider what experience or beliefs the coparents have about coparenting. If the family does not have models or experiences with intergenerational childrearing, role ambiguity, dissatisfaction, and disorganization are more likely to occur. Thus, the therapist should assess the history of generational coparenting and their expectations of the coparenting relationship. Additionally, the work should emphasize the needs of all three generations. It is important for each generation to feel heard and have a sense of power and responsibility in maintaining the family unit. The therapist serves as a cultural broker to help family members destigmatize therapy and understand cultural expectations, values, and beliefs within the family, with the hope that family members can better support one another.

Case Context: Characteristics, Culture, and Preferences

Riya and Biju were recently divorced after 13 years of marriage and have two children, daughter Anjali (10) and son Ashok (8). Riya and Biju are both Orthodox Christian and belong to a local South Indian Christian church. However, their attendance during the past 2 years had been limited owing to their marital stress. Biju at times attended church with the children to appease his mom, Mrs. Kurian. However, attendance was a source of strain between Biju and Mrs. Kurian, and he felt that his mother was critical of his parenting and never supported him in his marriage to Riya. After the divorce, Biju moved back in with his mom as opposed to getting his own apartment because it was closer to his work and she could help with childcare on his days with the kids. Mrs. Kurian often made the children's favorite traditional Indian dishes and told the children they can "always stay with her if they want good food." Subsequently, their son Ashok had frequent tantrums and wanted to go to grandmother's house to have "good food." Riya asked Biju to speak to his mother about this, but he replied, "there is nothing I can do about it." Riya said Biju's lack of assertiveness had always been an issue, while Biju believed his mother constantly questioned him and undermined his authority with the children. The family conflict also affected their daughter, Anjali, who had been acting out at school.

Clinical Decisions: Intervention Implementation

At the school's recommendation, Biju convinced his mother to attend therapy to discuss concerns about the children. The initial session provided psychoeducation about treatment because the family was uncomfortable talking to a therapist. Specifically, the therapist informed the family that she will inquire about the family's current stressors and related feelings. Further, the therapist encouraged the family to ask questions and the therapist would explain her rationale for seeking such information. After hearing the story of the family's struggles, she stated, "You have been through a lot the past few months, however, you seem invested in strengthening your family, which is the first step to helping your children and your relationship with one another." The therapist also asked them, "How is it to be a divorced family in the Indian Christian community?" Mrs. Kurian shared her experience of Biju moving back home and their conflicts because this was all very unexpected for her, especially given the cultural stigma against divorce. Biju expressed that he, too, was in unchartered territory and figuring things out, adjusting to a recent divorce and the **transition to coparenting**.

In the following sessions, the therapist first met with Mrs. Kurian as the matriarch of the family and as a way of recognizing her status in the home. Mrs. Kurian shared further detail about the conflicts with Biju and her wishes, hopes, and fears for their relationship. She expressed that Biju did not understand that this is new for her and something she had never personally experienced. She told the therapist, "I wish he would be more patient with me because this is all so new and overwhelming having him and the kids in my home." The therapist next met with Biju, who expressed his frustration with his mom's intrusiveness and unsolicited suggestions. The therapist then asked, "How do you end up responding to your mom when she asks too many questions?" and "How can your mom respond in ways that you find helpful?"

The next several sessions were with Biju and his mother together. The therapist worked collaboratively with the parent and grandparent to reframe their respective frustrating behaviors and served as cultural and emotional broker so that both mother/grandmother and son/father could see different perspectives. Instead of Mrs. Kurian being viewed as intrusive, the therapist suggested that she was concerned about her son, the cohesion of her family, and the unfamiliar territory. The therapist further explained that Biju was still learning to be a single parent.

The final phase of therapy focused on providing psychoeducation on the importance of healthy and clear ways of communicating to **reduce conflict**. This needs to be done sensitively and respectfully so as to not undermine culture and respect for the older generation. Biju agreed to be more respectful and open about what he needs from Mrs. Kurian to support him and children. Instead of offering unsolicited suggestions, Mrs. Kurian agreed she could first share her worry. Biju agreed that hearing that would make it easier for him to understand her suggestions and consider them in making parenting decisions. Through this process they agreed that their coparenting relationship should involve **open communication** that they could use should challenges arise in the future.

Clinical Expertise and Interpretation of Evidence: Coparenting Conflicts in Families With a Child on the Autism Spectrum

Coparenting is made even more complicated when a child has special needs. Children with ASD and their families (Family on the Spectrum [FotS]) are dependent on larger systems. The social and **communicative** deficits, as well as the hallmark rigidity of those with autism, transcend the individual with the diagnosis and impact the family unit as a whole. Parents are so often thrust into imbalanced **roles**, resulting in the job of caregiver becoming the predominant focus. Additionally, parents may be pulled between fully accepting their child's diagnosis and integrating their needs into the family system or trying to treat their child as more "typical." As a result, parents often endure the adversity of childrearing with an underwhelming amount of **support from extended family**. Tamara D. Afifi et al.'s research section can guide therapists in the development of clear and effective clinical practices to assist families. One particular area that Afifi and colleagues highlighted, Altiere and von Kluge's (2009) research addressing the challenge of involving extended family, is addressed here with specific attention to how clinical practice can assist in eliciting systemic support.

Clinical Experience: Observations of Common Interactional Patterns
With the challenge of experiencing rejection and exclusion from extended family, FotS often insulate themselves, leading to immense social isolation. This detached existence from the outside world results in poorer parental mental health and decreased marital satisfaction because one parent is always "on duty" with a child with ASD. These individuals may become so immersed within this autistic microcosm that they may feel entirely disconnected from their fellow parents of same-aged children, almost as if they are living on a different plane of existence.

This inability to find respite from the demanding nature of parenting cements these couples into their roles as caregivers, making it difficult for them to function as intimate partners and even parents of their neurotypical children. The disengagement from extended family varies drastically from system to system, with some extended family being embarrassed and intolerant of their relative with autism, and others being genuinely curious but unaware of how best to connect with that individual. Extended family members sometimes believe they lack the knowledge of how to help the FotS. Clinical intervention addressing these dynamics can serve as a catalyst for positive change, with both the couple and extended family expanding their familiar comfort zone and creating space to renegotiate their relationships with each other.

Case Context: Characteristics, Culture, and Preferences

James and Pam found themselves growing increasingly overwhelmed with "a pressure cooker of a household." Their son, Sam, is 9 years old and was diagnosed with autism a few weeks before his fourth birthday. Before his diagnosis, Sam exhibited concerning behaviors, such as extended bouts of hysterical crying, arm flapping, and having fewer than 20 words in his vocabulary. Although his communication has improved in recent years due to extensive speech therapy and applied behavior analysis (ABA) counseling, he is still prone to tantrums when denied his preferred activity, resulting in damaging property, uncontrollable screaming, and flinging himself to the ground. His mother, Pam, was recently diagnosed with depression, describing her life as "Groundhog Day." Both James and Pam feel guilty about the amount of attention they give Sam relative to his 7-year-old sister, Lucy. Additionally, they each expressed feeling alienated from external sources of support—namely, both of their extended families. James is an only child, and his father died before Sam's birth. However, his mother pulled away from the family in recent years, due to her difficulty in coping with Sam's outbursts. Initially, Pam's family had been much more involved in Sam's upbringing. However, Pam became distressed because arguing increased with her parents regarding what they described as "poor parenting." She found that her younger sister often offered unsolicited advice on how she parented her children and to "set better limits." As a result, Pam had distanced herself from both her parents and her sister.

Clinical Decisions: Intervention Implementation

The initial extended interview was conducted with Pam, James, Sam, and Lucy. In this way, the therapist conveyed that the child's issues exist within a family system. The intake assesses many of the typical areas addressed in a first meeting but with added focus on family history and current family patterns of functioning and support. The use of a genogram during this stage is essential because it serves as a map of the relationships in need of reparation. After identifying key extended family members on both sides of the family, the therapist asked Pam and James, "Ideally, what would you hope these relationships with extended family would look like?"

The potential increased involvement with extended family was discussed, and the therapist assessed for any potential reasons not to include specific family members in treatment, such as history of abuse or substance use. By the end of the first session, Pam and James identified which **extended family members** would be included in treatment.

In the second session, the therapist focused on processing the previous session with the parents and developing a strategy for contacting the previously identified extended family members. The therapist processed with Pam her concerns about having her sister involved. Pam stated, "My sister is always so critical of me. I'm really afraid of asking her for help and having her minimize the difficulty of raising Sam." The therapist responded, "Have you ever told your sister how much her help would mean to you and to have her as a source of support? How do you think she would respond?" James turned to Pam and said, "I know your sister loves you and really wants to be there for us. What if we approach her together?" The couple and the therapist brainstormed ways the couple could open the conversation with Pam's sister and then began discussing how to approach Sam's mother and ask for her support as well. "My mother is often overwhelmed by Sam, and I haven't really sat down with her to explain what happens when he gets upset," James explains to the therapist. "What if we met together and I helped you educate your mother about common behaviors of children like Sam?" asked the therapist. James and Pam agreed that having the therapist facilitate these conversations could lead to a deeper understanding and connection to their extended family.

Before the third session, the couple contacted the identified extended family members and developed appropriate plans for the subsequent sessions. Each extended family relationship warrants its own session because the couple can become overwhelmed by having multiple family members, potentially each with their own distinct past challenges, in the office at once. Pam decided the first extended family meeting with the therapist was between her, James, and her sister. In the next therapy session, the couple met with James's mother. After these two sessions, both Pam and James felt relieved that their relatives had responded with such compassion and willingness to learn more about how they could better support them in parenting Sam and Lucy.

This case study illustrates that extended family's disengagement from FotS is rarely an intentional abandonment but rather a complicated and sensitive dynamic with many layers. Both immediate and extended families need to be willing to make small yet powerful changes to improve the systemic functioning. Working within these systems requires a therapist to display a fair approach, highlighting the challenges on both sides in a validating, authentic manner. Helping these family members feel heard and understood can help them shift from a negative outlook to a more positive viewpoint in the future.

Conclusion

As this clinical section of the chapter has illustrated, regardless of family form, common factors emerge in clinical treatment with coparents when interventions are informed by empirical evidence. Foremost among these findings is the importance of prioritizing the needs of the child in addressing conflict between the adults who care for them. Effective therapy focuses on finding common ground between coparents and increasing mutual support despite their differences, uniting them in the mutual interest of raising well-adjusted children. Additionally, clinicians who understand the contexts within which coparenting relationships are embedded, as well as the typical stresses encountered in these families, can better support both parents and children through the process of change.

REFERENCES

Adler-Baeder, F., & Higginbotham, B. (2020). Efforts to design, implement, and evaluate community-based education for stepfamilies: Current knowledge and future directions. *Family Relations, 69*(3), 559–576. https://doi.org/10.1111/fare.12427

Afifi, T. D. (2003). "Feeling caught" in stepfamilies: Managing boundary turbulence through appropriate privacy coordination rules. *Journal of Social and Personal Relationships, 20*(6), 729–756. https://doi.org/10.1177/0265407503206002

Afifi, T. D., Granger, D., Joseph, A., Denes, A., & Aldeis, D. (2015). The influence of divorce and parents' communication skills on adolescents' and young adults' stress reactivity and recovery. *Communication Research, 42*(7), 1009–1042. https://doi.org/10.1177/0093650213509665

Altiere, M. J., & von Kluge, S. (2009). Searching for acceptance: Challenges encountered while raising a child with autism. *Journal of Intellectual & Developmental Disability, 34*(2), 142–152. https://doi.org/10.1080/13668250902845202

Amato, P. R. (2001). Children of divorce in the 1990s: An update of the Amato and Keith (1991) meta-analysis. *Journal of Family Psychology, 15*(3), 355–370. https://doi.org/10.1037/0893-3200.15.3.355

Amato, P. R., & Afifi, T. D. (2006). Feeling caught between parents: Adult children's relations with parents and subjective well-being. *Journal of Marriage and the Family, 68*(1), 222–236. https://doi.org/10.1111/j.1741-3737.2006.00243.x

Amato, P. R., Kane, J. B., & James, S. (2011). Reconsidering the "good divorce." *Family Relations, 60*(5), 511–524. https://doi.org/10.1111/j.1741-3729.2011.00666.x

American Psychiatric Association. (2013). *Diagnostic and statistical manual of mental disorders* (5th ed.).

Backhouse, J., & Graham, A. (2012). Grandparents raising grandchildren: Negotiating the complexities of role-identity conflict. *Child & Family Social Work, 17*(3), 306–315. https://doi.org/10.1111/j.1365-2206.2011.00781.x

Bámaca-Colbert, M. Y., Henry, C. S., Perez-Brena, N., Gayles, J. G., & Martinez, G. (2019). Cultural orientation gaps within a family systems perspective. *Journal of Family Theory & Review, 11*(4), 524–543. https://doi.org/10.1111/jftr.12353

Becher, E. H., Kim, H., Cronin, S. E., Deenanath, V., McGuire, J. K., McCann, E. M., & Powell, S. (2019). Positive parenting and parental conflict: Contributions to resilient coparenting during divorce. *Family Relations, 68*(1), 150–164. https://doi.org/10.1111/fare.12349

Beckmeyer, J. J., Krejnick, S. J., MacCray, J. A., Troilo, J., & Markham, M. S. (2020). A multidimensional perspective on former spouses' ongoing relationships: Associations with children's postdivorce well-being. *Family Relations, 70*(2), 467–482. https://doi.org/10.1111/fare.12504

Booth, A., & Amato, P. R. (2001). Parental predivorce relations and offspring postdivorce well-being. *Journal of Marriage and the Family, 63*(1), 197–212. https://doi.org/10.1111/j.1741-3737.2001.00197.x

Braithwaite, D. O., McBride, C., & Schrodt, P. (2003). "Parenting teams" and everyday interactions of coparenting in stepfamilies. *Communication Reports, 16*(2), 93–111. https://doi.org/10.1080/08934210309384493

Braithwaite, D. O., Olson, L., Golish, T. D., Soukup, C., & Turman, P. (2001). "Becoming a family": Developmental processes represented in blended family discourse. *Journal of Applied Communication Research, 29*(3), 221–247. https://doi.org/10.1080/00909880128112

Brown, M., Whiting, J., Kahumoku-Fessler, E., Witting, A. B., & Jensen, J. (2020). A dyadic model of stress, coping, and marital satisfaction among parents of children with autism. *Family Relations, 69*(1), 138–150. https://doi.org/10.1111/fare.12375

Caldwell, C. H., Antonucci, T. C., & Jackson, J. S. (1998). Supportive/conflictual family relations and depressive symptomatology: Teenage mother and grandmother perspectives. *Family Relations, 47*(4), 395–402. https://doi.org/10.2307/585270

Callander, E. J., & Lindsay, D. B. (2018). The impact of childhood autism spectrum disorder on parent's labour force participation: Can parents be expected to be able to re-join the labour force? *Autism: An International Journal of Research and Practise, 22*(5), 542–548. https://doi.org/10.1177/1362361316688331

Cartwright, C., & Gibson, K. (2013). The effects of coparenting relationships with ex-spouses on couples in step-families. *Family Matters, 92*, 18–28. https://aifs.gov.au/publications/family-matters/issue-92/effects-coparenting-relationships-ex-spouses-couples-step

Centers for Disease Control and Prevention (CDC). (2019, September 3). *Data & statistics on autism spectrum disorder*. https://www.cdc.gov/ncbddd/autism/data.html

Chan, G. W. L., & Goh, E. C. L. (2014). "My parents told us that they will always treat my brother differently because he is autistic"—Are siblings of autistic children the forgotten ones? *Journal of Social Work Practice, 28*(2), 155–171. https://doi.org/10.1080/02650533.2013.844114

Chang, J.-G., Hsu, C.-C., Shih, N.-H., & Chen, H.-C. (2014). Multicultural families and creative children. *Journal of Cross-Cultural Psychology, 45*(8), 1288–1296. https://doi.org/10.1177/0022022114537556

Chiang, Y.-L., & Park, H. (2015). Do grandparents matter? A multigenerational perspective on educational attainment in Taiwan. *Social Science Research, 51*, 163–173. https://doi.org/10.1016/j.ssresearch.2014.09.013

Cohrs, A. C., & Leslie, D. L. (2017). Depression in parents of children diagnosed with autism spectrum disorder: A claims-based analysis. *Journal of Autism and Developmental Disorders, 47*(5), 1416–1422. https://doi.org/10.1007/s10803-017-3063-y

Conn, B. M., Marks, A. K., & Coyne, L. (2013). A three-generation study of Chinese immigrant extended family child caregiving experiences in the preschool years. *Research in Human Development, 10*(4), 308–331. https://doi.org/10.1080/15427609.2013.846047

Fidler, B., & McHale, J. (2020). Building and enhancing efficacious coparenting in parenting coordination. *Family Court Review, 58*(3), 747–759. https://doi.org/10.1111/fcre.12510

Foody, C., James, J. E., & Leader, G. (2015). Parenting stress, salivary biomarkers, and ambulatory blood pressure: A comparison between mothers and fathers of children with autism spectrum disorders. *Journal of Autism and Developmental Disorders, 45*(4), 1084–1095. https://doi.org/10.1007/s10803-014-2263-y

Fruhauf, C. A., & Hayslip, B. J., Jr. (2013). Understanding collaborative efforts to assist grandparent caregivers: A multileveled perspective. *Journal of Family Social Work, 16*(5), 382–391. https://doi.org/10.1080/10522158.2013.832462

Ganong, L., & Coleman, M. (2017). *Stepfamily relationships: Development, dynamics, and interventions* (2nd ed.). Springer. https://doi.org/10.1007/978-1-4899-7702-1

Ganong, L., Coleman, M., Jamison, T., & Feistman, R. (2015). Divorced mothers' coparental boundary maintenance after parents repartner. *Journal of Family Psychology, 29*(2), 221–231. https://doi.org/10.1037/fam0000064

Gau, S. S., Chou, M., Chiang, H., Lee, J., Wong, C., Chou, W., & Wu, Y. (2012). Parental adjustment, marital relationship, and family function in families of children with autism. *Research in Autism Spectrum Disorders, 6*(1), 263–270. https://doi.org/10.1016/j.rasd.2011.05.007

Goodman, C., & Silverstein, M. (2002). Grandmothers raising grandchildren: Family structure and well-being in culturally diverse families. *The Gerontologist, 42*(5), 676–689. https://doi.org/10.1093/geront/42.5.676

Harper, A., Taylor Dyches, T., Harper, J., Olsen Roper, S., & South, M. (2013). Respite care, marital quality, and stress in parents of children with autism spectrum disorders. *Journal of Autism and Developmental Disorders, 43*(11), 2604–2616. https://doi.org/10.1007/s10803-013-1812-0

Hartley, S. L., Barker, E. T., Seltzer, M. M., Floyd, F., Greenberg, J., Orsmond, G., & Bolt, D. (2010). The relative risk and timing of divorce in families of children with an autism spectrum disorder. *Journal of Family Psychology, 24*(4), 449–457. https://doi.org/10.1037/a0019847

Hawkes, K., & Coxworth, J. E. (2013). Grandmothers and the evolution of human longevity: A review of findings and future directions. *Evolutionary Anthropology, 22*(6), 294–302. https://doi.org/10.1002/evan.21382

Hayslip, B., Jr., & Kaminski, P. L. (2005). Grandparents raising their grandchildren: A review of the literature and suggestions for practice. *The Gerontologist, 45*(2), 262–269. https://doi.org/10.1093/geront/45.2.262

Herrero, M., Martinez-Pampliega, A., & Alvarez, I. (2020). Family communication, adaptation to divorce and children's maladjustment: The moderating role of coparenting. *Journal of Family Communication, 20*(2), 114–128. https://doi.org/10.1080/15267431.2020.1723592

Hickey, E. J., Nix, R. L., & Hartley, S. L. (2019). Family emotional climate and children with autism spectrum disorder. *Journal of Autism and Developmental Disorders, 49*(8), 3244–3256. https://doi.org/10.1007/s10803-019-04037-6

Higgins, D. J., Bailey, S. R., & Pearce, J. C. (2005). Factors associated with functioning style and coping strategies of families with a child with an autism spectrum disorder. *Autism, 9*(2), 125–137. https://doi.org/10.1177/1362361305051403

Hoang, N., Haslam, D., & Sanders, M. (2020). Coparenting conflict and cooperation between parents and grandparents in Vietnamese families: The role of grandparent psychological control and parent-grandparent communication. *Family Process, 59*(3), 1161–1174. https://doi.org/10.1111/famp.12496

Höllinger, F., & Haller, M. (1990). Kinship and social networks in modern societies: A cross cultural comparison. *European Sociological Review, 6*(2), 103–124. https://doi.org/10.1093/oxfordjournals.esr.a036553

Jones, D. J., Zalot, A. A., Foster, S. E., Sterrett, E., & Chester, C. (2007). A review of childrearing in African American single mother families: The relevance of a coparenting framework. *Journal of Child and Family Studies, 16*(5), 671–683. https://doi.org/10.1007/s10826-006-9115-0

Karberg, E., & Cabrera, N. (2020). Children's adjustment to parent's breakup: The mediational effects of parenting and coparenting. *Journal of Family Issues, 41*(10), 1810–1833. https://doi.org/10.1177/0192513X19894347

Kelley, S. J., Whitley, D. M., & Campos, P. E. (2013). African American caregiving grandmothers: Results of an intervention to improve health indicators and health promotion behaviors. *Journal of Family Nursing, 19*(1), 53–73. https://doi.org/10.1177/1074840712462135

Kovshoff, H., Cebula, K., Tsai, H. J., & Hastings, R. P. (2017). Siblings of children with autism: The siblings embedded systems framework. *Current Developmental Disorders Reports, 4*(2), 37–45. https://doi.org/10.1007/s40474-017-0110-5

Lamela, D., Figueiredo, B., Bastos, A., & Feinberg, M. (2016). Typologies of post-divorce parenting and parental wellbeing, parenting quality, and children's psychological adjustment. *Child Psychiatry and Human Development, 47*(5), 716–728. https://doi.org/10.1007/s10578-015-0604-5

Landry-Meyer, L., & Newman, B. M. (2004). An exploration of the grandparent caregiver role. *Journal of Family Issues, 25*(8), 1005–1025. https://doi.org/10.1177/0192513X04265955

Leonce, T. E. (2020). The inevitable rise in dual income households and the intertemporal effects on labor markets. *Compensation & Benefits Review, 52*(2), 64–76. https://doi.org/10.1177/0886368719900032

Li, T., Lam, C. B., & Chan, K. K.-S. (2018). Grandparental involvement and young adults' cognitive and social adjustment: The moderating role of filial piety in Hong Kong. *Journal of Social and Personal Relationships, 35*(7), 999–1018. https://doi.org/10.1177/0265407517702011

Meadan, H., Halle, J. W., & Ebata, A. T. (2010). Families with children who have autism spectrum disorders: Stress and support. *Exceptional Children, 77*(1), 7–36. https://doi.org/10.1177/001440291007700101

Musil, C. M., Jeanblanc, A. B., Burant, C. J., Zauszniewski, J. A., & Warner, C. B. (2013). Longitudinal analysis of resourcefulness, family strain, and depressive symptoms in grandmother caregivers. *Nursing Outlook, 61*(4), 225–234.e2. https://doi.org/10.1016/j.outlook.2013.04.009

Nelson, J. G., Gibson, P. A., & Beauer, J. W. (2010). Kinship care and "child-only" welfare grants: Low participation despite potential benefits. *Journal of Family Social Work, 13*(1), 3–24. https://doi.org/10.1080/10522150903437466

Oburu, P. O., & Palmérus, K. (2005). Stress related factors among primary and part-time caregiving grandmothers of Kenyan grandchildren. *International Journal of Aging & Human Development, 60*(4), 273–282. https://doi.org/10.2190/XLQ2-UJEM-TAQR-4944

O'Mara, C., & Schrodt, P. (2017). Parents' negative relational disclosures and young adult children's perceptions of appropriateness and feelings of being caught. *Communication Quarterly, 65*(5), 565–579. https://doi.org/10.1080/01463373.2017.1321563

Papernow, P. L. (2018). Clinical guidelines for working with stepfamilies: What individual, couple, child, and family therapists need to know. *Family Process, 57*(1), 25–51. https://doi.org/10.1111/famp.12321

Perry-Fraser, C., & Fraser, R. (2018). A qualitative analysis of the stepparent role on transition days in blended families. *Open Journal of Social Sciences, 6*(8), 240–251. https://doi.org/10.4236/jss.2018.68020

Prendeville, P., & Kinsella, W. (2019). The role of grandparents in supporting families of children with autism spectrum disorders: A family systems approach. *Journal of Autism and Developmental Disorders, 49*(2), 738–749. https://doi.org/10.1007/s10803-018-3753-0

Pruchno, R. A., & McKenney, D. (2002). Psychological well-being of Black and White grandmothers raising grandchildren: Examination of a two-factor model. *The Journals of Gerontology: Series B. Psychological Sciences and Social Sciences, 57*(5), 444–452. https://doi.org/10.1093/geronb/57.5.P444

Pryor, J. (2004). Parenting in reconstituted and surrogate families. In M. Hoghughi & N. Long (Eds.), *Handbook of parenting: Theory and research for practice* (pp. 110–129). Sage Publications.

Raval, V. V., & Walker, B. L. (2019). Unpacking "culture": Caregiver socialization of emotion and child functioning in diverse families. *Developmental Review, 51*, 146–174. https://doi.org/10.1016/j.dr.2018.11.001

Rivers, J. W., & Stoneman, Z. (2003). Sibling relationships when a child has autism: Marital stress and support coping. *Journal of Autism and Developmental Disorders, 33*(4), 383–394. https://doi.org/10.1023/A:1025006727395

Saini, M. (2019). Strengthening coparenting relationships to improve strained parent–child relationships: A follow-up study of parents' experiences of attending the overcoming barriers program. *Family Court Review, 57*(2), 217–230. https://doi.org/10.1111/fcre.12405

Sandler, I., Ingram, A., Wolchik, S., Tein, J. Y., & Winslow, E. (2015). Long-term effects of parenting-focused preventive interventions to promote resilience of children and adolescents. *Child Development Perspectives, 9*(3), 164–171. https://doi.org/10.1111/cdep.12126

Schrodt, P. (2015). Coparental communication with nonresidential parents as a predictor of children's feelings of being caught in stepfamilies. *Communication Reports, 29*(2), 63–74. https://doi.org/10.1080/08934215.2015.1020562

Schrodt, P., & Afifi, T. D. (2018). Untying the ties that bind: Dispositional and relational patterns of negative relational disclosures and family members' feelings of being caught. *Journal of Family Issues, 39*(7), 1962–1983. https://doi.org/10.1177/0192513X17739050

Schrodt, P., & Braithwaite, D. (2011). Coparental communication, relational satisfaction, and mental health in stepfamilies. *Personal Relationships, 18*(3), 352–369. https://doi.org/10.1111/j.1475-6811.2010.01295.x

U.S. Census Bureau. (2011). *Living arrangements of children: 2009.* https://www.census.gov/prod/2011pubs/p70-126.pdf

van der Wal, R. C., Finkenauer, C., & Visser, M. M. (2019). Reconciling mixed findings on children's adjustment following high-conflict divorce. *Journal of Child and Family Studies, 28*(2), 468–478. https://doi.org/10.1007/s10826-018-1277-z

Vohra, R., Madhaven, S., Sambamoorthi, U., & St. Peter, C. (2014). Access to services, quality of care, and family impact for children with autism, other developmental disabilities, and other mental health conditions. *Autism, 18*(7), 815–826. https://doi.org/10.1177/1362361313512902

Wagner, A. C., & Diamond, R. M. (2017a). Divorce in couple and family therapy. In J. Lebow, A. Chambers, & D. C. Breunlin (Eds.), *Encyclopedia of couple and family therapy.* Springer International. https://doi.org/10.1007/978-3-319-15877-8_448-1

Wagner, A. C., & Diamond, R. M. (2017b). Families and divorce. In S. Browning & B. van Eeden-Moorefield (Eds.), *Contemporary families: At the nexus of research and practice* (pp. 15–18). Routledge Press.

Whitton, S. W., Nicholson, J. M., & Markman, H. J. (2008). Research on interventions for stepfamily couples: The state of the field. In J. Pryor (Ed.), *The international handbook of stepfamilies: Policy and practice in legal, research, and clinical environments* (pp. 455–484). Wiley. https://doi.org/10.1002/9781118269923.ch19

7

BOUNDARY AMBIGUITY

A Focus on Stepfamilies, Queer Families, Families With Adolescent Children, and Multigenerational Families

RESEARCH: MARILYN COLEMAN AND LAWRENCE GANONG
CLINICAL APPLICATIONS: SALVATORE D'AMORE, SCOTT BROWNING, DENA DINARDO, AND BINDU METHIKALAM

RESEARCH: MARILYN COLEMAN AND LAWRENCE GANONG

It has been more than 40 years since Pauline Boss (1977) created the concept of family boundary ambiguity. Boss (2002) defined *ambiguity* as "an inability to make sense of a contradiction between absence and presence" (p. 114). Boundaries define family or household composition or kinship ties. At the most basic level, they define who is in and who is not in a family. Boss (1980a) spoke of the construct of boundary ambiguity in relation to family stress—the stress of families with a member who was missing in action (MIA) during the Vietnam War; were the MIA soldiers still in the family, or not?

Both physical and psychological absence are part of boundary ambiguity theory (i.e., *physically present but psychologically absent*, as when a family member living at home has dementia; *physically absent but psychologically present*, as with the MIAs from Vietnam). Both types of absences create a sense of uncertain and ambiguous loss, unresolved or "frozen" grief

https://doi.org/10.1037/0000280-007
Treating Contemporary Families: Toward a More Inclusive Clinical Practice, S. Browning and B. van Eeden-Moorefield (Editors)

that is difficult to manage (Boss, 1999). Boss was a therapist–researcher who developed her theory of family boundary ambiguity from clinical observations, but she also emphasized the utility of the theory for studying dynamic, stressful changes in families across time (e.g., aging, births, remarriage, young adults leaving home; Boss, 1980b).

In an excellent review of family boundary ambiguity, Carroll et al. (2007) identified 37 studies primarily focusing on family membership changes due to death, divorce, remarriage, and stepfamily formation, Alzheimer's patients, and students leaving for college. These reviewers concluded that families with higher levels of boundary ambiguity had more dysfunction. They also concluded that "family boundary ambiguity has been found to be a useful family stress construct for researchers and family professionals in a wide array of disciplines" (p. 225). According to Boss et al. (2017), assumptions about boundary ambiguity include the following:

- Cultural diversity influences perceptions (e.g., deciding who is and is not a member of a family depends on the cultural background of the family). For instance, in the Maori culture, anyone who claims Maori genetic kinship is considered to be Maori.

- Outsiders cannot maintain a family's boundaries; each family must maintain their perceptions of membership and roles from the inside. For example, as much as people outside the family might want to dismiss former spouses from family membership, it is strictly up to the people within the family to decide whether former spouses are kin or not (Markham & Coleman, 2020).

- Boundary ambiguity is ubiquitous but is not necessarily a problem. Individuals gain and lose family membership for normative reasons, such as births, deaths, marriages, and so forth.

Boss et al. (2017) cautioned that boundary maintenance and boundary permeability are not the same as boundary ambiguity, although these concepts are related. In fact, she defined boundary maintenance as the opposite of **boundary ambiguity**. *Boundary maintenance* refers to family actions that promote clear boundaries developed through language, rituals, and rules. Those clear boundaries are most likely to become ambiguous when **developmental changes** happen within the family (e.g., someone dies, gets married, leaves the household for college).

These developmental changes mean that the family cannot go back to the way it was before. Transitions of individuals in and out of the family create boundary ambiguity—in some families this boundary ambiguity, if not addressed, creates increasing stress and dysfunction. Other families can reorganize and restructure their boundaries and manage the loss or addition of family members with resilience (Boss, 2002). In this chapter, we focus on stepfamilies, queer families, families with adolescents, and multigenerational families (see Table 7.1). We review relevant research evidence and follow that with descriptions of important psychoeducational points and clinical considerations and interventions. We use case examples for each family type to do this.

Research Evidence on Stepfamilies

A *stepfamily* is one in which at least one of the adults has a child or children from previous relationships (Ganong & Coleman, 2017). Long ago, Andrew Cherlin (1978) asserted that stepfamilies were **incompletely institutionalized** by societal norms, as evidenced by language, laws, and customs that did not work well for stepfamilies. For example, there is no term for the relationship between current and former spouses of an individual, even though those persons may have considerable influence on each other's lives. With neither *language* nor labels, it is difficult to think about or talk about such relationships. Stepparents, unlike biological parents, are unable to make health care decisions for stepchildren in emergency departments unless *legal steps* have been taken to allow them to do so. Because of *social norms*, children usually refer to their parents as Mom and Dad, but there are no social norms for what stepchildren call their stepparents. Incomplete institutionalization complicates traditional notions of family boundaries because blood lines and legal ties, the standard markers of kinship, do not apply to

TABLE 7.1. Boundary Ambiguity

Evidence-based area of clinical focus	Type of factor	Appropriateness for use across families	Selected references indicating evidence base
Levels of ambiguity	General	All	Boss, 1977, 1980a, 2002; Boss et al., 2017
Developmental change	General	All	Bengtson, 2001; King et al., 2015; Seltzer, 2019
Family belonging	General	All,[a] but more so in stepfamilies	King et al., 2015
Incomplete institutionalization	Unique	Stepfamilies	Cherlin, 1978
Social stigma	Unique	Stepfamilies, queer families	Ganong & Coleman, 2017; Goldberg & Allen, 2013

[a]This general factor could work for other family types included in this chapter but needs a small adaptation to ensure cultural relevance. Information about potential adaptations is included in the text.

step-relationships and may often stretch across multiple households. The absence of social norms contributes to boundary ambiguity for stepfamily members (Thorsen & King, 2016) and for outsiders who interact with step-families (e.g., schools, health care systems), which may in turn cause stress for stepfamily members and for others (Coleman & Ganong, 1995).

Every stepfamily must address the issue of family membership (who is in and who is out), and because of this incomplete institutionalization, the possibility of boundary ambiguity is greater for stepfamilies than for first-marriage nuclear families (Ganong & Coleman, 2017). Stewart (2005), in a study using the National Survey of Families and Households' nationally representative sample of American families, found that "boundary ambiguity is much more prevalent among stepfamilies than original two-parent families. Spouses or partners disagreed in their reports of each other's children in 25% of step-families compared to 8% of couples with only shared children" (p. 1014). In another study, Pasley (1987) reported that 40% of the remarried couples in her sample exhibited high physical or psychological boundary ambiguity (or both).

The extent to which stepfamilies experience boundary ambiguity is related to their structural complexity (Pasley, 1987). For example, which adult brings children from prior unions to the stepfamily, how many prior unions there were that produced children, and where those children reside all contribute to stepfamily structural complexity (Ganong & Coleman, 2017). Bearing children in the stepfamily also adds to the complexity of sibling relationships (Sanner et al., 2020)—and, therefore, to boundary ambiguity. Boundary ambiguity has been found to be greater when children from prior unions lived outside the stepfamily household (Ambert, 1986). Loss of both the original family and one's physical home may increase the ambiguity. Stewart (2005) found that boundary ambiguity was greatest when both parents in the remarriage had children living outside the household and lowest when the male partner only had children living outside the household. Other studies, however, have reported that boundary ambiguity was greater when the children of male part-ners lived elsewhere (Ambert, 1986).

Stepfamily boundary ambiguity is handled in multiple ways; one way is to consider only household members as family, a phenomenon called *exclu-siveness* (Castrén & Widmer, 2015). Those with exclusive boundaries limited their families to the people who shared their household, ignoring past family relationships. There is evidence that mothers in stepfamily households employ exclusive boundary definitions (in a sense "circling the wagon") more often than do fathers. Castrén and Widmer (2015) reported that mothers described their families almost solely in exclusive terms, as did their children (but not to the extent of the mothers). Other researchers have reported that children define stepfamily membership in multiple ways (Funder, 1991), likely using different criteria for kinship than do their mothers (DiVerniero, 2013). A study of British families described mothers in stepfamilies as presenting a "we-ness" to outsiders, including researchers, downplaying the fact that they were a stepfamily and focusing on the household only (Allan et al., 2011). When stepfamilies define themselves as consisting of household members only, this creates challenges for nonresidential parents and children, as well as for researchers (Sanner et al., 2021; Seltzer, 2019).

In contrast, other adults and children in stepfamilies manage boundary ambiguity by employing definitions of family membership that includes nonresidential parents and children (Castrén & Widmer, 2015). Adults with inclusive beliefs about stepfamily membership are more likely to be in complex family structures and have mothers with more education who work outside the home. There is some evidence that children are more likely than adults in stepfamilies to have family boundary definitions that include their nonresidential parents and siblings (Ganong et al., 2011); the absence of congruence between stepfamily members is not necessarily a problem, except when loyalty conflicts arise or parents and children conflict over managing "boundary turbulence" (Baxter et al., 2009).

Family belonging, a concept related to boundary ambiguity, means that individuals feel included in the family and that family members pay attention to them (King et al., 2015). A sense of family belonging is related to whether family boundaries are ambiguous, clear, or rigid. Adolescent stepchildren feel a sense of belonging when family boundaries are not ambiguous and the perceived quality of (step)parent-adolescent relationships are positive.

When adults use *exclusive* definitions, the new partnership or family is considered to replace the old family, or at least the part of it that is not in the household. When stepfathers do this, essentially replacing stepchildren they live with for biological children they may no longer see much, if at all, they are said to be *swapping families* (Manning & Smock, 2000). Ganong and Coleman (2017) asserted that this way of managing boundary ambiguity (by defining the household as the family) often creates problems for children and is only possible if everyone in the family agrees to embrace the new stepfamily household as the *only* family. Some remarried partners attempt to do this by adopting their stepchildren (Ganong et al., 1998), but that is unlikely to solve the problem of rigid boundaries if the children want to maintain contact with their nonresidential parent and extended kin or if they want to continue to include a deceased parent (and their extended kin) in their family. Permeable boundaries are easier on children in this case, although permeable boundaries are not always easy to maintain (Baxter et al., 2009).

Greater boundary ambiguity has been found among cohabiting stepcouples, those who had been together a shorter time, couples with younger children, persons of color, and those with a large age gap between the partners (Stewart, 2005). Boundary ambiguity is not limited to younger stepfamilies, however; later life remarriages (Chapman et al., 2018) and older stepfamilies (Van der Pas et al., 2013) grapple with defining kinship, as do older adults whose adult offspring acquire stepchildren through remarriage or repartnering (Sanner et al., 2019).

Boundary ambiguity is an issue that is not easily resolved in stepfamilies because kinship definitions change over time, and therefore boundaries must change as well. White (1998), in a longitudinal study of National Survey of Families and Households data, found that 15% of respondents added or subtracted children from inclusion in their stepfamilies in a 4-year-follow-up of data collected in the first year of the study. These changes were not due to birth, death, or adoption, nor was this a matter of measurement error. Instead, the changes were due to differences in how respondents defined who was in their stepfamilies. White cautioned that researchers should be clearer about the definition of terms so that participants' and researchers' definitions more closely match. Researchers more recently have argued, however, that clarity of definitions are not going to eliminate the discrepancies because family members have their own definitions of family (i.e., who they are; Sanner et al., 2020; Seltzer, 2019).

Research Evidence on Queer Families

The definition of stepfamilies presented earlier in this chapter fits most queer families (used as an umbrella term)—exceptions are when both partners adopt a child together (Ganong et al., 2015), when there are no children, or when the family consists of chosen members who are not legally or genetically connected to them. In queer families, often one or both partners have a child or children from previous relationships, which means only one of them has a biological and legal tie to the child (the parent), and the other adult does not (the stepparent). Potentially, the same boundary ambiguity dynamics can occur in queer families as in heterosexual stepfamilies (Bermea et al., 2020), particularly when queer couples divorce or separate (Ganong & Coleman, 2015; Goldberg & Allen, 2013). However, queer families have additional challenges related to boundary clarity and boundary setting, including **social stigma** (Catalpa & McGuire, 2018), poor concordance with how social systems and society in general defines family (Baumle & Compton, 2014; Jenkins, 2013), and the absence of norms to guide boundary negotiations (Goldberg & Allen, 2013; Jenkins, 2013).

Although there is relatively little research on boundary ambiguity in queer families, there is some evidence that adults (Bermea et al., 2020; Jenkins, 2013) and offspring (Catalpa & McGuire, 2018; Goldberg & Allen, 2013) in queer families experience boundary ambiguity. Boundary ambiguity in queer stepfamilies has drawbacks, such as stepparents who feel as if they are not really a part of the new queer stepfamily. This is a consequence of boundary ambiguity for all stepfamilies, however, not just queer stepfamilies.

The resolution of family boundary ambiguity has been found to have both positive and negative consequences. Open boundaries, for example, can support frequent communication and emotional closeness in a variety of family relationships (a good thing), or open boundaries can promote continued hostility between former partners attempting to coparent (a bad thing; Bermea et al., 2020). Closed boundaries, on the other hand, may indicate that former partners have developed independence from each other (a good thing) or that former partners refuse to communicate about their shared children (a bad thing).

Boundary ambiguity has potentially serious implications for transgender youth. Family acceptance and connectedness were resilience factors that helped transgender youth, whereas ambiguity about being part of the family was related to financial, physical, and psychological well-being of these youth (Catalpa & McGuire, 2018). Offspring from queer families, however, identified advantages as well as disadvantages in resolving the boundary ambiguities they faced when parent and stepparent dissolved their unions (Goldberg & Allen, 2013). Clearly, much more research is needed on queer families and how they have experienced boundary ambiguity.

Research Evidence on Families With Adolescents

Boss (1999) conceived boundary ambiguity as a developmentally normative problem facing families when adolescents left the family household to pursue education, military service, marriage, or employment. In these contexts, the issue is whether the family members consider an absent adolescent to be in the family. Family boundary ambiguity in these families has rarely been investigated, however. Instead, concepts such as **family belonging** and connectedness, adolescent autonomy-seeking, and independence have been studied (e.g., King & Boyd, 2016). The few studies on boundary ambiguity in families with adolescents have examined changes in family structure, where a parent may be either physically or psychologically absent due to parental divorce, remarriage, or repartnering (Buehler & Pasley, 2000). Other studies have explored boundary ambiguity when youth have chronic illnesses (Russell et al., 2016) or when a parent has been deployed due to military obligations (Drummet et al., 2003).

Life course theory would suggest that when adolescents leave home, it creates a family crisis of sorts (Wood et al., 2017). This is often the beginning of more ambiguous boundaries for the family. Whether the adolescent leaves home to marry, attend college, join the military, or to establish independence through a job or career, the notion of whether they are still in the family or not creates confusion. Commonly, families claim they are still emotionally close to their adolescent and thus they still are a member of the family, which raises the notion of whether a child can be a member of two families at once. This is a regular theme of stepchildren who maintain ties with nonresidential parents as well as those sharing their household. Flexible boundaries allow the stepchild to go back and forth between households. Boundaries of adolescents who leave the household for any of the reasons just described benefit from flexible family boundaries as well. The well-being of a child who feels guilty for not making it home to Sunday dinner, for example, may be damaged if they feel they are not living up to their family's standards for being a family member.

Research Evidence on Multigenerational Families

Increased longevity means that there are more multigenerational families than ever in history and that individuals share a greater proportion of their lives with grandparents and even great-grandparents (Park, 2014). Moreover, these multigenerational families have changed shape (Bengtson, 2001), from pyramids (i.e., few elders at the top linked to greater numbers of children and grandchildren below) to beanpoles or rectangles (i.e., nearly the same numbers of family members in each generation, a function of both increased longevity and lower rates of reproduction). These rectangular-shaped families are more complex and diverse than in the past because of increases in divorce, cohabitation, remarriages, and multiple partner fertility (Bengtson, 2001). Rather than nuclear family households being linked generationally to other nuclear family households, multigenerational families in the 21st century are households representing diverse family forms linked to other diverse family households. As such, extremely complex multigenerational families form that may contain great-grandparents, stepgrandparents, grandparents, half-siblings, stepsiblings, full biological and adoptive siblings, single-parent-headed households, cohabiting households, queer households, individuals living alone, and households that contain nonbiological kin (Seltzer, 2019). Family gerontologists have observed for decades that multigenerational families, and really all families, have become increasingly important sources of emotional support (Bengtson, 2001; Park, 2014). Multigenerational families are also relied on to provide tangible types of resources (e.g., financial, caregiving).

Investigations of boundary ambiguity in multigenerational families have seldom focused on boundary ambiguity per se (see Suanet et al., 2013, for an exception). Instead, related concepts such as intergenerational solidarity, conflict, and ambivalence have been examined extensively. As families have become more structurally complex, researchers have begun to explore the importance of boundary ambiguity to family members' well-being and to families' resilience (Van der Pas et al., 2013). Issues such as caregiving of older individuals, inheritance, and intergenerational responsibilities for assistance and resource exchanges highlight the relevance of families' beliefs about who is and who is not part of the kin network. Marital transitions—divorces, remarriages, cohabitations—have stimulated the need for families to grapple with boundary ambiguity (Chapman et al., 2018; Sanner et al., 2019; Van der Pas et al., 2013).

As members of the oldest generation die (i.e., physical absence but psychological presence) or become cognitively impaired (i.e., physical presence but psychological absence), it is certain that every multigenerational family will have to address ambiguous losses as a result of boundary ambiguity (Boss, 1999). Scholars are focusing on these types of normative losses and how other kin manage unresolved grief. As industrialized societies age, it seems likely that these boundary ambiguity issues will become more important for larger groups of families. There is some evidence that multigenerational boundaries are expanding (Suanet et al., 2013), but more research is needed in this area.

CLINICAL APPLICATIONS: SALVATORE D'AMORE, SCOTT BROWNING, DENA DINARDO, AND BINDU METHIKALAM

Clinical Expertise and Interpretation of Evidence: An Overview

Boundaries are crucial in helping a system define and maintain its unique identity. Certainly, research has helped produce significant information about the role of boundaries in family life. Indeed, the term *family boundaries* proposed by Minuchin (1974) refers to the family rules that define which individuals participate in a family, and it continues to influence the practice of couple and family therapy today. Boss (1999) added complexity to this definition when she described *boundary* ambiguity as a "state in which family members are uncertain in their perception about who is in or out of the family and who is performing what roles and tasks within the family system" (p. 2). Green and Mitchell (2008) expanded on boundary ambiguity by suggesting the term *relational ambiguity*, which refers to an unclear definition of a relationship where roles and boundaries tend be undefined if there is a lack of social support and acceptance. Relational ambiguity includes boundaries and roles but also indicates that intention should be part of relationships, as should couple and family commitment. However, where there is an absence of social norms and full legal standing (e.g., queer families and stepfamilies), individuals involved face uncertainty about what it means to commit to a relationship. Ambiguity has a cultural dimension (Boss et al., 2017), but it is important to remember that boundaries are also defined in a sociocultural context. Thus, no concept of boundary has universal meaning or represents an intrinsic property of all systems (Green & Mitchell, 2008). Here, we approach different boundary aspects among multigenerational families, families with adolescents, gay-parented families, and stepfamilies. In these families, ambiguity is a relational phenomenon that all experience in varying forms. Ambiguity creates confusion about boundaries (who is inside or outside the family) and family identity (we exist as a couple and a family, but we are not recognized outside) in certain cultural, religious, and sociopolitical contexts. Also, ambiguity creates stress, low resilience, rigidity, loss of purpose, mastery, flexibility, and adequacy. Ambiguity also creates immobility, loss of hope, and psychological sufferings.

Clinical Expertise and Interpretation of Evidence: Stepfamilies

In the research section of this chapter, Coleman and Ganong wrote of the supporting research for the concept of exclusiveness in stepfamilies. They articulated that this phenomenon results in a heightened sense of family within the structural boundaries of a stepfamily. Thus, when a new stepfamily is formed, the adult members, particularly the female members of a stepfamily (as suggested by Castrén & Widmer, 2015, cited in the research section of this chapter), tend to draw a tight boundary around the stepfamily, thus suggesting that the previous spouse is no longer part of the family. There are two aspects of this narrowing the definition of "the family." The first is that this effect often leads the adults in a stepfamily to pursue a sense of closeness that does not match with the **developmental stage** of this relatively new stepfamily. The second effect is that the nonresidential parent is treated as an unwelcome stranger, rather than a legitimate member of the family.

The blurring of relational boundaries often sees the biological mother pushing her new spouse and child (or children) to rapidly become close. At the same time, the child's relationship with their biological father is challenged as unimportant. Thus, these two forces shifting the boundaries of the stepfamily cause a premature attempt to make the immediate stepfamily an "instant family." This level of togetherness metaphorically suffocates the family. Too much togetherness increases volatility. So, the desire to create closeness quickly often backfires.

Clinical Experience: Observations of Common Interactional Patterns

What this interpersonal problem looks like in practice may vary, but commonly it involves the adolescent becoming frustrated with both his or her residential parent, as well as the stepparent. The parent, frequently the mother, is perplexed by her child's increased anger at her new spouse, feeling that spending time together (as a group) will make things better. At the same time, the residential parent has little interest in supporting the child's desire to connect with the nonresidential parent.

Once the push for "family time" becomes a demand, especially of teenagers, it can generate significant anger. The stepparent feels angry that his stepchildren don't seem interested in him, and they certainly don't seem to like him. The biological parent is committed to seeing their child get to know what a good person their new spouse is. The child/stepchild is adjusting to the ambiguous loss of a parent, having a new disciplining authority figure sleeping with his or her parent and a reduction of closeness with the resident parent, all while going through adolescence. Adding to this stress is the child's sense that they are not encouraged to connect with a nonresidential parent because that person is "not part of the family."

Case Context: Characteristics, Culture, and Preferences

Jim (age 14) knows his mom, Beth, wants him to feel close to Pablo (his new stepfather). However, the more time Jim spends in "family time," the more he feels betrayed by his mom—and a growing dislike for Pablo. Jim also feels pushed away from his father. Pablo is deeply in love with Beth (his wife and Jim's mom), and he came into this stepfamily with a positive relationship with Jim. Beth is a good mother and a good wife. But Beth wants proof that they are all "coming together" as a family.

Beth has requested that the three eat together every night and do at least two "family activities" on the weekends (e.g., take an outing, play a game at home, watch a movie together). Pablo is more interested in spending time with Beth, but he agrees that this new family does not feel very comfortable. Pablo is not sure if Jim is a difficult adolescent or if Beth is too needy, but either way, Pablo has become disappointed about the limited sense of "family."

Jim has a few friends and is permitted to have a normal social life during the week, but come Friday night, his mom really wants him around a lot.

He can go out with his friends sometimes, but between the outings, movies, and family dinners, Jim does not get to spend much time with friends, even online.

Clinical Decisions: Intervention Implementation

The first session is with the couple. The key goal for this session is to hear from the couple about their concerns. A clear understanding of their view, combined with some basic psychoeducation, often defines the initial session. There are many interactional problems common to stepfamilies, but for the sake of the intervention discussed in this section, the therapist is looking for evidence that the parent and stepparent are pushing for a rapid sense of togetherness among the stepfamily entirely. If this pattern exists, then this intervention is strongly recommended. The goal is to loosen the narrow definition of family so that natural relationships can build and Jim's father is not perceived as an outsider.

The next session is the presentation of a specific research-based intervention. The couple is informed that the pattern they are attempting—quickly connecting the stepfamily together—and acting as if the nonresidential father is not part of the extended family, although understandable, is frequently not helpful in the stepfamily formation process. One possible way for the therapist to describe this intervention is this:

> A clash of developmental cycles often occurs in the recently formed stepfamily with an adolescent. The adolescent is seeking to connect with the outside world at the same time the parent or stepparent wish to solidify the new stepfamily. Rather than leading to closeness, this pattern often achieves the opposite effect, making the new stepfamily more volatile and less stable.

The parent (and stepparent) is taught to view their stepfamily as a collection of subsystems (Beth and Pablo; Beth and Jim; Pablo and Jim; Jim and his father, Bill). The couple needs to leave the session with a clear mandate to increase time spent across subsystems. Pablo and Beth will initiate a date night. Beth is going to spend quality time with Jim. Pablo is going to reconnect with a family member (his sister, Cara), and Jim is encouraged to reach out to his dad. The therapist explains, "Many stepfamilies try to blend too quickly, and the effort often explodes. Stepfamilies need stable subsystems to withstand the difficulties that come with normal stepfamily development."

What needs to be made clear is that the notion of improving subsystems within the stepfamily is intended to assist the full stepfamily to come together, but that sense of unity can take years. Thus, the therapist assists the stepfamily in becoming stronger, one subsystem at a time, to withstand the pressures of stepfamily life. It is important for relational connections to be stable across the extended stepfamily; while the divorced couple may never be close, the goal of forcing a wedge between a child and parent is strongly challenged, and the idea that all members of this stepfamily, including former spouses, are still family, is reinforced.

Commonly, the adolescent is grateful to have a little more one-on-one time with their own parent. The therapist needs to normalize this occurrence and ensure the stepparent that this reality does not indicate that the adolescent has no interest in a relationship with the stepparent. Rather, a relationship between adolescent and stepparent is much easier to accomplish when that adolescent feels secure in their connection to their own parents, both residential and nonresidential.

Clinical Expertise and Interpretation of Evidence: Queer Families

In the research section, Coleman and Ganong underline that the same boundary **ambiguity** dynamics can occur in queer families as in heterosexual-identified stepfamilies, particularly those related to divorce or dissolution. However, queer families face additional challenges related to boundaries, including homophobia, heterosexism, and heteronormativity. As Coleman and Ganong further suggest, for these couples, there is poor concordance with how social systems and society define family in general and the absence of norms to guide their boundary negotiations.

Relational ambiguity affects diverse couples, families, and minority groups (Green & Mitchell, 2008): Queer couples and families physically exist but often are not considered valid relational or psychological systems. Consequently, boundary construction and management is complicated for queer couples and families. Given homonegative and heterosexist biases, these couples and families are not even recognized in some sociopolitical and cultural contexts. Moreover, because certain queer couples are not treated as legitimate, these couples' existence can come under attack from society, culture, and religion as well. Additionally, as there are not readily available models of how to form and maintain such relationships, the procedure to follow when living as both a queer couple and parents can be problematic. Some parents are also not recognized as "viable" because they are not the biological or genetic parent with a gestational or adoption-based link to their children.

Clinical Experience: Observations of Common Interactional Patterns

In our clinical experience with same-gender couples and parents, we discovered seven common (negative) systemic patterns in same-gender couples and families regarding boundaries. The first pattern indicates that social and cultural models to be a couple and family are less clear. In opposition to different-gender couples, for whom there is a traditional script to follow with explicit and implicit rules, there is no prescribed way of being a same-gender couple. This situation can then generate confusion and conflict among individuals in same-gender relationships.

Second, coming-out differentials (i.e., when one member is out and the other is not) affect relational and intimate couples' boundaries. If one partner is out and the other is closeted, this affects the couple's social and relational boundaries: The couple may exist in certain contexts but not in others because the closeted partner may be afraid of others' reactions. This situation refers to a second type of ambiguous loss (Boss, 1999): The partner exists physically but not psychologically because their true identity is hidden or denied.

Third, the lack of legal nonbiological parent recognition may rigidify some parent and family boundaries. Nonbiological or nonlegal coparents may face much stress due to the absence of alternative parenting models. Sometimes these parents may also be rejected or excluded by their partner's family of origin, schools, medical settings, and institutional contexts because they do not have a biological or legal link with their children. They thereby suffer from rigid, exclusionary boundaries.

Fourth, homonegativity, both internal and external, influences lesbian and gay couples' boundaries. The auto- and hetero-rejection of homosexuality attacks couple and family identity. As such, in certain contexts these couples and families have to become "invisibles" or use "passing strategies."

Fifth, ethnicity and culture play a role in boundary **ambiguity** and may affect boundary function quality. In some countries and cultures, to be in a same-gender relationship or have children with a same-gender partner is considered inconceivable, an illness, or a sin. Therefore, same-gender couples and families may not exist "psychologically" when they interact with their country of origin and its cultural models and codes.

Sixth, some same-gender filiations, such as alternative insemination with anonymous donors, adoption, or surrogacy, could increase boundary ambiguity. Alternative insemination and surrogacy introduce ambiguous boundaries in the lives of intended parents (couples or single parents). They must engage with important persons, including genetic donors and gestational carriers, who are physically absent but psychologically present. Both children and parents have to decide who to include or not include in their family boundaries. For instance, a child from a same-gender family may ask the following questions: Is my surrogate my mother? Is a genetic donor part of my family?

The seventh and final pattern states that to be a single queer parent may increase boundary ambiguity. Heteronormative life models prescribe that a normal family is biparental and composed of different-gender parents.

For example, to be a single gay father triggers ambiguity because this father is expected to coparent with a wife.

Case Context: Characteristics, Culture, and Preferences
This same-gender family sought family and couples counseling. In this family, there is Daddy Benoit, the biological father, aged 39, who works full time in a finance company; Daddy Charles, aged 41, who works full time in a fashion company; and Lilli, aged 8, born via surrogacy in Ukraine with a Ukrainian surrogate, Ivana, and a semianonymous egg donor. Benoit and Charles got married in 2016, after which Charles could legally adopt Lilli, which he has done. Ivana is married with a son and supportive husband. However, surrogacy is illegal and widely unaccepted in Ukraine, so sadly, after her surrogacy, Ivana lost several friends and her job. Still, Lilli and her parents remain in contact with Ivana via social media and photos. The family live in a large French city, about 600 km away from Benoit's parents.

Benoit grew up in France in an affluent, White, Catholic, conservative community. His father is a lawyer who often traveled abroad for extensive periods of time. His mother is a homemaker who raised Benoit and another son. Benoit is closeted at work. After he came out (at 26), his relationship with his father became complicated. Overall, though, being queer has been well-accepted by his parents, and they are involved in Lilli's life. Charles, meanwhile, is Chinese–Burmese. His entire family lives in China. He has two brothers and two sisters, and his parents have been separated since he was 15. Born into a Catholic family, Charles lived his childhood under strong religious influence and came out at 19. He developed a conflicted relationship with his parents—in particular, with his father—when he came out, which has lasted even to today. Lilli has no contact with Charles's father, although her grandmother (Charles's mother) is involved in her life, despite their physical distance (she lives 9 months in China and 3 months in France). For a long time, Charles experienced discrimination, rejection, and microaggressions from his family. His father and one of his brothers never ask about him, his relationship with Benoit, or Lilli, as if they do not exist. Visits from his siblings often result in conflict, and he perceives an attitude of "tolerance" from them (especially his brother) rather than acceptance.

Benoit and Charles commented in the intake that the therapy requested is for Lilli because her participation and attention at school are not consistent among different activities, and sometimes she has separation anxiety, especially with Charles. In the first therapy session, it is observed that Lilli found it difficult to focus on a play activity, and she tends to avoid talking. Benoit spoke often, whereas Charles had more trouble doing so due to frequent interruptions from his husband.

Clinical Experience: Observations of Common Interactional Patterns

Upon meeting the couple, the ambiguous boundary in relation to Benoit and Charles's roles and coparenting functions was evident. Benoit was present and excessively underlined his paternal function but not so much his coparental one (i.e., he was less psychologically present for Charles), whereas Charles was physically present but did not take a coparental stance. Rather, he read his phone (i.e., he was less psychologically present for Benoit and Lilli). There was also palpable tension between the couple during the session, but no conflict occurred.

In their second session, Benoit and Charles were visibly in conflict, and Charles had requested a separation. Charles blamed Benoit for not doing enough to talk about the couple: Benoit was not out at work and did not discuss Charles and Lilli there, and Benoit blamed Charles for not recognizing him for all his efforts to be more publicly out. Intimacy between the couple was also rare at the time of this session because they were so "busy" with work and parenting. Accordingly, the couple suffered major relational **ambiguity**. In particular, they were affected by coming-out differentials. Specifically, Benoit could not demonstrate his personal, couple, or family identity at work, and Charles's father does not recognize him.

Clinical Decisions: Intervention Implementation

Addressing Family Needs. Charles questioned his parental role and the absence of a genetic link with Lilli. However, the couple addressed this concern and tried to reduce this parental gap. In addition, Lilli reported that in different activities at school, many times only heterosexual coupling and parenting models were represented and valued. She said to the therapist, "Too many moms, dads, and sons . . . and what about me and us?" She would have liked to talk about Ivana at school, but she felt that there was no way to do so. After that, Lilli questioned her birth origins and, in particular, Ivana's place and role in her life. Benoit, too, was concerned about his role given the couple's dysfunction and his frequent feelings of loneliness despite their relationship. Benoit was also Lilli's only legally recognized parent for a long while, so he assumed the role of her sole caregiver. Accordingly, the sessions alternated between the whole family and just the parental couple, the goal being to listen to the needs of everyone in the family and the couple subsystem, as well as to understand Lilli and the family's difficulties.

Strengthening Coparental Roles and Reducing Ambiguity. The intervention illustrated here is based on both clinical expertise and evidence-based research, which documented how relational **ambiguity** among same-gender couples affects their security and dynamism and ultimately weakens their positive coparenting. The first objective was for Benoit and Charles to find a united front as coparents in the face of the difficulties Lilli presented. The therapist emphasized the importance of focusing on problematic interactions that can generate parental overload (Benoit) and parental withdrawal (Charles); as such, our assessment was that the couple suffered from an imbalance of recognition and support, as Benoit, the biological father, received more support from his family than Charles, who was rejected by his family and emigrated from China. Additionally, until French law recognized same-gender marriage and adoption, Benoit was Lilli's only recognized parent, and Charles had to cope with many situations where he lacked parental recognition and endured isolation. Benoit, for his part, gradually left the position of sole caregiver and let Charles take the parental initiative.

Promoting Social Support. The intervention's second objective was to identify additional support for the family. Benoit and Charles had become isolated from each other and focused more on work and parenting. It was important to intensify their social network by increasing the number of family members of choice (an instrumental and affective belonging system that substitutes family of origin when it is absent or unavailable). This was intended as a means for them to reconnect through others. In their therapy sessions, we thus generated a sociogram and thought together about the concept of family of choice. Surprisingly, after this intervention, Benoit spoke to a coworker about his relationship and family and invited him and his wife to a Sunday brunch. He and Charles later invited more people and friends to their house.

Socializing Family and Family Origins. For the third objective, we created an opportunity for Benoit and Charles to support Lilli in discussing her family at school. With the help of both her parents, Lilli organized a presentation on Father's Day in the form of a small booklet, where she spoke about her birth story and family. Lilli through her parents also contacted Ivana via Skype and mail to ask for her help. The reactions from her friends and teachers were very positive and supportive. The booklet was further reproduced for more of Lilli's school friends and acquaintances.

The family's therapist explained,

> Becoming a same-gender family involves deconstructing heterosexual models and externalizing judgment in order to regain a possibility of freedom without having to justify oneself or ask permission to exist. You are parents and a courageous family because you have had to put up with a lot. What you should not miss is the support of the couple, above all else.

What was important, then, was to reduce **ambiguity** where possible and, when this was not possible, learn how to deal with it with the therapist's help. Reinforcing Charles's hypofunctional parental role, increasing the family's social network density to strengthen their family of choice, supporting Benoit coming out at work and showing how coming-out differentials generate conflict and discomfort in the couple, affirming Lilli's identity at school by addressing her origins through clear conveyance of the different ways of being and doing family, and trying to increase the connection between Ivana and the family ultimately allowed Benoit, Charles, and Lilli to move forward as a family.

As the family's and couple's degree of security increased, Lilli became more fulfilled. One therapy session after the summer holidays, the therapist learned that the family had visited Ivana, which went well. Benoit and Charles also decided to reduce their work time to create more time together as a family and a couple and started a date-night cycle. Further, Charles renewed contact with his father. He wrote a letter to him in which he expressed his feelings of joy and pride about his relationship and his daughter. He also held frequent Skype sessions with his mother and family of origin. A follow-up 6 months after the last session showed better adjustment for Lilli, Benoit, and Charles's coparental subsystem and for the couple.

Clinical Expertise and Interpretation of Evidence: Families With Adolescents

Boundary **ambiguity** increases as elementary-school-age children transition into adolescence. This process can be both supported and compromised by a variety of factors, including how the family has transitioned boundaries in earlier stages of the family life cycle and levels of differentiation amongst family members at the time of the shift into adolescence. Coleman and Ganong's research section supports the phenomenon that the more ambiguous the boundary, the more dysfunctional the family (Carroll et al., 2007), it is noted that inflexible adherence to rigid boundaries can also create dysfunction. Clinical intervention should consider that such ambiguity is often experienced as a difficult and overwhelming process marked by significant trial and error in parent–child interactions. As a result, families become vulnerable to challenges associated with ambiguity, such as not knowing what to carry over from phases in their younger to older years, how to recognize oneself as a parent in the family, and misunderstanding how and why the boundaries need to shift and evolve. To ensure an effective and functional transition, clinicians and family members must attend to the mental and emotional flexibility that this phenomenon requires. Moreover, the clinician must remain consciously aware of how to best support the family in the context of their unique circumstances.

Clinical Experience: Observations of Common Interactional Patterns
It is important that parents are educated about the inherent **ambiguity** of the transition into adolescence and the need for discontinuing dichotomous and linear thinking. Generally, in the childrearing process, parents find themselves identifying with rigid thinking that sounds like "there is a wrong and a right way of deciding and implementing rules," especially when a firstborn enters adolescence. Parents also find themselves thinking in this linear way: "if I do x, the result will be y." Both styles of thinking can leave the parent feeling frustrated or disappointed because neither mentality tends to support a functional transition. Once the parents are faced with the process of engaging with ambiguity and they have started experiencing the difficulties associated with it, they generally seek to exert more control to stave off the new challenges, often times unintentionally, in an attempt to return the system to a prior homeostasis.

With adolescence, children are usually seeking greater personal individuation and healthy identity development while trying to balance **family belongingness** and connectedness (e.g., Gavazzi, 2011; King & Boyd, 2016). Because ambiguity promotes fear and uncertainty, parents may cling even more vigilantly to what feels safe for their own selves, which is often at odds with promoting a growing sense of autonomy and independence in their adolescent child. A lack of control or a sense of losing control can be deeply embedded in the parent's psyche, undermining their ability to navigate boundaries with their adolescent children. Parents worry both about doing a good job and keeping their children safe. As such, trust becomes a linchpin between the parent and adolescent; the parent must trust their parenting of the adolescent before the adolescent **stage of development** enough to believe that they have effectively and functionally guided their child toward a beginning of being capable of making "good" decisions. If the parents find themselves unable to increase their flexibility, their own level of differentiation (how enmeshed they are with their child) becomes an important point of awareness and possible treatment.

Parents had at one time been the child-turned-adolescent and experienced boundary ambiguity in their family of origin. As such, parents often find themselves wishing to replicate or repudiate the style in which their own parents constructed and enforced boundaries, which socially and traditionally involved a top-down approach. This can cast a bright light, for the clinician, on the need to discern between the systemic patterns of previous generations and the uniqueness of the current parent and child personalities, attributes, and idiosyncrasies as it relates to boundary ambiguity. There is typically a great deal of information about what is motivating the parent to think, feel, and behave in the ways they do before seeking treatment. Unfortunately, conversations about boundaries typically are not engaged until there is a matter at hand. When an adolescent seeks an increase in autonomy, the parent must determine whether accepting that bid for autonomy is deserved. A parent and child relationship with a healthy level of differentiation supports a greater sense of appropriate autonomy. Also, it fosters the opportunity for the parent to proactively engage and encourage their adolescents to participate in a series of conversations that clarify the ratio of instruction and freedom in their evolving relationship. Adolescents having "a say" or "options" and opportunity for compromise can prove beneficial for both parents and the adolescents. However, to the parent who is not well differentiated, this can feel like a disregard of their position in the family, a disloyalty to their own family of origin, or a threat to their ability to cope with a decreased experience of control.

Case Context: Characteristics, Culture, and Preferences

Mom, Gloria, 38; Dad, Gregory Jr., 42; son, Gregory III, 16; daughter, Gaby, 12. Both Gloria and Gregory grew up in an affluent White Protestant community. Gloria's father was an engineer who worked long hours and often traveled for extensive periods of time. Her mother was a homemaker who was in charge of raising her five children, of which Gloria was the eldest, as well as tending to the household. Gloria is also a homemaker. Gregory Jr. is an attorney who took over his father's (Gregory Sr.) law firm after his retirement. His father attended law school after serving in the Vietnam War. His mother, who was also a stay-at-home Mom, raised Gregory. His interactions with his father were limited to discipline regarding his academic performance and occasionally being reprimanded if he didn't obey his mother. Gregory Jr. had a younger sister, who passed away at 16 in a car accident; a friend was driving.

Gloria reached out to a therapist for help for her daughter who was experiencing "intense anxiety" attacks. She reported that her daughter, an extrovert, marched to the beat of her own drum; she was unable to share why she felt this way and did not know how to help her daughter. They were referred to this therapist by their pediatrician, who the daughter had visited six times in the last 3 months for shortness of breath and stomach cramping with no identifiable medical diagnoses. After several visits with Gaby, it became clear that her anxiety started when her older brother, an introverted, meticulously obedient son, received his driver's permit. Around that time, she also noticed that her mother seemed to be "more intense" and more closely monitoring Gaby and her activities outside of the home. In fact, she started saying no to her daughter much more as a result of her husband's increase in checking in on Gaby and what she was up to.

Given Gregory III's introverted and obedient nature, challenges to the boundary structure were not inherently obvious with the firstborn child, and difficulties did not seem apparent. Therefore, conversations about increasing boundary permeability were not necessary. Being a different child, boundary ambiguity was a more prominent issue with Gaby, an extrovert seeking to gain more independence while moving into adolescence. Both parents were triggered to consider their own parenting, which was rule-based; rules were meant to be followed and not questioned. Both parents continued to think this way, and because they felt this "worked" with Gregory III, they were unable to understand why it was not working with Gaby. Neither parent had experience or felt prepared to have a different kind of conversation with Gaby. She either follows the rules or she does not (dichotomous thinking), and because this worked with her brother, it should also work with her (linear thinking). Furthermore, both parents were unaware that their parenting had become stricter since their son learned to drive. Although the increased parental worry and attempt to strengthen control over their children may seem obvious to the systemic clinician, it is often the case that it is motivated by the unconscious drives of the parents. Specifically, it may not be in either parent's conscious awareness that their teenage driving concerns are triggered by the tragic loss of Gregory Jr.'s younger sister in a motor vehicle accident involving teenage drivers.

Clinical Decisions: Intervention Implementation
This family would be well served by inviting all four members to the initial session. The therapist would first attend to the "presenting problem," which in this case is concern about Gaby. A casual, but character comprehensive, three-generational genogram would be created throughout the intake in which the therapist would become aware, early on, that Dad's younger sister died in a teenage driver motor vehicle accident. Each family member would have their turn to express their perspective of "the presenting problem" as well as their thoughts and feelings about attending sessions together. The therapist would take the opportunity to join with each member by listening to, reflecting, clarifying, and validating each of their perspectives. This might sound like the therapist saying to the parents, "I can imagine that your daughter not following the rules in the same way as your son has caused difficulty and confusion for you both." It might also sound like the therapist asking Gaby, "What sense do you make out of the way your parents are thinking and feeling about you?" This question to Gaby neither supports nor condemns the parent's perspective but acknowledges it. The question also gives Gaby an opportunity to learn early on that she is welcome to have an independent, differentiated voice in the therapy sessions as she struggles to secure that for herself outside of the therapy sessions.

The therapist could either invite all four members back for a follow-up or schedule individual sessions with each family member before holding a second session with all four family members. The benefits of the individual sessions include increasing rapport and joining with each individual by developing a refined understanding of the perspective and personality of each family member as a part of their system. Each family member would experience the therapist acknowledging, understanding, and validating their position, as well as understanding the conflict between them in a privatized, nuanced way. The benefits of continued joint sessions include more immediate relief for the identified patient (Gaby) and an increased sense of connectedness among family members desiring a more functional, loving flow of communication. Whichever path the clinician and family collaboratively choose, the clinician engages in genuine validation and empathic psychoeducation on the normalcy and difficulty associated with families transitioning children to adolescence, regardless of whether this is being identified as the presenting problem from the family.

After the first six sessions (if they are family–individual combination) or the first four sessions (if they are exclusively full family), the therapist begins to draw connections between the increase of symptoms and the challenges that the family has been facing, possibly unbeknownst to them. By this point, Gregory III would have shared that he was becoming a new driver, and the therapist would make the connection between this milestone and Dad's loss of his sister. Specifically, the clinician highlights the trauma of the father losing his youngest sister in a car accident as he supports his son in becoming an independent, safe driver. Gaby's sensitivity, care, and concern for her brother's driving, along with her knowledge of her father's having lost his sister in a teenage driving accident, becomes a point of attention and consideration for the family as they work to increase their understanding of Gaby's somatic symptoms. Mother's challenges associated with "doing a good job" as a full-time homemaker are highlighted, and relief is offered to her for ways that she sees her daughter's struggling as a "failure" on her part. Finally, the differences in the personalities of each of the adolescents are attended to to provide a clearer understanding of how different parenting styles and boundaries may be warranted to support a more functional transition through this stage of the family life cycle.

Clinical Expertise and Interpretation of Evidence: Multigenerational Families

As stated previously, increased life expectancy means that there is an increase in the presence of multigenerational families (Park, 2014). Although there are many advantages to multigenerational families, the increase in coexisting generations also increases the complexity of relationships (Duffy, 1984). The three most common (negative) systemic patterns occurring in relational **ambiguity** are confusion around caretaking, hierarchy and cultural differences within families, and a lack of communication between family members. These three issues are not mutually exclusive and, in many cases, can overlap with one another depending on the context of the multigenerational family.

Clinical Experience: Observations of Common Interactional Patterns
Multigenerational families vary in their composition, and boundary **ambiguity** can ensue because of life changes that occur (Boss et al., 2017). Studies support the notion that the greater boundary ambiguity, the more likely dysfunction may occur (Carroll et al., 2007). The lack of role clarity in roles and tension between the various generations might warrant the need for treatment interventions. All members of the family have a role and serve a purpose; however, when boundary maintenance is disrupted, stress ensues and often highlights which family members are present and which are absent (whether physically or psychologically) from the family (Boss, 1977).

   In many collectivistic groups, it is the responsibility of various generations to take care of one another, whether that be financially, emotionally, or physically. There is an unspoken rule that the caretaking will occur to some degree. This might mean taking care of elderly parents, giving money to siblings, or being present for family events. However, when there is cultural heterogeneity within the family and members are not familiar with the cultural expectations of caretaking, it can cause conflict between members. Additionally, there is often a hierarchy in multigenerational households. In many families, either the elders or the males in the group hold more power and therefore are consulted more by younger family members. These hierarchal patterns of interacting and communicating are set, and once again, if other family members are not familiar with this expectation, it can cause tension in relationships and the family unit. Furthermore, in traditional homes, respect is expected to be given to the elders. Depending on factors such as acculturation and cultural values, this expected deference might not be offered to all members in the family, which may also cause conflicts. Finally, if there are many generations living in the household, then communication can become a problem. Information can go to one or two family members, which can lead to communications with the rest of the family, and family members can develop resentment if information is not relayed consistently.

Case Context: Characteristics, Culture, and Preferences
Priya (44) and Roshan (47) are a professional Indian American couple. They have been married for 17 years and have two children, Sindhu (16)

and Suresh (13). Priya and Prashant's (her brother) father passed away before Priya met Roshan. Ms. Geetha, Priya's mother, recently moved in with the family due to her advanced cancer diagnosis. To help take care of Ms. Geetha, Prashant also moved in with them. Prashant, 48, is a computer engineer who works from home and is a single male. Before Prashant moved in, he was living about 3 hours away but always made time for Priya and her family. Prashant and Priya are the only children of their parents' union and are close siblings. Prashant is an active uncle and Priya's best friend. They talk often and became closer after the sudden loss of their father to a heart attack 23 years earlier. Priya often found that Prashant was more available given Roshan's increased work hours. Roshan's parents were both in India before their recent deaths. Roshan left India to attend college in the United States and had a complicated and distant relationship with his parents, which continued until they passed away. He felt close to Ms. Geetha and Priya's family; however, more recently Roshan feels that the work he does for the family goes unnoticed, and due to his demanding work schedule, Priya, Prashant, Ms. Geetha, and the kids often spend more time together and make plans leaving him out. More recently, Sindhu has been preparing for the SATs and Priya signed her up for SAT classes but did not discuss this with Roshan. He found out when Priya, Prashant, and Sindhu were discussing her first practice test. Roshan became upset because this is just another example of how he is left out of decisions. The couple decided to seek treatment after Roshan stated that he "can't keep doing things like this as a family."

Clinical Decisions: Intervention Implementation
The work with multigenerational families should emphasize the needs of all the various generations. All members of the system have a role in the preservation of a healthy multigenerational system. The therapist assists in helping families understand and elucidate the roles and responsibilities of the system such that the family can function in a healthy manner. Often when families move in with one another, it is due to an emergency and is unexpected and sudden, which does not allow much time to process and discuss boundaries. This poses many challenges and can lead to **ambiguity** around who has authority. Hence, it is important to start with the adults with the most power as boundary ambiguity in families can have an impact on children and cause greater distress. Therefore, the therapist will start with the three members whose roles cause the most confusion within the system—in this case, Priya, Roshan, and Prashant.

The initial session focused on building a therapeutic alliance through active listening, providing psychoeducation about the process, and acknowledging the struggles of each of the family members. The therapist heard from each of the three members of the family and specifically around all the recent stressors, transitions, and loss the family had experienced. The therapist introduced the sessions as a space where a wide range of issues might be discussed and welcomed the three family members to ask questions. It should be noted that therapy was Roshan's suggestion, and the therapist was uncertain about Priya's and Prashant's thoughts on seeking services. The therapist started by asking each member about their thoughts on therapy and the issues from their perspective. It is important for the therapist to know how comfortable and familiar each member is with therapy to answer any questions and provide psychoeducation about the therapeutic process. The clients can then also share their hopes and wishes for treatment. Roshan shared that he felt his role as a father and husband were being ignored and that he was being sidelined. Priya and Prashant shared that this was not their intention; however, they were trying to take care of their mother and the needs of the children, while managing anticipatory grief. The family collectively shared their hesitation about seeking therapy. Because other Indian families rarely seek such help, the expectations of therapy are unclear. The therapist can use this time to normalize and join the family regarding cultural **stigma** around therapy and further provide information on the nature of therapy and what they can expect. Once the family has an understanding of the process, the therapist moves to gathering relevant information about the family, specifically the role of extended family in caretaking and cultural expectations. For example, the therapist asked, "How is caregiving handled within the culture?" Additionally, the therapist inquired about how they have dealt with all the changes in the family with the recent losses of Roshan's parents, Prashant's moving in, and the recent diagnosis of Ms. Geetha. This was an ideal time to do a cultural genogram so that the therapist and family members could visualize and discuss how problems were handled across generations and how the family communicates. The therapist tried to emphasize the losses and emotionally charged transition that the family was experiencing. Additionally, the therapist tried to provide some psychoeducation and validation, explaining that these are all complex situations and that they were all doing the best they can considering the circumstances. Doing so made the process more tangible and allowed the family members to feel heard and realize that although they were going through a stressful time, they were figuring out ways to manage, thereby also instilling hope that therapy was a way to address these issues. This intervention acknowledged the family's recent stressors and their strengths as a family, which is important to acknowledge early in treatment. Finally, the initial session would address the mutual goals that these three adults shared for the family. The therapist stated, "You all are doing a lot for the family and somehow it is getting missed, so we will work on how you can be stronger together so you can help the children and Ms. Geetha."

Subsequent sessions focused on patterns of communication, expectations, and inquiry about how decisions are made. The family needed more support and familiarity during this stressful time of Ms. Geetha's illness, and it was a joint decision for Prashant to move in with the family, however, the limits and expectations of this decision had not been discussed. Prashant, who is the older brother, had always been in the caretaking role after his father passed, and he continued in this role when he moved back in with Priya and her family. Although this was a familiar role to Priya, it was not comfortable for Roshan because he had never lived or interacted with Prashant for an extended period of time. The therapist discussed how the family composition and expectations have changed since the father's passing more than 20 years ago. It is important to make clear what expectations are realistic and unrealistic given how the family has evolved because unrealistic expectations can jeopardize the family's development (Michaels, 2007; Papernow, 1993). The therapist helped the family to see how roles can be fluid and change depending on the situation and circumstances. Further, as new members emerge in the family, new responsibilities and strengths are also part of the process. The therapist invited discourse between the three family members on how things have changed and how caretaking has differed since the passing of Priya and Prashant's father, as well as what was needed in their new circumstances, so that they can note the differences realistically. For example, Priya disclosed that she was only 21 and a graduating senior living 5 hours from home when her father passed, which required Prashant to step in as a father figure at that time. Although she loves him very much, she also realized that currently she is a working professional woman, wife, and mother who has gone through her own life experiences, so Prashant does not have to constantly manage things for her the way he did after the loss of their father. At this point in the therapy process, it is important for the family to negotiate roles and expectations in a constructive manner.

When issues of **relational ambiguity** occur in families, it is important for family members to recognize each individual's involvement and how they can be more active and deliberate in making visible each of the other members' contribution to the family structure. The joint sessions should focus on each member sharing how they see themselves working with the others toward the common goal and how they can contribute to the overall family system. Roshan shared his appreciation for Prashant stepping in to help the family on such short notice, and he recognized that although he had to take on more hours because Priya reduced some of her work hours, when he is home, we would try to be more active in the children's lives.

Similarly, Priya appreciated the different ways she was being supported by both Roshan and Prashant and acknowledged the need to make a greater effort to communicate clearly to Roshan about the children and what she needs from him. Finally, Prashant was grateful to have this time to be with the family and take care of his mother but also realized that he did not have to be the "sole caretaker," a role he had assumed as the male after his father's death.

Further, the therapy helped the family strengthen their communication with one another, so that they could better manage future stressors (e.g., the death of Ms. Geetha). Future sessions should focus on allowing the family to share their emotional experiences in a healthy manner. Finally, a few sessions should address strengthening and nurturing the marital system and protecting the boundary of the married couple so that they communicate clearly, invest time in one another, and resolve any issues in a timely manner. Additionally, it is important to discuss boundaries with Prashant and how to support his desire to be an active son, brother (in-law), and uncle. He shared how much he values his family and wants to be present for each of them but realized the importance of not overextending himself and that each adult has distinct responsibilities. This was a new way of engaging for the family and would take time. However, they started to see that they did not fail as a family unit but need to take time to discuss and understand the roles and expectations of each family member and find new ways to see each other and communicate with one another.

Conclusion

Boundary ambiguity is a state in which family members are uncertain as to whom, exactly, is considered a full member of the family or what their exact roles are within the family system. This state of confusion or sense that one may not be fully in a family results in predictable chaos. Without the security of stable, agreed-on family boundaries, stress pervades the system. Clinicians are able to assist in addressing this concern by helping the family understand why overtly defining membership is a necessary developmental process. The very act of agreeing on boundaries and roles can mitigate familial conflict and create a path forward rooted in closeness and understanding.

REFERENCES

Allan, G., Crow, G., & Hawker, S. (2011). *Stepfamilies*. Palgrave. https://doi.org/10.1057/9780230308671

Ambert, A. M. (1986). Being a stepparent: Live-in and visiting stepchildren. *Journal of Marriage and the Family*, *48*(4), 795–804. https://doi.org/10.2307/352572

Baumle, A. K., & Compton, D. R. (2014). Identity versus identification: How LGBTQ parents identify their children on census surveys. *Journal of Marriage and Family*, *76*(1), 94–104. https://doi.org/10.1111/jomf.12076

Baxter, L. A., Braithwaite, D. O., Kellas, J. K., LeClair-Underberg, C., Normand, E. L., & Routsong, T. (2009). Empty ritual: Young-adult stepchildren's perceptions of the remarriage ceremony. *Journal of Social and Personal Relationships*, *26*(4), 467–487. https://doi.org/10.1177/0265407509350872

Bengtson, V. (2001). Beyond the nuclear family: The increasing importance of multi-generational bonds. *Journal of Marriage and the Family*, *63*(1), 1–15. https://doi.org/10.1111/j.1741-3737.2001.00001.x

Bermea, A. M., Khaw, L., & Hardesty, J. L., Rosenbloom, L., & Salerno, C. (2020). Mental and active preparation: Examining variations in women's processes of preparing to leave abusive relationships. *Journal of Interpersonal Violence*, *35*(3–4), 988–1011. https://doi.org/10.1177/0886260517692332

Boss, P. (1977). A clarification of the concept of psychological father presence in families experiencing ambiguity of boundary. *Journal of Marriage and the Family*, *39*(1), 141–151. https://doi.org/10.2307/351070

Boss, P. (1999). *Ambiguous loss*. Harvard University Press.

Boss, P. (2002). *Family stress management: A contextual approach* (2nd ed.). Sage Publications. https://doi.org/10.4135/9781452233895

Boss, P., Bryant, C., & Mancini, J. (2017). *Family stress management: A contextual approach* (3rd ed.). Sage Publications.

Boss, P. G. (1980a). Normative family stress: Family boundary changes across the life-span. *Family Relations*, *29*(4), 445–450. https://doi.org/10.2307/584457

Boss, P. G. (1980b). The relationship of psychological father presence, wife's personal qualities, and wife/family dysfunction in families of missing fathers. *Journal of Marriage and the Family*, *42*(3), 541–549. https://doi.org/10.2307/351898

Buehler, C., & Pasley, K. (2000). Family boundary ambiguity, marital status, and child adjustment. *The Journal of Early Adolescence*, *20*(3), 281–308. https://doi.org/10.1177/0272431600020003002

Carroll, J., Olson, C., & Buckmiller, N. (2007). Family boundary ambiguity: A 30-year review of theory, research, and measurement. *Family Relations*, *56*(2), 210–230. https://doi.org/10.1111/j.1741-3729.2007.00453.x

Castrén, A.-M., & Widmer, E. D. (2015). Insiders and outsiders in stepfamilies: Adults' and children's views on family boundaries. *Current Sociology*, *63*(1), 35–56. https://doi.org/10.1177/0011392114551650

Catalpa, J. M., & McGuire, J. K. (2018). Family boundary ambiguity among trans-gender youth. *Family Relations*, *67*(1), 88–103. https://doi.org/10.1111/fare.12304

Chapman, A., Kang, Y., Ganong, L., Sanner, C., & Coleman, M. (2018). A comparison of stepgrandchildren's perceptions of long-term and later-life stepgrandparents. *Journal of Aging Studies*, *47*, 104–113. https://doi.org/10.1016/j.jaging.2018.03.005

Cherlin, A. (1978). Remarriage as an incomplete institution. *American Journal of Sociology*, *84*(3), 634–650. https://doi.org/10.1086/226830

Coleman, M., & Ganong, L. (1995). Insiders' and outsiders' beliefs about stepfamilies: Assessment and implications for practice. In D. Huntley (Ed.), *Understanding step-families: Implications for assessment and treatment* (pp. 101–112). American Counseling Association Press.

DiVerniero, R. (2013). Children of divorce and their nonresidential parent's family: Examining perceptions of communication accommodation. *Journal of Family Communication*, *13*(4), 301–320. https://doi.org/10.1080/15267431.2013.823429

Drummet, A., Coleman, M., & Cable, S. (2003). Military families under stress: Implications for family life education. *Family Relations, 52*(3), 279–287. https://doi.org/10.1111/j.1741-3729.2003.00279.x

Duffy, P. R. (1984). Cybernetics. *The Journal of Business Communication, 21*(1), 33–41. https://doi.org/10.1177/002194368402100104

Funder, K. (1991). Children's construction of their post-divorce families: A family sculpture approach. In K. Funder (Ed.), *Images of Australian families* (pp. 73–101). Longman Cheshire.

Ganong, L., & Coleman, M. (2017). *Stepfamily relationships: Development, dynamics, and intervention* (2nd ed.). Springer. https://doi.org/10.1007/978-1-4899-7702-1

Ganong, L., Coleman, M., Fine, M., & McDaniel, A. K. (1998). Issues considered in stepparent adoption. *Family Relations, 47*, 63–72. https://doi.org/10.2307/584852

Ganong, L., Coleman, M., & Jamison, T. (2011). Patterns of stepchild–stepparent relationship development. *Journal of Marriage and the Family, 73*(2), 396–413. https://doi.org/10.1111/j.1741-3737.2010.00814.x

Ganong, L., Coleman, M., & Russell, L. (2015). Children in diverse families. In M. H. Bornstein & T. Leventhal (Eds.), *Handbook of child psychology and developmental science: Volume 4. Ecological settings and processes in developmental systems* (pp. 133–174). John Wiley & Sons. https://doi.org/10.1002/9781118963418

Gavazzi, S. M. (2011). *Families with adolescents: Bridging the gaps between theory, research, and practice.* Springer Science + Business Media. https://doi.org/10.1007/978-1-4419-8246-9

Goldberg, A., & Allen, K. (2013). Same-sex relation dissolution and LGB stepfamily formation: Perspectives of young adults with LGB parents. *Family Relations, 62*(4), 529–544. https://doi.org/10.1111/fare.12024

Green, R.-J., & Mitchell, V. (2008). Gay and lesbian couples in therapy: Minority stress, relational ambiguity, and families of choice. In A. S. Gurman (Ed.), *Clinical handbook of couple therapy* (pp. 662–680). Guilford Press.

Jenkins, D. (2013). Boundary ambiguity in gay stepfamilies: Perspectives of gay biological fathers and their same-sex partners. *Journal of Divorce & Remarriage, 54*(4), 329–348. https://doi.org/10.1080/10502556.2013.780501

King, V., & Boyd, L. M. (2016). Factors associated with perceptions of family belonging among adolescents. *Journal of Marriage and Family, 78*(4), 1114–1130. https://doi.org/10.1111/jomf.12322

King, V., Boyd, L. M., & Thorsen, M. L. (2015). Adolescents' perceptions of family belonging in stepfamilies. *Journal of Marriage and the Family, 77*(3), 761–774. https://doi.org/10.1111/jomf.12181

Manning, W., & Smock, P. (2000). "Swapping" families: Serial parenting and economic support for children. *Journal of Marriage and the Family, 62*(1), 111–122. https://doi.org/10.1111/j.1741-3737.2000.00111.x

Markham, M., & Coleman, M. (2020). "Part-time parent": Mothering in the context of shared physical custody. *Family Relations, 69*(5), 1128–1142. https://doi.org/10.1111/fare.12491

Michaels, M. L. (2007). Remarital issues in couple therapy. *Journal of Couple & Relationship Therapy, 6*(1/2), 125–139. https://doi.org/10.1300/J398v06n01_11

Minuchin, S. (1974). *Families & family therapy.* Harvard University Press.

Papernow, P. L. (1993). *Becoming a stepfamily: Patterns of development in remarried families.* Jossey-Bass.

Park, S. (2014). Theory of intergenerational ambivalence: Is it the perfect new lens for studying intergenerational relationships? *Population Ageing, 7*(4), 323–334. https://doi.org/10.1007/s12062-014-9106-7

Pasley, K. (1987). Family boundary ambiguity: Perceptions of adult stepfamily members. In K. Pasley & M. Ihinger-Tallman (Eds.), *Remarriage and stepparenting: Current research and theory* (pp. 206–224). Guilford Press.

Russell, L. T., Coleman, M., Ganong, L. H., & Gayer, D. (2016). Divorce and childhood chronic illness: A grounded theory of trust, gender, and third-party care providers. *Journal of Family Nursing, 22*(2), 252–278. https://doi.org/10.1177/1074840716639909

Sanner, C., Coleman, M., & Ganong, L. (2020). Shared children in stepfamilies: Experiences living in a hybrid family structure. *Journal of Marriage and the Family, 82*(2), 606–621. https://doi.org/10.1111/jomf.12631

Sanner, C., Ganong, L., Chapman, A., Kang, Y., & Coleman, M. (2019). Building family relationships with inherited stepgrandparents. *Family Relations, 68*(4), 484–499. https://doi.org/10.1111/fare.12381

Sanner, C., Ganong, L., & Coleman, M. (2021). Families are socially constructed: Pragmatic implications for researchers. *Journal of Family Issues, 42*(2), 422–444. https://doi.org/10.1177/0192513X20905334

Seltzer, J. A. (2019). Family change and changing family demography. *Demography, 56*(2), 405–426. https://doi.org/10.1007/s13524-019-00766-6

Stewart, A. (2005). Boundary ambiguity in stepfamilies. *Journal of Family Issues, 26*(7), 1002–1029. https://doi.org/10.1177/0192513X04273591

Suanet, B., Van Der Pas, S., & Van Tilburg, T. (2013). Who is in the stepfamily? Change in stepparents' family boundaries between 1992 and 2009. *Journal of Marriage and the Family, 75*(5), 1070–1083. https://doi.org/10.1111/jomf.12053

Thorsen, M. L., & King, V. (2016). My mother's husband. *Journal of Social and Personal Relationships, 33*(6), 835–851. https://doi.org/10.1177/0265407515599677

Van der Pas, S., Tilburg, T., & Silverstein, M. (2013). Stepfamilies in later life. *Journal of Marriage and the Family, 75*(5), 1065–1069. https://doi.org/10.1111/jomf.12054

White, L. (1998). Who's counting? Quasi-facts and stepfamilies in reports of number of siblings. *Journal of Marriage and the Family, 60*(3), 725–733. https://doi.org/10.2307/353541

Wood, D., Crapnell, T., Lau, L., Bennett, A., Lotstein, D., Ferris, M., & Kuo, A. (2018). Emerging adulthood as a critical stage in the life course. In N. Halfon, C. B. Forrest, R. M. Lerner, & E. M. Faustman (Eds.), *Handbook of life course health development* (123–143). Springer.

Wood, K. (2017). Families beyond boundaries: Conceptualising kinship in gay and lesbian adoption and fostering. *Child & Family Social Work, 23*(2), 155–162. https://doi.org/10.1111/cfs.12394

8

AMBIGUOUS LOSS

A Focus on Immigrant Families, Postincarceration Family Life, Addiction and Families, and Military Families

RESEARCH: CATHERINE SOLHEIM AND ANNE WILLIAMS-WENGERD
CLINICAL APPLICATIONS: CHRISTINE KODMAN-JONES, KYLE BURKE, CAMILLE ST. JAMES, MIGUEL LEWIS, AND MICHELLE SHERMAN

RESEARCH: CATHERINE SOLHEIM AND ANNE WILLIAMS-WENGERD

For both researchers and practitioners, the framework of ambiguous loss provides an informative and meaningful foundation for understanding family losses that are unclear. Since Pauline Boss first conceptualized ambiguous loss theory, it has been applied to the study of numerous types of family situations such as families who care for a family member with dementia, families in which someone is missing in action or has been kidnapped, and transnational families. In these and other loss situations, families experience the physical absence yet psychological presence or conversely, the physical presence yet psychological absence of their family member. Differing from

We acknowledge the work of Anran Zhou, who worked on the literature review for this chapter.

https://doi.org/10.1037/0000280-008
Treating Contemporary Families: Toward a More Inclusive Clinical Practice, S. Browning and B. van Eeden-Moorefield (Editors)

grief theories that focus on an individual's experience of loss, the ambiguous loss framework is inherently relational, based on an assumption that families experience grief systemically and interdependently (Boss, 1999; Solheim & Ballard, 2016).

A more traditional experience of loss, such as the death of a loved one, is typically marked at a particular point in time and is often ritualized and socially recognized by a wake or funeral. In contrast, an ambiguous loss is ongoing; it may "defy resolution" by having no foreseeable ending (e.g., losses related to substance use, incarceration, chronic illness). There is no ritual to mark that a loss has occurred, and others may not even recognize it as loss (Boss, 1999, 2016). Boss (2016) asserted that the lack of finality and recognition can block natural coping and grieving processes, making it the most stressful kind of loss for a family to endure.

In this chapter, we explore the use of ambiguous loss theory and its key constructs that have been used in recent research focused on four specific family experiences: families experiencing incarceration, families with a member dealing with substance use disorder, military families who experience deployment, and immigrant families, particularly those who have family members at risk of deportation (see Table 8.1). In all four contexts, families experienced either one or both types of ambiguous loss: **physical absence with psychological presence** or **psychological absence with physical presence**. Although all of these family experiences involve some overlapping core elements of ambiguous loss (such as boundary ambiguity), there are also unique factors that may reduce or exacerbate the stress caused by the ambiguity of the loss, such as the degree of social recognition, degree of control, and psychosocial factors. After presenting some of the core research evidence, we present a clinical case for each family type with an intervention articulated. Psychoeducation suggestions also are described.

Research Evidence on Immigrant Families

It is safe to say that all immigrants experience ambiguous loss to some degree. Regardless of their migration path, whether they are refugees due to **forced migration** from armed conflict or natural disasters, privileged migrants with employer-sponsored work visas, or desperate migrants seeking work to provide for their family's survival, migrants leave family, friends, and "home" behind when they move to a new country. Thus, when they arrive in their new country, immigrants experience the type of ambiguous loss that involves the **physical absence** of loved ones who stay behind yet closely hold their **psychological presence** as they navigate their new environment.

TABLE 8.1. Ambiguous Loss in Families

Evidence-based area of clinical focus	Type of factor	Appropriateness for use across families	Selected references indicating evidence base
Types of loss: physical presence/ psychological absence and physical absence/ psychological presence	General	All[a]	Boss, 1999; Faber et al., 2008; Solheim, 2016
Boundary ambiguity	General	All[a]	Boss, 2006
Deportation and forced separation effects	Unique	Immigrant families	Gulbas et al., 2016; Solheim et al., 2016
Socioemotional health	Unique	Families dealing with substance use	Winstanley & Stover, 2019
Children's coping abilities	Unique	Families dealing with substance use	Fraser et al., 2009; Mechling et al., 2018
Ambiguous absence and maintenance paradox	Unique	Families experiencing military deployment	Faber et al., 2008; Maguire et al., 2013
Role and relational adaptations across incarceration and reintegration	Unique	Families with an incarcerated family member	Arditti, 2005; Bocknek et al., 2009; Easterling et al., 2019
Frozen grief	Unique	Families with an incarcerated family member	Bocknek et al., 2009; Boss, 1999

[a]The general factor could work for other family types included in this chapter but needs a small adaptation to ensure cultural relevance. Information about potential adaptations is included in the text.

Their move creates a family void; their absence initiates **family boundary ambiguity** that requires adjustment in roles and relationships. For example, historically, the typical migration pattern from Central and South America to the United States involved an adult male who migrated for work. Their remaining partner assumed all family responsibilities out of necessity. Women became more independent when men were absent (Suárez-Orozco et al., 2002), but they described this work as difficult and stressful when the head of the household was not there (Solheim et al., 2016). Psychological presence was maintained through phone or internet communication, although often information was withheld to protect one another from worry, something Solheim et al. (2016) described as "ambiguous communication" (p. 347).

There is also ambiguous loss experienced with regard to the immigrant's parental role. Feelings of guilt arise as a result of not knowing what is going on in their children's lives. Children can feel abandoned by their parents, especially if the promise to return soon is not fulfilled (Jerves et al., 2020; Solheim et al., 2012). Suárez-Orozco et al. (2002) found that if the person who steps into the caretaker role in a parent's absence speaks positively about the parent and keeps the child informed of what is happening, the relationship between the child and the absent parent is better. They suggested that the range of depression experienced by children in their study could be attributed to the ambiguous nature of the loss during separation. Some children viewed their parents' absence as a more permanent loss, whereas other children considered their absence a more temporary separation and were able to keep them psychologically present.

A more recent trend is for entire families to migrate to the United States due to dire economic and safety conditions in their countries of origin. Currently, U.S. immigrant families from the global south are often composed of children born in the United States and who are therefore U.S. citizens, yet their parents do not have legal documentation. These families are referred to as *mixed-status immigrant families*. According to the American Immigration Council (Orcés & Ewing, 2019), 4.1 million children under age 18 live with at least one parent who is unauthorized; the number grows to 5.9 million if children under age 18 living with an unauthorized family member are included. Children in these families worry constantly that their parents will be taken away. That fear is grounded in reality; there were approximately 256,000 removals (deportations) and returns (voluntary deportations) in the United States in 2018 and 267,000 in 2019. This means that tens of thousands of children have experienced the apprehension, detention, or deportation of at least one parent. Rosas (2020) described the fear of separation and deportation that influences how mixed-status immigrant families must live their daily lives with the "knowledge of an impending loss" (p. 2) as anticipatory loss (Rolland, 1990).

A growing body of literature documents the tremendous and long-lasting detrimental effects that deportation (**separation effects**), and even the risk of deportation, have on families, especially children. Although most studies on the impact of deportation on children have not explicitly used an ambiguous loss theoretical framework, losses are clearly evident and often quite ambiguous. Living with the fear of a family member's deportation contributes to children's depression; anxiety; traumatic stress; internalizing and externalizing behaviors; poor educational outcomes; and food, income, and housing insecurity (see Gulbas et al., 2016, 2017; Lovato, 2019; Van Hook & Glick, 2020). Here, we illustrate the family vulnerabilities, specifically those related to ambiguous loss, created by forced separation. Dreby (2012) documented stories that describe both real and ambiguous losses caused by detention and deportation. She noted that when one parent is detained, an income is lost. That income is often connected to a family role such as provider or breadwinner, particularly if the deported parent is father or husband. As a result, roles and relationships must shift; wives/mothers must now assume or increase their income-producing role, leaving less time and energy for parenting. This can lead to children's confusion over parental roles and relationships—**boundary ambiguity** in ambiguous loss terminology— sometimes due to their father's changing perception of his family role. If providing for one's family is closely aligned with fathering, then the inability to fulfill the former may result in a distancing from the latter (Dreby, 2012). Moreover, children wonder if their parent's absence is temporary and there is hope for reunification, or if detention will result in deportation and their absence will be permanent. Ambiguity permeates the losses these children experience—their parent is physically absent but psychologically present.

Research Evidence on Families Experiencing Military Deployment

Researchers studying the family experience of military deployment have found that multiple factors impact the stress that families experience during deployment, including the military rank of the family member, the race/ethnicity of the deployed, and parental status (Gewirtz et al., 2018; Pittman et al., 2004). Additionally, researchers have approached the experience of military deployment not only from individual family members' perspectives, such as the deployed (Walsh, 2017) or the children of the deployed (Lester & Flake, 2013), but also from the couple and family perspective (Allen et al., 2010), which includes the interaction of two or more family members. Due to the tremendous complexity involved in the impact of military deployment on the family, there is a small but growing body of literature that applies the model of ambiguous loss to this family experience.

From an ambiguous loss perspective, there appear to be two types of possible loss experienced by families in military deployment: loss involved from deployment and loss involved in reunion. During deployment, the deployed family member is **physically absent** and is often **psychologically present** (typically through virtual communication via phone or computer); however, in reunion, the previously deployed family member is physically present but may be psychologically absent. The change that occurs in families from deployment to reunion has been documented by Faber et al. (2008), who found that those whose deployed family members participated in active combat experienced both of these types of losses.

Faber et al. (2008) identified the experience of deployment (where there was physical absence and psychological presence) as that of "ambiguous absence" (p. 225). Thus, while deployed, family members left behind struggled to manage the loss of the deployed member's physical presence, as well as their intermittent psychological presence. Managing this "ambiguous absence" often includes worry about the safety of the deployed family member and not knowing if or when they may see them again. In particular, the concept of boundary ambiguity was a particularly salient experience for the remaining family members during deployment. Boundary ambiguity, a concept defined by Boss (2006, p. 12) in which family members struggle to know who is in and out of the family at any given point, was uniquely heightened when the families were alerted to concerns about the safety of their deployed family member. Families also noted that ambiguity permeated their considerations of how they might reconfigure family roles and function if the worst-case scenario occurred and their family member died while deployed.

Maguire et al. (2013) identified that, during a time of ambiguous absence, spouses and partners had to work to manage what they called a "**maintenance paradox**" (p. 253). More specifically, spouses struggled to manage their technologically mediated communication with their spouses during deployment and during occasional face-to-face visits. Although spouses enjoyed and anticipated their virtual interactions, too much of this communication could trigger unanticipated feelings of grief and loss. Maintenance strategies (both interpersonal and dyadic) used by spouses, consistent with coping strategies often cited in the ambiguous loss literature, include prayer, thinking of the future, seeking social support, intentional communication (through phone, email, etc.), and providing reassurance. These maintenance strategies helped couples cope with deployment.

The paradox of balancing communication and connection with the family member who was physically absent while deployed appears to continue after families are reunited postdeployment. They must again deal with boundary ambiguity, albeit with a different type of struggle—that of reintegrating the deployed family member into a family system that had adjusted to their absence. Faber et al. (2008) called this "ambiguous presence" (p. 226). Although now physically present, the soldier/family member's psychological presence may be different than it had been before their tour of duty. Families in Faber and colleague's study found that a different person had returned; they noted that the person who returned was "psychologically absent" (p. 226). The fluctuation between feelings of relief and happiness that their loved one had returned created ambiguity; feelings of not knowing who that person was any more triggered stress that significantly affected relationships.

Boundary ambiguity became apparent in the reunion experience, where the now reunited family must relearn how to be a family and also adjust to the changes in the person who has returned.

The transition between deployment and reintegration can be particularly difficult for youth who may be struggling developmentally with their own growing sense of identity. Huebner et al. (2007) found that when a parent was deployed, the youth were often required to take on some of the deployed parent's roles. However, when that parent returned, parents expected the youth to transition back somewhat automatically to being a child again, without acknowledgment of the change or direct communication of clear expectations. Due to the ambiguity and complexity surrounding unspoken and changing family role expectations, this period of reintegration can be especially stressful for youth.

Other research that has applied the framework of ambiguous loss to the experience of military deployment has studied the impact of deployment on parents of deployed adult children. Similar to spouses and children of deployed individuals, parents of deployed individuals also experience grief and loss that involves not only a lack of clarity about the absence of their child but also ambivalence about their child participating in military deployment. Although military service in the United States is often socially supported and carries noble connotations, not all families support the use of military force. In a study by Crow et al. (2016), parents indicated feeling highly ambivalent about their adult child's decision to engage in military service in Iraq and Afghanistan, making it difficult for them to receive positive community recognition for their child's service. Their ambivalent feelings, and the ambiguity surrounding the physical absence yet psychological presence of their deployed adult child, complicated their personal experience of stress and grief.

Research Evidence on Families Dealing With Substance Use

In her 1999 book, Boss used drug and alcohol addiction as an example of the physical presence–psychological absence type of ambiguous loss in which "the sick family member is present but his or her mind is not" (p. 16). Despite an epidemic proportion of individuals experiencing a substance use disorder in the United States (Lipari & Van Horn, 2017), little published research on substance use disorders in families has applied ambiguous loss theory. An abundance of research has demonstrated many negative social-emotional impacts of parental substance use on children (Comiskey, 2013; Kroll, 2004; Ostler et al., 2007; Winstanley & Stover, 2019). Following are examples of studies that have explicitly used an ambiguous loss lens and others for which ambiguous loss ideas are present.

One example of an explicit use of ambiguous loss theory is a paper by Mechling et al. (2018) that described children's experiences of a parent's opioid use disorder (OUD). More specifically, the authors suggested how the two types of ambiguous loss could be present for children of parents with OUD: **physical presence–psychological absence** and **physical absence–psychological presence**. When a parent is under the influence of a drug or is intoxicated, their drug use may render the parent physically present but psychologically absent. There could also be times when a parent could be physically absent due to hospitalization, in-patient treatment, incarceration, or missing due to drug use but psychologically present to the child. For children experiencing both of these types of ambiguous loss, the child may lack clarity about the parent's ongoing role in their life (characterized as boundary ambiguity) as well as their ability to be present on a day-to-day basis. These changes and the resulting experience of ambiguity in the parent–child relationship can affect the child's development and their **coping**.

In a 2018 study, Mechling et al. explicitly explored the importance of children's coping abilities. More specifically, the authors noted the importance of **meaning making** and the development of dialectical thinking. Citing a previous research study (Fraser et al., 2009), they noted that children of parents with substance use disorders often must hold two opposing beliefs in their minds: "My parent may be physically here, but at times their illness prevents them from being here emotionally or psychologically" (Mechling et al., 2018, p. 58). Additionally, they found that children show a tremendous capacity for staying connected and also anticipating an improved relationship with their parent in the future.

Parents of adolescent or adult children who have a substance use disorder also experience grief, which is likewise complicated by presence and absence. Although we found no explicit application of the ambiguous loss framework on parents' experiences, it is clear that these parents experience ongoing stress and ambiguous loss as they struggle to grieve the often changing presence of their children (Butler & Bauld, 2005; Zucker et al., 2015). Substance abuse is often a hidden secret in families. Therefore, parents lack social recognition of what they are experiencing and may even receive negative judgement or feel socially stigmatized because of what is happening with their child (Butler & Bauld, 2005; Zucker et al., 2015). The ongoing ambiguity surrounding absence–presence, as well as the lack of social recognition in substance use disorders, may contribute to a blocked or frozen grieving process. Evidence in the literature also points to the importance and effectiveness of coping strategies, specifically, meaning making and receiving social support and recognition.

Research Evidence on Families With an Incarcerated Family Member

We have seen a significant increase in the number of families experiencing the incarceration or imprisonment of a family member over the past 30 years (Arditti, 2016); this shift to mass incarceration has disproportionately affected families of color. Researchers have studied the experiences of family members with incarcerated family members, as well as those who are incarcerated. Similar to reunification of deployed family members, studies have also examined family reintegration postincarceration. They have noted two different yet interrelated experiences that involve ambiguity and loss: incarceration (leaving and absence from the family) and reintegration (returning to the family). Thus, although families experience the physical absence and psychological presence of their incarcerated loved one while they serve their sentence, they also experience the **physical presence and psychological absence** when released, return to live with their family, and reintegrate into family and community life.

Easterling et al. (2019) used an ambiguous loss lens to describe ways that incarcerated mothers experienced their inability to perform their role as mother. They wanted to learn how mothers responded to and negotiated their feelings of loss, particularly due to the ambiguity surrounding communication with their children, involvement in making decisions and disciplining their children, and presence in their children's lives. They found that mothers negotiated their feelings of loss by modifying their mothering identities in three ways. One group adapted their mothering role as "modified mom"; they accepted their limited ability to parent their children and recognized that other people were now stepping into their parenting role. A second group of mothers tried very hard to keep things as if nothing had changed; the researchers identified them as using a "same mom" strategy. These mothers worked hard to maintain their same role with their children over the phone or on weekend visits. "Suspended mom" was the label for a third group of mothers who no longer saw themselves as a mother while in prison. They ceded their parenting role to the current caregivers of the child. The unresolvable grief and loss due to incarceration and the social stigma of being incarcerated as women exacerbated their struggle to redefine their mothering role.

A predominant theme of children's experiences with an incarcerated parent was documented in a study by Bocknek et al. (2009). Findings revealed that children experienced a tremendous lack of clarity regarding the status of their relationship with their incarcerated parents. Without accurate information about parents' incarceration status or sufficient external support from family and society, children struggled to make sense of their parent's absence.

Many of them reported feeling isolated, tended to internalize the distress by avoiding others, blocked their feelings, and relied on symbolic relationships to cope. This experience of grief is consistent with the concept of **frozen grief**, as defined by Boss (1999, p. 1), in which an individual is not able to acknowledge and work through their loss and grief. Additionally, the stigma associated with incarceration contributed to children's experience of ambiguous loss and further disrupted their grieving process, as the participants struggled to choose between getting clarification about their parent's situations and identifying their parents as criminals.

A study by Johnson and Easterling (2015) of 10 adolescents (ages 11–16) with an incarcerated parent found slightly different themes than Bocknek et al. (2009). Participants in both studies reported that children engaged in avoidance of the incarcerated parent as a way to manage their loss. However, in the Johnson and Easterling study, some of the adolescent participants attempted to make meaning out of their parent's incarceration by helping others through sharing their experiences and developing plans for how they would make a difference in the future. Thus, while some children may experience "frozen grief" others have found ways in which they can acknowledge and make sense of their loss.

The process of accepting their loss and moving forward is only one aspect of the grief experienced by children of parents who are incarcerated. There is also ambiguous loss associated with reintegration after incarceration. Although there is limited research on the reintegration process, Few-Demo and Arditti (2014) interviewed 10 mothers who had been or were incarcerated with a focus on examining their relational vulnerabilities and how those vulnerabilities may impact reentry. Specifically, the researchers found that the relational vulnerabilities most impactful on participants engaging in reentry included ambiguous and ambivalent relationships, as well as unresolved grief and loss. For example, participants in this study indicated experiences of ambivalent relationships with their parents, as well as experiences of ambivalent and ambiguous intimate relationships. Six of the 10 participants noted their own experiences of being children of parents who were incarcerated, and three of the 10 participants reported having intimate partners who were incarcerated. It also contributed to loss in their relationships with their children. Participants described pain when reengaging with their children after they were incarcerated. Chronic relational vulnerabilities contributed to depression and relational difficulties postincarceration. However, if family relationships were consistent, reentry was more likely to be successful and further involvement with the criminal adjustment system was more likely avoided. Thus, incarceration created significant relational ambiguity across generations that had important ramifications for individual, family, and societal well-being over time.

Summary: Ambiguous Loss Across Family Experiences

Experiences of ambiguous loss across the four family situations highlighted in this chapter are woven with threads of commonality and uniqueness. Key points from theory and research that have implications for clinicians are summarized as follows:

- All these families experience either **physical presence–psychological absence**, **psychological presence–physical absence**, or both types of ambiguous loss and multiple times, the latter due to the cyclical nature or the "in and out" of family members' presence and absence.

- Boundary ambiguity, or confusion about roles and relationships, is inherent in all of these family situations that create experiences of ambiguous loss. Ongoing relational adjustment is required in these families, particularly due to the aforementioned cyclical nature of family members' presence and absence. This is confounded by the absent person's psychological presence, which may inhibit adjustments needed for optimal family functioning.

- Conversely, boundary ambiguity reemerges when a family member physically returns. The reintegration process may be confounded by the now physically present person's psychological absence—if they have been affected by deployment, substance use, detention, for example.

- Families experiencing ambiguous loss often engage in "ambiguous communication" (Solheim et al., 2016, p. 347); that is, they avoid discussions about difficult things that are occurring in their respective situations. They use this as a coping strategy—a way to protect one another when separated.

- Families will vary in the extent of social support or social stigma they experience depending on whether society frames their situation as "noble" or problematic. This affects whether they will receive positive social support or be cut off from critical coping resources.

- Whether or not families perceive they have choice or agency in what has happened influences the meaning they ascribe to their loss and affects their ability to cope with the ambiguity of their situation.

- Children are affected tremendously by the ambiguity surrounding their parent's absence. They experience tremendous stress as they wonder why their parent is gone, if their parent is safe, how long their parent will be away, and how they should relate to the absent parent vis-à-vis other caregivers who may step in to fulfill roles.

When an ambiguous loss theoretical lens has been applied in research with families who are dealing with substance abuse, incarceration of a family member, immigration and, specifically, a threat of deportation, and military-related deployment, scholars have focused on ways that the ambiguity surrounding the physical absence–psychological presence or physical presence–psychological absence (or both) of a loved one has contributed to boundary ambiguity in roles, relationships, and communication patterns. This ambiguity creates stress that is ongoing, loss that is unrecognized by others, and sometimes social stigma that adds a dimension of shame or guilt to their stress. Moreover, the nature of the role ambiguity changes as families move between physical absence–psychological presence and physical presence–psychological absence.

The literature seems to focus primarily on describing these experiences of ambiguous loss. This is an important first step—name the experience, conceptualize it as relational, highlight ways in which it differs from other **types of loss**, identify the effects of ambiguous losses for family members, and note meaning making and coping strategies that families use to deal with ambiguous losses. In conversations with our clinical collaborators, we concluded that more research is needed to better understand the latter dimensions, meaning making, and coping strategies, particularly those that involve belief structures, that is, religious beliefs and community resources such as therapists, faith communities, and affinity-based support groups.

Pauline Boss (1999) conceptualized her ambiguous loss theory based on clinical practice experience. It is not surprising that it resonates with people and helps them articulate experiences of loss that, due to the ambiguity that surrounds them, seem to defy explanation. It is also a powerful theoretical lens to guide research involving experiences of ongoing stress; framing the stressor as an ambiguous loss and attending to the effect that the stressor has not only on the individual but also on their family relationships, can create a more holistic understanding of what is happening. In turn, intervention and treatment to deal with the stressor or alleviate the stress will be more effective.

CLINICAL APPLICATIONS: CHRISTINE KODMAN-JONES, KYLE BURKE, CAMILLE ST. JAMES, MIGUEL LEWIS, AND MICHELLE SHERMAN

Clinical Expertise and Interpretation of Evidence: An Overview

Consistent with the research section of this chapter, ambiguous loss, as Boss (1999) defined it, is a complicated loss characterized by an illogical, chaotic, unbelievably painful situation that families with a missing loved one endure.

Losses can be physical and/or psychological. A different way to describe this type of loss is that the psychological family is different from the physical family that is present, and the reverse is also true. This complicated loss can occur in any family, although some family types are more vulnerable to this experience. Solheim and Williams-Wengerd's research review in the previous section focuses on four family types: families with an undocumented immigrant member, families with a member who has an addiction, families with a member who is incarcerated, and families with a military member who is deployed. Their review of these four family types offers insight into common family patterns associated with the challenges of having to adapt to either having a family member psychologically present and physically absent or physically present and psychologically absent. Despite the ambiguous loss, these families' lives continue to evolve and change, facing various typical life transitions among and across family members. These transitions are not always predictable or acknowledged. As the research review reveals, a family can destabilize without sufficient community support (Arditti, 2005; Doka, 1989; Zucker et al., 2015). There is an emerging body of research on this type of complicated loss. For example, Solheim and Williams-Wengerd's review elucidates important trends that can alert therapists on how to guide and foster adjustments with families who regroup and remain together as they traverse this difficult-to-discuss experience of ambiguous loss (Van Hook & Glick, 2020).

Clinicians' awareness of common interactional family patterns, as members respond to complex grief or ambiguous loss, is key to assessment and treatment planning. In particular, ambiguous loss can create a cascade of ambiguous communication patterns, **boundary confusion/ambiguity**, and role confusion (Boss, 2006; Easterling et al., 2019; Faber et al., 2008; Falicov, 2002; Solheim et al., 2016). These families struggle with how to discuss their concerns and with whom to include in these discussions. Such families may experience a range of emotions connected to the ambiguous loss, while simultaneously working to contain and edit their overt emotional response. The isolation experienced by many of these families may be due to social stigma or genuine confusion. These families may regroup and adjust as they struggle with the stress of change. Many times, the families have fewer resources because the complicated loss of the family member can drain the members. Adults in these families often struggle with determining how much information is to be shared with children or even extended family. Additionally, information often changes frequently, thereby adding another layer to communication exchanges and choices. Often, ambiguous loss is not easily remedied. Disclosing to one's children may only lead to numerous questions for which no answer exists. If the situation is chronic, how does a family adjust?

Knowing the typical therapeutic questions and what interactional patterns families might adopt can guide the family therapist's approach. Therapists may provide a holding place to safely address the family's ability to discuss, relate, and develop an important story that captures the family emotional experience and needs. Psychoeducation is predicated on knowing patterns and the fallout of family decisions. Although psychoeducation is not the only therapeutic tool that the therapist offers to families, it is a strong intervention providing predictability.

Clinical Expertise and Interpretation of Evidence: Undocumented Immigrants and Deportation

Families who migrate to another country such as the United States, and who then become undocumented, either because they arrive illegally or they overstay a visa, live with the ongoing threat they will be discovered by Immigration and Customs Enforcement (ICE). When a family member who is undocumented is arrested, detained, or returned to their country of origin, it is a forced separation that not only is traumatic for the family but also creates an ongoing ambiguous loss. Boss (2016) described an ambiguous loss as one that lacks clarity, social recognition, or finality, all of which interfere with the family's natural coping and grieving processes. **Deportation** is the type of ambiguous loss described in Solheim and Williams-Wengerd's research review in which a family member is physically absent but psychologically present. The research review found studies documenting long-lasting detrimental effects of detention and deportation on families, especially children. The findings by Van Hook and Glick (2020) are particularly relevant for clinicians because they describe how deportation of a parent changes both the remaining parent's **role** and the overall family structure. Some families with deportation experience are in transition from a stable two-parent unit to a single-parent one. This new unit is often quite fragile, vulnerable, and isolated in their suffering. Not only is there a sudden loss of family income when a parent is detained or deported, particularly if it is the father, but the remaining parent is often depressed and overwhelmed. The result is that the physical and emotional availability of the remaining parent for supporting the children drops precipitously at a time when the children are most vulnerable. Communication between family members is indirect and ambiguous. Addressing this interactional pattern through opening communication and building connection between family members is an important focus when clinicians or other professionals encounter immigrant families with a parent who is in detention or has been deported.

Clinical Experience: Observations of Common Interactional Patterns

The remaining parent and children usually lose their financial security when a parent is detained or deported. The family may need to move to find affordable housing. Often, the move involves a change to a school system with fewer resources, and the children lose their neighborhood and school friends. Immigrant families are typically traditional in family **roles** and structure. The father is frequently the breadwinner and the mother the homemaker; if the father is disabled, the reverse is true. This means that the remaining parent, who is often the mother, is typically unskilled, so their jobs bring a lower income. Not only does this parent now have to struggle with earning an income and keeping the family together, she may experience symptoms of posttraumatic stress disorder from trauma occurring in the family's country of origin. There may be little emotional bandwidth available to take care of the children's emotional needs, leaving them isolated and having to cope on their own.

The emotional and behavioral impact on children of losing a parent through detention or deportation typically first shows up outside the home, at school. As described in Solheim and Williams-Wengerd's research review, children often respond to a caregiver's removal with anxiety, intense sadness, and depression. This can create performance issues at school. The child may appear distracted and unmotivated or overly emotional. Although children may be in great pain, Solheim and Williams-Wengerd's research review suggests that they are not likely to tell anyone at school about the detention or deportation because of fear that it will create more problems for their family. Children also are unlikely to tell either of their parents about their difficulties. They can see that the remaining parent in the home is stressed and overwhelmed and do not want to add to the distress. In addition, they may not want to worry the deported parent during their weekly calls home because they know it will make them feel more powerless and accentuate their loss.

Case Context: Characteristics, Culture, and Preferences

Gloria is the remaining parent in this family following the **deportation** of her husband, Juan. He was deported back to Mexico 3 months earlier. While traveling to work in Pennsylvania, Juan was picked up by ICE and charged with driving without a license and being undocumented. In Mexico, Juan is searching for work in his village in an area that is primarily agricultural. Regular work is scarce. Juan acquired some seasonal farm work. There are no funds to send to his wife and family; surviving is his primary focus. The regular phone calls from Juan to Gloria hardly assuage the day-to-day stress for his family. The children, a boy, age 8 years, and a girl, age 10 years, cry when they hear their father's voice on the phone. Both children are Americans by birth, which means the family is mixed status; both parents are undocumented. Often, the mother decides not to tell the children about the phone call because it takes hours for them to settle back down. There are gangs and thieves that Juan must avoid, and Gloria fears for his safety. Gloria finds work with a cleaning service, and her initial hours are 4 days per week with the hopes of working 5 days. She heads the home as a wage earner and mother of two depressed children who share little about how scared and sad they feel. They hesitate to share their worries with her because they hear her crying at night and feel such discussions will be too much for her. Gloria is coping with depression too.

In one incident, the daughter cried uncontrollably at her school, and a teacher sent her to the guidance counselor. The daughter declined to talk to the counselor because she does not want to reveal any of the family's struggles. The children tend either not to sleep at night or they try to crawl in bed with their mother for reassurance. The two children, unable to focus on homework, wait for their mother to return home. They fear losing the remaining parent. Since school has started, Gloria leaves early and tries to return when the children come home. They have moved to a new, unfamiliar, lower rent neighborhood, and so they stay indoors. Typically, they are home alone for about 30 to 60 minutes. They phone Gloria repeatedly until she arrives. They are scared she will be taken away by ICE. When Gloria arrives, they cling to her. She has received a call from the school to attend a meeting about her daughter.

Clinical Decisions: Intervention Implementation

Gloria was contacted by the guidance counselor about her daughter's crying. The school requested that Gloria obtain counseling for her daughter outside of school and provided her with several Spanish-speaking family therapists. Gloria was fortunate because referrals tend to slant toward individual child therapy, and the family's language and cultural background may not be considered sufficiently when recommending therapists. The therapist's approach to treatment was guided by ecosystemic structural family therapy (Jones, 2019), which makes stabilizing and supporting parents in their family leadership **role** a top priority. The therapist worked with Gloria collaboratively, assisting her in locating community resources that could help meet the family's immediate concrete needs and helping her to organize a routine for her children at home. The mother's church stepped up and became a valuable natural support for the family, offering an after-school program for the children while their mother was working.

Based on Boss's (2016) work and the studies reviewed by Solheim and Williams-Wengerd, one important intervention in this case was to address the ambiguous communication between family members, particularly that surrounding the father's deportation and the resulting family changes. Gloria asked each child how they felt about their father's absence and what they understood about his leaving the family. She asked additional questions such as, what is it like for each of you in this new neighborhood. She stated,

> I had to make decisions that you may not understand and may feel unfair. I wonder if you are disappointed in these choices that I made? The neighborhood does not feel as friendly as the last one; do you sense the difference too?

The children were slow to respond at first, saying little. They were not accustomed to their mother being this open. The children became more responsive in these conversations because they sensed that their mother was not alone and was trusting the therapist. The therapist also involved the father, Juan, by telephone, helping him and Gloria talk more directly and honestly about the challenges they were facing and clarifying how they could help one another. To reduce Gloria's isolation, she was encouraged to stop protecting Juan from information he should have as the children's father.

One result of the opening of direct communication between Gloria and Juan was a plan to reduce each family member's isolation from their community, particularly the school. This helped Gloria to feel more informed and on top of her children's needs, even though she was working a lot of hours. She brought the information back to Juan so he could have input into how best to support their girls. Another important topic of discussion between the parents was how to acquire a pro bono immigration lawyer to address Gloria's undocumented status.

Clinical Expertise and Interpretation of Evidence: Postincarceration Families

As Solheim and Williams-Wengerd note, incarcerated families struggle with the ambiguous loss of a family member who is incarcerated. Although physically absent, the family member in prison has a powerful psychological presence in the family. On a practical level, the incarcerated person contributes to the system in a number of ways, including helping financially and with parenting responsibilities. The partner who remains at home demonstrates both resiliency and a sense of being overwhelmed, as they typically assume additional responsibilities once performed by the incarcerated partner. An additional stressor involves children missing opportunities to be parented by the incarcerated partner. Families typically struggle negotiating and renegotiating the subsequent shifts in relational responsibilities at the time of imprisonment, during the **incarceration**, and upon the **reunion**.

Easterling et al. (2019) further indicated that incarcerated mothers struggle balancing dual identities of "mother" and "inmate" and are often at a loss with respect to this balancing act. Families tend to have overly optimistic expectations for the reunion and fail to consider the real and significant barriers that contribute to the high rate of recidivism. Failure to consider and plan how to contend with the obstacles they will face increases the likelihood of a number of unwanted outcomes for the family, up to and including reincarceration. Whether due to the desire to protect family members from their struggles—at home or in jail or prison—families coping with imprisonment often shield each other from their day-to-day feelings because they tend to focus on future goals rather than present feelings of loss, sadness, anger, confusion, and so on. Avoiding these conversations, although well intentioned, serves to create a sense of isolation for each member. In addition, children are often hurt and angry by their parents' absence, but they do not get to express these feelings. In part, this is due to the loss of the relationship with their incarcerated parent and because children do not want to add to the burden the of their incarcerated parent.

Clinical Experience: Observations of Common Interactional Patterns
Each incarcerated family's experience is unique; however, **roles** within the family change due to the incarcerated family member's inability to perform tasks for which they were previously responsible. The incarcerated family member will likely struggle to navigate their dual role of parent and prisoner, while their partner assumes more family responsibility. Children are often left to cope alone with their new reality in a single-parent-led household. Partners will often avoid having difficult conversations about feeling overwhelmed. The parent left to take on additional duties in the home tends to feel resentful. Aware of the burdens of **incarceration**, the remaining parent will often avoid sharing the tribulations of home life. Although again well intentioned, the goal of protecting their partner and not wanting to further burden them can result in unexpressed negative affect, which will likely make it more difficult to foster their relationship. In addition, children of incarcerated families will feel a range of emotions including sadness, confusion, and anger. Further, the ambiguous loss of a parent is highlighted by that parent's absence at important events in the child's life. Often, in an effort protect each other, negative feelings are kept to oneself. It is this desperate silence in the midst of family grief that belies the sense of ambiguous loss for incarcerated families. Family members experience the absence of their incarcerated family member, and, at the same time, they work to "hold space" for the absent family member while struggling to operate "as if" they were still present. Family therapy with incarcerated families should help

them take a broader, systemic perspective. Family members can hold each other accountable without assigning blame, express their thoughts and feelings throughout their shared experience of incarceration, and work toward understanding and improving how they function as a unit.

Case Context: Characteristics, Culture, and Preferences

Charles was recently charged with drug possession and distribution and is currently awaiting trial in the local county jail because his family was unable to afford his bail. His longtime girlfriend, Kuma, and their two children, Amir (age 13 years) and Casandra (age 17 years), have been making weekly visits to the jail. Before his **incarceration**, Charles was working full-time and was the primary breadwinner in the family, while Kuma worked part-time and took care of most of the parenting and household duties. Charles was actively involved in his children's activities. He helped coach Amir's basketball team occasionally and encouraged Casandra to continue excelling at school as she prepared to apply for college. Charles had a history of incarceration when he was younger, but he had not been involved with the legal system for 7 years. Kuma recently required surgery that the family could not afford, and Charles decided to sell drugs to provide additional income for his family. He did so without consulting Kuma.

Charles's incarceration left Kuma feeling shocked initially, which gave way to extreme anger. Amir was devastated because he idolized his father; Casandra was livid with her father and felt embarrassed because all of her friends knew. After the initial shock and disruption, the family settled into a pattern. Charles kept a low profile in jail and communicated with Kuma and their children through weekly phone calls and visits, during which they would bring him money for food and phone calls. Kuma began working full time at her current job and leaned on her extended family to help provide caregiving for Amir and Casandra. Charles soon began to expect both visits and money and became angry when his family could not call or attend visits. Kuma quickly became overwhelmed with the additional responsibilities and was resentful of Charles for putting her in a position to ask for help from his family with whom she did not get along. Amir stopped attending his basketball practices, and his coach kicked him off the team. Casandra stopped attending visits or speaking with Charles because she was angry with him. The family avoided talking about how they felt, which only further served to entrench the above pattern.

Kuma tentatively discussed with Charles some of the concerns that she and her children had. As a part of his plea agreement, Charles agreed to participate in weekly therapy, and he requested family therapy to address how his incarceration affected his family. The family began participating in therapy sessions 90 days before Charles's release from jail, with an entrenched family pattern of Charles maintaining a low profile in prison and assuming that Kuma will provide him with all the support he needed, while Kuma assumed more responsibility, was overwhelmed, and became angry in response to Charles's need for more financial and emotional support. Although the case example addresses a father-incarcerated family with unexpressed negative affect and shifts in family member roles, this phenomenon is also noted in mother-incarcerated families.

Clinical Decisions: Intervention Implementation

Research clearly indicates that incarcerated families struggle with shifts in roles, managing additional responsibilities, receiving enough social support, and effective expression of thoughts and feelings regarding the experience of incarceration. The therapy discussed here uses a clinical approach with the various subsystems within the family. Presessions will be conducted with Charles individually, then with Kuma, and finally the children. The assessment presession meetings focus on identifying current hierarchies (Minuchin, 1974) and interactional patterns that include gathering information for a genogram to guide the session structure and direction. In addition, the assessment includes asking family members to identify their concerns and goals for therapy.

Given the struggles incarcerated families have navigating the "as if" nature of incarceration, uncertainty dominates the family's reality. A child in these families is not sure if a punishment prescribed by dad has to be followed. Family therapy with this population should focus on helping discuss their sense of ambiguous loss. As noted, family members are likely to struggle with living both "as if" the incarcerated parent is still present in day-to-day life and their very real absence. Family members often do not have the opportunity to discuss how they navigate this sense of loss, and they are likely to avoid conversations about how they feel. This type of avoidance comes from the inability to reconcile the real status of the missing person. "Am I mad at Dad, am I sad because he is not here, or both?" Communication tends toward ambiguity from this avoidance. Family therapy with incarcerated families should facilitate conversations about how all members of the system have been and continue to be affected by the experience of incarceration. The therapist should help Charles and Kuma express how they have been affected by Charles's incarceration, with particular emphasis on the emotional impact of each of their experiences. The therapist uses psychoeducation to explain systems thinking, especially with respect to how patterns emerge within families and how unhelpful it is to assign blame to one party while ensuring that the result of therapy, a stronger, more connected and open family will still allow members to hold each other accountable appropriately.

Following similar steps described earlier, the therapist should make space for the children to express how they have been affected by their father's incarceration. As Solheim and Williams-Wengerd note in their review, the research indicates that the age and developmental level of children in incarcerated families is another critical factor to consider. The children may be reluctant to participate in the treatment. The family therapist should work with Kuma to help her empower the children to take ownership of their part in the therapeutic process. Additional cultural and systemic considerations that may affect therapy, including family roles and hierarchies, should be considered as needed.

The therapist should encourage open, honest, and nonblaming communication. The therapist, when needed, will remind the family of the broader, systemic perspective. These interventions should help the family understand what occurred between them in systemic terms. The unexpressed negative affect will be understood within a pattern that developed in response to Charles's incarceration. Additionally, Charles should model holding himself accountable for his children, along with empathy by acknowledging that everyone in the family is entitled to their feelings.

In addition, the therapist should guide the family in discussing their strengths as a system and talk about potential barriers that may hinder their communication and growth. The therapist should use psychoeducation regarding the need to be hopeful yet realistic about a successful reunion. Using the literature, they should discuss barriers to successful reentry and reunification that the family does not bring up on its own. Linking the family to postincarceration services is critical for promoting this family's success.

Clinical Expertise and Interpretation of Evidence: Families With a Member With an Addiction

As indicated by Solheim and Williams-Wengerd's research review, there is a persistent thread of ambiguous loss experienced by the family when a member is struggling with addiction. As Solheim and Williams-Wengerd point out, ambiguous loss associated with substance use disorders is the sense of uncertainty for all involved caused by ambiguous presence and ambiguous absence (Hogan, 2007; Landau & Garrett, 2014; Mechling et al., 2018). Role **ambiguity** (Hogan, 2007; Mechling, et al., 2018) adds to systemic instability and arises when children take on emotional or physical caretaking roles or when grandparents become primary caregivers to grandchildren. Role confusion also occurs when a child has an addiction, engaging in behaviors that are out of sync with developmental norms. The child feels a sense of loss, such as a loss of childhood, loss of self, and loss of relationship. Finally, the shame and stigma surrounding addiction magnifies alienation and isolation within the family, increasing the sense of ambiguous loss (Hogan, 2007; Landau & Garrett, 2014).

Clinical Experience: Observations of Common Interactional Patterns

A range of family scenarios arise when a family member has an addiction. Ambiguous presence/loss occurs when the individual with the addiction is **physically absent and psychologically present**, such as when a parent is in inpatient treatment. Also common is the physically present addicted member who is psychologically absent. Addicted parents often use their child to cloak their addiction, sometimes hanging out with their children so that their altered state is not noticed by their romantic partner. Additionally, ambiguity is correlated to addiction. First, the person is often parenting when drunk or stoned. Second, at some point, if recovery is to occur, there will need to be a detoxification intervention. And even in early recovery, the addicted person needs to be "self-centered" to avoid relapse. All of these factors increase the ambiguous interpersonal connection.

Case Context: Characteristics, Culture, and Preferences

Cathy is a 41-year-old mother of two daughters, Lisa, age 9, and Kala, age 13. Her substance use started socially in college, abated slightly during child-bearing years, and escalated as work demands increased and her children matured and needed less hands-on care. Cathy's recovery journey started 3 years ago when she went to her first inpatient rehabilitation facility for 28 days to save her job. Since then, she has been away for treatment on three more occasions. Soon after the first two inpatient stays, Cathy relapsed, and with each relapse, her substance use became more severe. She would disappear for days at a time. Six months ago, after a 4-day binge, Cathy lost her job, and her husband filed for divorce. Cathy's parents, believing this to be a temporary situation, welcomed her and her daughters into their home.

Since that time, Cathy's use increased in frequency and intensity. Her soon-to-be ex-husband largely withdrew from the family due to anger and resentment. Her parents became involved, providing childcare and financial support. In addition, both children had been model students but are now struggling academically and behaviorally. Kala has been missing assignments due to helping her younger sister with homework, taking care of Cathy when she is incapacitated, and spending time with friends. The younger child has withdrawn from friends and recently expressed feeling depressed. The family was referred to family therapy as part of Cathy's aftercare program subsequent to her latest inpatient stay. She will also engage in intensive outpatient treatment and attend 12-Step meetings.

Clinical Decisions: Intervention Implementation

The following intervention is based on research and clinical experience in the field of addiction treatment and is informed by both feminist and structural approaches to family therapy. A feminist perspective supports rebalancing power dynamics through collaboration (Hare-Mustin, 1984). A structural approach also supports rebalancing by addressing boundaries and **roles** within the system and by engaging all family members to be a part of the solution (Crnkovic & Delcampo, 1998; Micucci, 2009). Although there is ample evidence in support of family involvement in treating those with a substance use disorder, one factor stands out: The more family members involved in treatment the better the outcome for the individual (McNabb & DerKarabetian, 1989). As indicated by Solheim and Williams-Wengerd's research review, **role ambiguity** contributes to the ambiguous loss experienced by families affected by addiction. Clinical experience suggests that once addressed, healthier roles and boundaries promote clearer communication and assuage the impact of ambiguous presence and ambiguous absence that accompanies addiction.

During the initial assessment, a detailed genogram was created that illuminated problematic interactional patterns and systemic dynamics present within the family and were further perpetuated during Cathy's active addiction. Producing a detailed genogram allows the focus to shift off of Cathy and onto the family system associated with ambiguous loss and, in particular, role ambiguity experienced by Cathy's daughter and parents. Also, during the early stages of treatment, age-appropriate psychoeducation was provided to address issues of shame and stigma, highlight the value of social support (Fraser et al., 2009; Zucker et al., 2015), and introduce the family to resources including the suggestion that they attend AlAnon. In this way, psychoeducation supported a systemic exploration of addiction as a family disease.

In one session with Cathy, her daughters, and her parents, the issue of role ambiguity was addressed using an enactment—a structural family therapy technique to create healthier interpersonal interactions during the session. Kala expressed her frustration about her mother's absence "even when she is here" and her anger about having to care for her younger sister and miss out on time with her friends. The therapist encouraged Kala to tell her family how she felt and what she needed. Kala shared, "I just want time with my friends." Immediately, the grandparents objected, stating she should not be allowed to socialize until her schoolwork is done. To rebalance the power dynamics, the therapist focused on Kala and asked her again what she needed and what a solution would look like. Kala became emotional and stated, "I want to be a normal kid!" She went on to explain how she felt like an adult with her mother and sister and like a young child with her grandparents. The therapist then turned to Cathy and asked for her input. Cathy apologized to Kala for putting her in this difficult situation, thanked her for all her support, committed to be a more engaged parent, and specifically offered to oversee Lisa's schoolwork. Kala spontaneously acknowledged that this would free her up to have more time to socialize and attend to her own schoolwork, would help her to see her mother as capable, and recognize that her mother was there for her also. This ultimately promoted greater psychosocial wellness (Mechling et al., 2018) for Kala.

The therapist encouraged Cathy to share with her family the likely impact of retaking the role as primary caregiver. She acknowledged it would be an adjustment but that ultimately it would bolster her self-esteem (Hogan, 2007), reduce her resentment toward her parents, and allow her to feel more connected to her daughters. Cathy also recognized that she would only be able to accept this responsibility and follow through in her roles as mother and daughter if she stayed sober. The therapist then engaged Cathy's parents by asking them how their roles would change. They acknowledged that they would be able to reclaim their roles as grandparents to Kala and Lisa, worry about Cathy less, and resume healthier roles as her parents.

Consistent with the findings outlined in Solheim and Williams-Wengerd's review, by redefining healthy roles within the family, Cathy's daughters developed coping strategies that allowed them to remain connected to their mother while Cathy continued to address her addiction and enabled her parents to connect to additional support and reclaim their roles as parents and grandparents. By facilitating a process that focused on roles, the family was able to address issues of ambiguous loss and establish healthier dynamics throughout the system that supported Cathy's recovery.

Clinical Expertise and Interpretation of Evidence: Military Deployment and Reunion in Families

The often cyclical pattern of deployment and reunion among military families can involve many features of ambiguous loss. Pauline Boss (2002) described two types of ambiguous loss: ambiguous absence and ambiguous presence. Ambiguous absence happens when a family member is perceived as physically absent but psychologically present, which can occur during military deployment. At home, family members sometimes become preoccupied with the absent relative, partly due to predictable systemic change. The role of each family member can also become unclear. For example, children may wonder if their deployed parent is actually weighing in on discipline decisions. In addition, partners of deployed military personnel often experience loneliness, role overload, and concern about the safety and well-being of their military member as the ambiguous absence extends over time (Vormbrock, 1993; Wood et al., 1995).

Ambiguous presence occurs when a family member is physically present but psychologically absent; this phenomenon can occur when the deployed military member returns home to the family unit. Everyone has changed during the deployment, so it takes time and effort for family members to get to know one another again. Generally, reintegration involves four key tasks including redefining roles, expectations, and division of labor; managing strong emotions; abandoning emotional constriction and creating intimacy in relationships; and creating shared meaning (Bowling & Sherman, 2008). Renegotiating roles, responsibilities, and boundaries in an intimate relationship can be challenging. When a veteran has experienced a traumatic event during deployment, they may be preoccupied with combat experiences upon homecoming, making reconnecting with the family difficult. The partner and children may then struggle with the military personnel's physical presence but emotional absence.

Clinical Experience: Observations of Common Interactional Patterns

Military families, like all families, can develop various systemic patterns that can create friction in relationships. For example, couples can enact a pursue–withdrawal pattern, which can be exacerbated by military deployments. That is, one partner may pursue their need for connection as a result of feeling alone. Yet they do so by criticizing their partner by stating, "You are never here. You are always at work." As a result of the criticism, the other partner may tend to feel inadequate and think, "I can never get it right with her." Then, that partner withdraws emotionally during conflicts to manage strong feelings. When the military member is deployed, these patterns may be exacerbated, and reconnecting as a couple may take more time.

Other patterns can emerge when the military personnel have experienced trauma or has posttraumatic stress disorder (PTSD). For example, many with PTSD experience hypervigilance, general irritability, and angry outbursts; rates of interpersonal violence are, in fact, elevated among dyads in which the veteran has PTSD (Taft et al., 2011). Partners and children of these veterans may tend to walk on eggshells, never knowing when the veteran will explode verbally or physically. Some children personalize these angry outbursts, wondering what they did wrong to cause them. Partners can find themselves in difficult situations because they want to present a united parenting front to the children yet also want to protect them from the potentially abusive behavior. If the partner defends the veteran, the children can feel misunderstood. If the partner sides with the children, the veteran becomes upset.

As noted earlier, the veteran's return from deployment can also introduce stress to the family system. While the veteran was deployed, the children took on new roles and responsibilities within the family. When the veteran returns, the children are expected to give up these roles and return to how the family functioned prior to the deployment. This situation is ripe for confusion, especially when families avoid open discussions about the changes and include the children in these conversations. This reintegration process can be especially challenging for National Guard and Reserve families who generally have fewer deployments, more established families, and families with members in existing nonmilitary careers that are affected by prolonged absences from home.

Case Context: Characteristics, Culture, and Preferences

Mark and Judy have been married for 15 years. They have two teenage sons aged 17 and 12 years. Mark was in the Army Reserves for nearly 10 years; his first combat deployment occurred recently, lasted 8 months, and involved considerable exposure to combat, including an especially upsetting incident when a good friend was badly injured by an improvised explosive device. Although Judy and their two teenagers were relieved and happy upon Mark's return from Iraq, these feelings quickly dissipated as he become more irritable and withdrawn due to his PTSD. In addition, Judy and her children are also growing tired of him not leaving the home or participating in family outings. Mark no longer participates in family outings to the park due to his hypervigilance and belief that the world is not safe. As a result, Judy feels lonely and isolated and misses the "old Mark" she loved before his deployment. His two teenage sons also miss their old father, who had always attended outings with them.

Clinical Decisions: Intervention Implementation

Focusing on Boss's work and the studies reviewed by Solheim and Williams-Wengerd, one important intervention could focus on communication about the ambiguous loss as to why Mark is different now—namely, his lack of interest in family outings, displays of irritability, yelling, and a lack of patience toward his family. The intervention could focus on how the family can learn more through family therapy about how Mark's PTSD has changed him. The discussion between Mark and Judy provides a possible avenue to address this couple's distance.

JUDY: (*In an angry and loud tone*) Mark, you are always on your own, away from the family. It's so selfish. You never do anything with us.

MARK: There you go again. Always criticizing me. I hate it. Can't you ever say anything nice about me?

THERAPIST: (*In a soft, slow-paced voice*) Let's slow down here, as a lot is going on between you. I can tell this is probably what happens at home between the two of you. I want something different to happen here so we can create a better bond where there is safety and trust. I would like to eventually see more vulnerability of the softer emotions with both of you because this can create a different pattern—a pattern where both of you can be more responsive to each other in an empathic way.

   I'm going to start with Judy and then I may have time to get to you, Mark, later. Judy? When Mark does not spend time with the family, what does that mean to you?

JUDY: Hmm . . . it means that he's being selfish.

THERAPIST: Okay, I can understand that. It's painful for him to not be with you and your children. You miss the old Mark. I can see that clearly. And when you say it means he is selfish, that's talking about him. I want to hear about you and your experience today. What does it mean to you when he is not with the family?

JUDY: (*Pauses for about 5 seconds*) Um . . . it means he does not care about me.

THERAPIST: Yes, that makes sense. (*Therapist validates her experience*) It's so important for him to care about you. I am hearing how important Mark is to you in those moments when he does not go to the park with you. It's important for him to be with you right there by your side like he used to be on these family outings. It sounds very painful.

JUDY: It is. Yet, he is still selfish!

THERAPIST: (*Again in a slow and soft voice*) It's easier to be angry than it is to talk about your tender feelings, huh? It makes sense you are angry. It's what you know, and Mark also knows this side of you. Yet he doesn't know the side of you that misses him. That longs for him to be with you and care about you. He doesn't know about that part, that painful part that sounds deeply sad.

As this dialogue highlights, much of what assists these families is an awareness of the process connected to trauma. One's partner who is wrestling with trauma-based symptoms is both there and not there. This tenuous relational connection needs to be understood; thus, all involved parties are less likely to misinterpret protection as rejection. Family therapy can give military families a chance to learn and openly talk about the impacts of deployment and trauma on the family. For example, the therapist can help Mark explain his triggers to his wife and kids, so they can understand how challenging the Fourth of July is for him because of the fireworks. The therapist can explain how irritability and challenges with anger are common elements of PTSD, but Mark is still held responsible and expresses his commitment to working on how he handles strong emotions. Everyone has changed during the deployment, so family therapy can be a chance for family members to get to know each other again and reestablish positive bonds. Mark is also supported in expressing his appreciation to his family of their patience and support.

Conclusion

Ambiguous loss is painful and confusing, and it often leaves a family without known language to define their experiences. Naming the phenomenon and explaining this loss to the family experiencing this pain can lead to insight and healing. The individual who is "lost" either psychologically or physically is no longer a member of the family in the way they once were, leaving the overall family unit in limbo. Often, the family in one of the situations that result in ambiguous loss is "frozen" in their grief. The relationship with that individual is changed, yet the person is still a presence, thus the ability to mourn the altered relationship does not occur. Clinicians need to offer these families a roadmap to address the person missing from the home—whether their absence is psychological or physical—and allow the family space to acknowledge the pain resulting from this altered familial state that is often overlooked.

REFERENCES

Allen, B., Cisneros, E. M., & Tellez, A. (2015). The children left behind: The impact of parental deportation on mental health. *Journal of Child and Family Studies*, *24*(2), 386–392. https://doi.org/10.1007/s10826-013-9848-5

Allen, E. S., Rhoades, G. K., Stanley, S. M., & Markman, H. J. (2010). Hitting home: Relationships between recent deployment, posttraumatic stress symptoms, and marital functioning for Army couples. *Journal of Family Psychology*, *24*(3), 280–288. https://doi.org/10.1037/a0019405

Arditti, J. A. (2005). Families and incarceration: An ecological approach. *Families in Society*, *86*(2), 251–260. https://doi.org/10.1606/1044-3894.2460

Arditti, J. A. (2016). A family stress-proximal process model for understanding the effects of parental incarceration on children and their families. *Couple & Family Psychology*, *5*(2), 65–88. https://doi.org/10.1037/cfp0000058

Bocknek, E. L., Sanderson, J., & Britner, P. A., IV. (2009). Ambiguous loss and post-traumatic stress in school-age children of prisoners. *Journal of Child and Family Studies, 18*(3), 323–333. https://doi.org/10.1007/s10826-008-9233-y

Boss, P. (1999). *Ambiguous loss: Learning to live with unresolved grief.* Harvard University Press.

Boss, P. (2002). *Family stress management.* Sage Publications.

Boss, P. (2006). *Loss, trauma, and resilience: Therapeutic work with ambiguous loss.* W. W. Norton & Company.

Boss, P. (2016). The context and process of theory development: The story of ambiguous loss. *Journal of Family Theory & Review, 8*(3), 269–286. https://doi.org/10.1111/jftr.12152

Bowling, U. B., & Sherman, M. D. (2008). Welcoming them home: Supporting service members and their families in navigating the tasks of reintegration. *Professional Psychology, Research and Practice, 39*(4), 451–458. https://doi.org/10.1037/0735-7028.39.4.451

Butler, R., & Bauld, L. (2005). The parents' experience: Coping with drug use in the family. *Drugs Education Prevention & Policy, 12*(1), 35–45. https://doi.org/10.1080/0968763042000275308

Comiskey, C. M. (2013). A 3 year national longitudinal study comparing drug treatment outcomes for opioid users with and without children in their custodial care at intake. *Journal of Substance Abuse Treatment, 44*(1), 90–96. https://doi.org/10.1016/j.jsat.2012.04.002

Crnkovic, A. E., & DelCampo, R. L. (1998). A systems approach to the treatment of chemical addiction. *Contemporary Family Therapy, 20*(1), 25–36.

Crow, J. R., Myers, D. R., Ellor, J. W., Dolan, S. L., & Morissette, S. (2016). Military deployment of an adult child: Ambiguous loss and boundary ambiguity reflected in the experiences of parents of service members. *Marriage & Family Review, 52*(5), 481–509. https://doi.org/10.1080/01494929.2015.1115454

Doka, K. (1989). *Disenfranchised grief.* Lexington Books.

Dreby, J. (2012). The burden of deportation on children in Mexican immigrant families. *Journal of Marriage and the Family, 74*(4), 828–845. https://doi.org/10.1111/j.1741-3737.2012.00989.x

Easterling, B. A., Feldmeyer, B., & Presser, L. (2019). Narrating mother identities from prison. *Feminist Criminology, 14*(5), 519–539. https://doi.org/10.1177/1557085118773457

Faber, A. J., Willerton, E., Clymer, S. R., MacDermid, S. M., & Weiss, H. M. (2008). Ambiguous absence, ambiguous presence: A qualitative study of military reserve families in wartime. *Journal of Family Psychology, 22*(2), 222–230. https://doi.org/10.1037/0893-3200.22.2.222

Falicov, C. J. (2002). Ambiguous loss: Risk and resilience in Latino immigrant families. In M. Suarez-Orozco & M. Paez (Eds.), *Latinos: Remaking America* (pp. 274–288). University of California Press.

Few-Demo, A. L., & Arditti, J. A. (2014). Relational vulnerabilities of incarcerated and reentry mothers: Therapeutic implications. *International Journal of Offender Therapy and Comparative Criminology, 58*(11), 1297–1320. https://doi.org/10.1177/0306624X13495378

Fraser, C., McIntyre, A., & Manby, M. (2009). Exploring the impact of parental drug/alcohol problems on children and parents in a Midlands county in 2005/06. *British Journal of Social Work, 39*(5), 846–866. https://doi.org/10.1093/bjsw/bcn016

Gewirtz, A. H., DeGarmo, D. S., & Zamir, O. (2018). Testing a military family stress model. *Family Process*, *57*(2), 415–431. https://doi.org/10.1111/famp.12282

Gulbas, L. E., & Zayas, L. H. (2017). Exploring the effects of U.S. immigration enforcement on the well-being of citizen children in Mexican immigrant families. *The Russell Sage Foundation Journal of the Social Sciences*, *3*(4), 53–69. https://doi.org/10.7758/rsf.2017.3.4.04

Gulbas, L. E., Zayas, L. H., Yoon, H., Szlyk, H., Aguilar-Gaxiola, S., & Natera, G. (2016). Deportation experiences and depression among U.S. citizen-children with undocumented Mexican parents. *Child: Care, Health and Development*, *42*(2), 220–230. https://doi.org/10.1111/cch.12307

Hare-Mustin, R. T. (1984). A feminist approach to family therapy. In P. P. Rieker & E. Carmen (Eds.), *The gender gap in psychotherapy* (pp. 301–318). Springer.

Hogan, D. M. (2007). The impact of opiate dependence on parenting processes: Contextual, physiological and psychological factors. *Addiction Research & Theory*, *15*(6), 617–635. https://doi.org/10.1080/16066350701663698

Huebner, A. J., Mancini, J. A., Wilcox, R. M., Grass, S. R., & Grass, G. A. (2007). Parental deployment and youth in military families: Exploring uncertainty and ambiguous loss. *Family Relations*, *56*(2), 112–122. https://doi.org/10.1111/j.1741-3729.2007.00445.x

Jerves, E., Rober, P., Enzlin, P., & De Haene, L. (2020). Ambiguous loss in transnational families' adolescents: An exploratory study in Ecuador. *Family Process*, *59*(2), 725–739. https://doi.org/10.1111/famp.12453

Johnson, E. I., & Easterling, B. A. (2015). Coping with confinement: Adolescents' experiences with parental incarceration. *Journal of Adolescent Research*, *30*(2), 244–267. https://doi.org/10.1177/0743558414558593

Jones, C. W. (2019). *Setting the stage for change: An ecosystemic approach to in-home family-based treatment*. Center for Family Based Training.

Kroll, B. (2004). Living with an elephant: Growing up with parental substance misuse. *Child & Family Social Work*, *9*(2), 129–140. https://doi.org/10.1111/j.1365-2206.2004.00325.x

Landau, J., & Garrett, J. (2014). Neurobiology and addiction: Assisting the family and support system to get resistant loved ones into treatment. In T. Nelson & H. Winawer (Eds.), *Critical topics in family therapy* (pp. 93–102). Springer.

Lester, P., & Flake, E. (2013). How wartime military service affects children and families. *The Future of Children*, *23*(2), 121–141. https://doi.org/10.1353/foc.2013.0015

Lipari, R. N., & Van Horn, S. L. (2017). Children living with parents who have a substance use disorder. *The CBHSQ Report*. Substance Abuse and Mental Health Services Administration. https://www.samhsa.gov/data/sites/default/files/report_3223/ShortReport-3223.pdf

Lovato, K. (2019). Forced separation: A qualitative examination of how Latino/a adolescents cope with parental deportation. *Children and Youth Services Review*, *98*, 42–50. https://doi.org/10.1016/j.childyouth.2018.12.012

Maguire, K. C., Heinemann-LaFave, D., & Sahlstein, E. (2013). "To be so connected, yet not at all": Relational presence, absence, and maintenance in the context of a wartime deployment. *Western Journal of Communication*, *77*(3), 249–271, https://doi.org/10.1080/10570314.2012.757797

Martínez Rosas, G. (2020). Critically accommodating "illegality": Anticipatory losses within mixed-status immigrant families. *Journal of Loss and Trauma, 25*(5), 488–500. https://doi.org/10.1080/15325024.2020.1716162

McNabb, J., & DerKarabetian, A. (1989). Family involvement and outcome in treatment of alcoholism. *Psychological Reports, 65*(3, Part 2), 1327–1330.

Mechling, B. M., Ahern, N. R., & Palumbo, R. (2018). Applying ambiguous loss theory to children of parents with an opioid use disorder. *Journal of Child and Adolescent Psychiatric Nursing, 31*(2–3), 53–60. https://doi.org/10.1111/jcap.12209

Micucci, J. A. (2009). *The adolescent in family therapy: Harnessing the power of relationships* (2nd ed.). Guilford Press.

Minuchin, S. (1974). *Families & family therapy*. Harvard University Press.

Orcés, D. M., & Ewing, W. A. (2019). *The role of contact and values in public attitudes towards unauthorized immigrants* [Special report]. American Immigration Council. https://www.americanimmigrationcouncil.org/sites/default/files/research/the_role_of_contact_and_values_in_public_attitudes_toward_unauthorized_immigrants.pdf

Ostler, T., Haight, W., Black, J., Choi, G. Y., Kingery, L., & Sheridan, K. (2007). Case series: Mental health needs and perspectives of rural children reared by parents who abuse methamphetamine. *Journal of the American Academy of Child & Adolescent Psychiatry, 46*(4), 500–507. https://doi.org/10.1097/chi.0b013e3180306298

Pittman, J. F., Kerpelman, J. L., & McFadyen, J. M. (2004). Internal and external adaptation in army families: Lessons from Operations Desert Shield and Desert Storm. *Family Relations, 53*(3), 249–260. https://doi.org/10.1111/j.0197-6664.2004.0001.x

Rolland, J. S. (1990). Anticipatory loss: A family systems developmental framework. *Family Process, 29*(3), 229–244. https://doi.org/10.1111/j.1545-5300.1990.00229.x

Rosas, G. M. (2020). Critically accommodating "illegality": Anticipatory losses within mixed-status immigrant families. *Journal of Loss and Trauma, 25*(5), 488–500. https://doi.org/10.1080/15325024.2020.1716162

Solheim, C., Zaid, S., & Ballard, J. (2016). Ambiguous loss experienced by transnational Mexican immigrant families. *Family Process, 55*(2), 338–353. https://doi.org/10.1111/famp.12130

Solheim, C. A., & Ballard, J. (2016). Ambiguous loss due to separation in voluntary transnational families. *Journal of Family Theory & Review, 8*(3), 341–359. https://doi.org/10.1111/jftr.12160

Solheim, C. A., Rojas-Garcia, G., Olson, P. D., & Zuiker, V. S. (2012). Family influences on goals, remittance use, and settlement of Mexican immigrant agricultural workers in Minnesota. *Journal of Comparative Family Studies, 43*(2), 237–259. https://doi.org/10.3138/jcfs.43.2.237

Suárez-Orozco, C., Todorova, I. L. G., & Louie, J. (2002). Making up for lost time: The experience of separation and reunification among immigrant families. *Family Process, 41*(4), 625–643. https://doi.org/10.1111/j.1545-5300.2002.00625.x

Taft, C. T., Walling, S. M., Howard, J. M., & Monson, C. (2011). Trauma, PTSD, and partner violence in military families. In S. M. Wadsworth & D. A. Riggs (Eds.), *Risk and resilience in US military families* (pp. 195–212). Springer. https://doi.org/10.1007/978-1-4419-7064-0_10

Van Hook, J., & Glick, J. E. (2020). Spanning borders, cultures, and generations: A decade of research on immigrant families. *Journal of Marriage and the Family, 82*(1), 224–243. https://doi.org/10.1111/jomf.12621

Vormbrock, J. (1993). Attachment theory as applied to wartime and job-related marital separation. *Child Development, 114*(1), 122–144.

Walsh, T. B. (2017). Mothers and deployment: Understanding the experiences and support needs of deploying mothers of children birth to five. *Journal of Family Social Work, 20*(2), 84–105. https://doi.org/10.1080/10522158.2017.1279576

Winstanley, E. L., & Stover, A. N. (2019). The impact of the opioid epidemic on children and adolescents. *Clinical Therapeutics, 41*(9), 1655–1662. https://doi.org/10.1016/j.clinthera.2019.06.003

Wood, S., Scarville, J., & Gravino, K. (1995). Waiting wives: Separation and reunion among Army wives. *Armed Forces & Society, 21*(2), 217–236.

Zucker, D. M., Dion, K., & McKeever, R. P. (2015). Concept clarification of grief in mothers of children with an addiction. *Journal of Advanced Nursing, 71*(4), 751–767. https://doi.org/10.1111/jan.12591

9

LOSS AND BEREAVEMENT

A Focus on Cancer and Families, Death of a Parent, Death of a Young Child, and Sudden or Violent Death in Families

RESEARCH: JACQUELYN J. BENSON, ABIGAIL J. ROLBIECKI, AND TASHEL C. BORDERE
CLINICAL APPLICATIONS: CADMONA A. HALL, ALLIE ABRAHAM, DENA DINARDO, MARIANNE CELANO, AND ILEANA UNGUREANU

RESEARCH: JACQUELYN J. BENSON, ABIGAIL J. ROLBIECKI, AND TASHEL C. BORDERE

All individuals will undoubtedly experience losses of both minor and major magnitude across their life course (Harvey & Weber, 1998). When a major loss occurs, particularly the loss of a loved one through death, the bereaved are commonly thrust into a period of grieving. *Bereavement* is a broad term used to describe the period of time that occurs after a loss during which grief is experienced. *Grief*, however, is primarily the intrapsychic, emotional response an individual experiences as a reaction to loss (Stroebe et al., 2008). Typical grief reactions can include sadness, numbness, shock, disbelief or denial, anxiety, mourning (i.e., external, public expressions of grief), changes in appetite, lethargy, apathy, intrusive thoughts, difficulty concentrating, and preoccupation with the deceased (e.g., Stroebe et al., 2008). Although grief reactions often overlap with symptoms of depression, anxiety, or posttraumatic stress disorder (PTSD), research suggests these are unique

https://doi.org/10.1037/0000280-009
Treating Contemporary Families: Toward a More Inclusive Clinical Practice, S. Browning and B. van Eeden-Moorefield (Editors)

(Shear, 2012). How a person grieves in response to the loss of a loved one is contingent on several factors, including the personality of the bereaved person; their **coping skills**, support network, psychiatric history, and relationship to the deceased; any unresolved conflict or unfinished business with the deceased; socioeconomic status; and cultural and religious beliefs (Yamashita et al., 2017).

Several stage models of typical grief have been proposed to suggest that grieving is a linear process involving specific and ordered emotional reactions from those who become bereaved or experience loss (Stroebe et al., 2017). However, these models have largely been contested due to a lack of empirical support. Most grief and bereavement scholars do agree that most grief dissipates over time as the loss is gradually accepted and typical daily activities resume (Jacobs, 1993). Although a number of consistent thoughts, feelings, and behaviors typify typical grief reactions (e.g., sadness, yearning, disinterest in daily activities), the patterning of these reactions, as well as the degree of intensity, varies across individuals (Shear, 2012). In many grief responses, intense, omnipresent, and painful feelings of sadness transform into what Shear (2012) described as "acceptance of the inevitability of the loss, integration of its reality into ongoing life, and reimagining a future with the possibility of joy and satisfaction" (p. 2).

Complicated grief, also referred to as abnormal, chronic, traumatic, pathologic, or disordered grief, occurs in individuals who continue to experience elevated levels of grief after approximately 6 to 12 months (PDQ Supportive & Palliative Care Editorial Board, 2020). Complicated grief occurs in about 15% to 30% of bereaved individuals (Bonanno, 2004). Risk factors for complicated grief can include histories of a mood or anxiety disorder, previous trauma or accumulated loss, or an insecure attachment style (Shear, 2012). Certain **types of losses** (e.g., loss of a child, suicide or homicide loss) are associated with higher rates of complicated grief. Ambiguous losses (i.e., those that lack clarity) and the disenfranchisement (i.e., minimization or stigmatization) that can accompany such losses may contribute to a complicated grief experience (e.g., Boss, 2004). Moreover, circumstances of the death can also increase the risk for developing complicated grief, such as being absent at the time of death, ambivalence or conflict surrounding medical decision making, feelings of insecurity or disappointment regarding one's ability to provide comfort to the deceased, or managing their pain before death (Shear, 2012).

Anticipatory grief is another type of grief reaction that occurs in individuals anticipating the impending death of a loved one or their own death. Although anticipatory grief includes many of the same symptoms of grief experienced by bereaved individuals, it can include heightened feelings of ambiguity, frustration or anger, disenfranchised loss, and guilt (e.g., Coelho & Barbosa, 2017). Anticipatory grief may be experienced differently depending on illness and the various types of loss associated with each illness. For example, in a study comparing family caregivers of individuals with cancer to those caring for individuals with dementia (Johansson et al., 2013), cancer caregivers were more preoccupied with thoughts about the illness, found it more difficult to concentrate on work, reported more sleeping problems or episodes of tearfulness, and felt less interested in day-to-day activities. Conversely, dementia caregivers reported feeling more detached from their ill relative.

In this section, we provide a brief review of research on loss and bereavement in families that have experienced loss from cancer, the death of an older parent, the death of a child, or the sudden, violent death of a family member. Specifically, each section includes a description of the loss, including prevalence, and the types of grief associated with the loss. Variation and prevalence in grief types or grief response by age, gender, marital status, personality, and relationship type are also included when data were available (see Table 9.1). The clinical applications section presents a case and

TABLE 9.1. Loss and Bereavement

Evidence-based area of clinical focus	Type of factor	Appropriateness for use across families	Selected references indicating evidence base
Coping skills (problems-based and emotions-based coping)	General	All	Yamashita et al., 2017
Meaning-making	General	All	Neimeyer et al., 2010
Social networks/formal external support	General	All	Robson & Walter, 2013
Circumstances of death (cause; timing; end-of-life environment)	General	All	Walsh & McGoldrick, 2004
Family life-cycle stage	General	All	Malkinson, 2001; Walsh & McGoldrick, 2004
Family-level bereavement (disparate grieving processes among family members)	General	All	Morris et al., 2016
Disenfranchised grief	Unique	Sudden death[a]	Doka, 2002
Anticipatory grief	Unique	Cancer, death of a parent, death of a young child[a]	Overton & Cottone, 2016

[a]The general factor could work for other family types included in this chapter but needs a small adaptation to ensure cultural relevance. Information about potential adaptations is included in the text.

intervention for each family type, and consistent with the research evidence. Psychoeducation plays an important role and is also referenced.

Research Evidence on Loss Associated With Cancer

As the second leading cause of death globally, cancer affects the lives of millions of people; there were an estimated 9.6 million deaths worldwide due to cancer in 2018 (World Health Organization, 2018). In the United States, approximately 16.9 million people were living with a history of cancer at the beginning of 2019. This number is expected to grow to 22.1 million by 2030 (American Cancer Society, 2019). The 2030 projection for the number of U.S. cancer survivors—defined as any persons with a history of cancer from the time of diagnosis through the remainder of their life—is largely due to the growth and aging of the population, as well as early detection and advances in treatment. Indeed, recent statistics suggest that 67% (10.3 million) of cancer survivors in the United States live at least 5 years or more from the time of their diagnosis (Bluethmann et al., 2016). Over the next decade, this number is projected to increase 33%, indicating approximately 15.1 million people.

Grief and loss are a fundamental part of the cancer experience for both the person living with cancer and their family members. In the wake of a cancer diagnoses, patients and their families are faced with the major task of learning how to cope with multiple losses (Block, 2001). The disease itself, treatments, and the side effects of treatments take both a physical and emotional toll on patients and their family caregivers. Common losses associated with living with cancer include a patient's loss of their ability to function independently, loss of professional identity, changes in role definition in the family, cognitive and psychological functioning, aspects of the self, hopes about the future, and the ability to complete plans and projects (Hottensen, 2010). Physical losses—whether symptoms of the cancer itself or side effects of treatment—are particularly numerous and troubling for patients and their caregivers. For example, many patients experience sensory loss or distortion, hair loss, dental problems, weight loss, and diminished muscle tone and bone density (National Cancer Institute, 2020). Relational losses associated with sexual and physical intimacy are also reported (National Cancer Institute, 2020). The most common sexual change for patients is an overall loss of desire, the primary culprit being several common side effects of treatment, such as fatigue, nausea, diarrhea, and constipation (MD Anderson Cancer Center, 2020).

For most cancer survivors and their family members, grief responses are typical (PDQ Supportive and Palliative Care Editorial Board, 2020). Many individuals, including those diagnosed with advanced cancer, report positive consequences as a result of their cancer experience, such as an increased sense of personal growth or **meaning making** (Moreno & Stanton, 2013). For others, the cancer experience can be associated with various patterns of chronic or complicated grief (PDQ Supportive and Palliative Care Editorial Board). As many as 40% of family caregivers experience complicated grief after losing a family member to cancer (Guldin et al., 2012). Some research suggests family caregivers of cancer patients can experience symptoms of complicated grief even before their family member dies (Tomarken et al., 2008). Anticipatory grief, which can be indicative of complicated grief, has been studied among both family caregivers and cancer patients. Approximately 25% of patients with incurable cancer experience anticipatory grief, which commonly mirrors the reactions and signs of distress associated with normal grief (Johnson et al., 2017). However, as many as 26% of family caregivers of cancer patients have been found to be at high risk of complicated, anticipatory grief (Areia et al., 2019).

Age is a common factor in anticipatory grief responses, with both younger caregivers and younger patients reporting higher ratings of anticipatory grief (Tsilika et al., 2009). Several studies have shown that older spouse and nonspouse cancer caregivers report fewer symptoms of anticipatory grief compared with adult child caregivers (e.g., Johansson et al., 2013). Other factors, including being female, having less education, neuroticism, relational dependency, and discomfort with closeness and intimacy, have been shown to place individuals at risk for anticipatory grief (e.g., Burke et al., 2015). However, these studies included samples of individuals and families that were battling other terminal diagnoses besides cancer, such as dementia, and include samples of both adults and children as patients. Moreover, in terms of gender differences, it is important to note that research comparing mothers' and fathers' anticipatory grief responses is largely mixed. Some studies suggest mother's anticipatory grief is significantly greater than father's (Benfield et al., 1976), whereas others report no significant differences (Valizadeh et al., 2013). In light of these findings, it is important to note that empirical investigation on the topic of anticipatory grief has been fraught with controversy and contradiction. Some researchers have argued that the phenomenon does not exist because grief is only experienced in response to a loss by death (Glick et al., 1974). Others have argued that anticipatory grief is adaptive and serves to mitigate grief reactions that will occur after death (e.g., Zisook, 2000). Some, including Lindemann (1994), who introduced the concept in 1944, have argued that anticipatory grief is actually associated with negative outcomes for caregivers (e.g., Levy, 1991). Other studies have demonstrated that anticipatory grief is unrelated to the grief reactions that occur during bereavement (Hill et al., 1988; Roach & Kitson, 1989). Inconsistent findings have been attributed to conceptual confusion, disparate operational definitions, and methodological differences and shortcomings involving untested assumptions, varying samples, instrument validity, and variation in data gathering techniques (Reynolds & Botha, 2006).

Research Evidence on Death of an Older Adult Parent

Although the death of an older adult parent is a common experience and often perceived as a "normative" event, the emotional toll that parental death can exact on adult children can be profound (Umberson, 2003). "Ties between parent and child are often among the longest of the life course. They have spent decades sharing experiences and developing joint views of reality" (Moss & Moss, 1997, p. 347). Thus, although an older parent's death may seem normative or expected due to advanced age, Umberson (2003) argued that the death of a parent "imposes an unexpected crisis for most healthy, well-functioning adults" (p. 7). Umberson (2003) also described how parental death can result in "high levels of psychological distress, increased risk for depression, impaired physical health, or increased alcohol consumption" (p. 7). Research has also shown that gender, age, and marital status can have an effect on these outcomes (Hayslip et al., 2015; Umberson & Chen, 1994). Data from one prospective longitudinal study revealed that a father's death led to more negative outcomes for sons compared with daughters, and daughters experienced more adverse effects as a result of their mother's death compared with sons (Marks et al., 2007). Over a 5-year period, however, having one or both parents deceased was more problematic for daughters' overall well-being compared with sons. Compared with those whose parents were both still alive, sons with one or both parents deceased reported greater declines in physical health over time, whereas daughters reported poorer psychological well-being over time. Regarding age of the adult child, results are mixed, with some studies reporting that younger adults are more affected by parental death than middle-aged adults (Hayslip et al., 2015) and other studies reporting the opposite (Umberson & Chen, 1994). These inconsistent results may be attributed to differential operationalizations of well-being as some researchers used measures assessing hedonic components of well-being (e.g., alcohol consumption) versus others who used measures assessing eudaimonic components (e.g., self-esteem) or self-assessed physical health (Marks et al., 2007). As well, some evidence exists that single or separated adult children experience greater personal distress than their married counterparts (Hayslip et al., 2015). However, decline in marital quality following the death of a parent has been revealed as a significant quantitative and qualitative consequence (Umberson, 1995).

Unfortunately, the perception of parental death as expected and timely for older adults can result in undue suffering on behalf of bereaved adult children if they feel their loss devalued by members of their support network (i.e., **disenfranchised grief**; Robson & Walter, 2013). Indeed, several researchers have argued that the deaths of older people are thought to be less socially disruptive or tragic (e.g., Cortese, 1999). Although the death of an older parent typically brings about adverse psychological effects for most adults, some report experiencing improved functioning or reduced levels of distress (e.g., Umberson & Chen, 1994). Some positive changes in health behaviors (e.g., reduced alcohol consumption, smoking cessation) may result in reaction to a parent's death because an adult child wishes to avoid the same fate as the parent. Moreover, adult children who reported negative childhood memories or characterized their past relationships with parents as dysfunctional or abusive were also more likely to report improved functioning and well-being after experiencing a parental death (Umberson & Chen, 1994).

Research Evidence on Death of a Child

The death of a child is arguably one of the most life-shattering events a family can experience. Bereavement after a child's death is associated with heightened risk for parental depression, anxiety, substance abuse, and other psychiatric morbidities (Rogers et al., 2008). Research has underscored the impact of parental bereavement on socioeconomic factors, citing increased rates of divorce among bereaved parents and early exit from the workforce (Weitzman & Smith-Greenaway, 2020). The unique parent–child relationship, combined with deeply rooted beliefs that parents should not outlive their children, makes bereaved parents particularly vulnerable to complicated grief, which is an intense form of grief that disrupts one's ability to cope after the death (e.g., Lichtenthal et al., 2010).

The experience of bereavement after a child's death is enduring for parents and influences how the family copes and functions cohesively after the death (Nadeau, 2001). That said, the death of a sibling during childhood is also associated with psychological and social consequences, such as depression, anxiety, behavioral health problems, academic issues, relational problems, and increased risk of early mortality (Rostila et al., 2017). Many bereaved siblings have expressed that they feel pressured to suppress their own feelings of grief as a way to protect their parents from further suffering (Horsley & Patterson, 2006). Consequently, bereaved siblings are often referred to as "forgotten mourners" because they are left to navigate not only their own grief but also the weight of their parents' grief (Horsley & Patterson, 2006).

The ways in which parents model their grieving behavior have been found to directly affect the way surviving children react to the death of their sibling (Morris et al., 2016). When bereaved parents choose not to disclose their feelings about the illness or death experience, it affects their ability to make sense of the death, which can have deleterious effects on surviving siblings' postloss functioning (Steffen & Coyle, 2017). Research suggests that family communication about death and illness has been shown to be a protective factor for surviving family members during bereavement. When parents openly express their feelings of sadness with surviving children and discuss how to manage their feelings, it enables them to learn effective ways of communicating about and **coping** with the death and encourages the family to begin the meaning-making process (Davies & Limbo, 2010).

A family's search for meaning in the illness or death experience has been implicated as a key component of the grieving process and is linked to improved post-loss functioning (Nadeau, 2001). Bereavement scholars have increasingly focused their work on the ameliorative impact of family meaning-making following the death of a family member (Lichtenthal & Breitbart, 2015; Nadeau, 2001). These studies demonstrate that when bereaved family members can make meaning of the death, they have a restored sense of purpose and order in their world and are thus better able to cope with the death. Despite this understanding, few researchers have examined the therapeutic benefit of interventions designed to foster family meaning-making through increased communication about the death experience and feelings of grief.

Bereavement care in the United States is underresourced, resulting in a lack of quality and consistent recommendations for how to best support bereaved families. Government-funded research tends to focus on curative relief, rather than large-scale epidemiological studies designed to examine the prevalence and outcomes of bereavement (Mulheron & Inouye, 2020). This contributes to a lack of an evidence base for bereavement interventions in general and more specifically for bereaved families. One way to address this gap is to support agencies in the advancement of the science of family bereavement care.

Additionally, there are numerous societal and cultural norms in the United States that may contribute to our inability to understand the lived experiences of bereaved family members. This, of course, influences our ability to meet the needs of families who are grieving the death of a child. Moreover, grief is generally considered a healthy response to bereavement, and some bereavement experts believe that intervening with the normal grieving trajectory can actually cause unnecessary harm for the bereaved (Jordan & Neimeyer, 2003). There are a minority of people, however, whose grief extends beyond the normal time of healing and who experience prolonged complicated grief (Rosner, 2015). Due to these norms and lack of quality evidence-based bereavement care, these individuals and families fall through the cracks. Despite these limitations, there is a growing body of literature that suggests early, targeted intervention for bereaved families is the best source of prevention for complicated grief postdeath (Jordan & Neimeyer, 2003; Rosner, 2015).

Research Evidence on Sudden, Violent Loss

Grief related to sudden, violent deaths in homicide and suicide must be contextualized in understanding outcomes for bereaved children and families. Deaths by gun violence are highest among youth residing in urban and rural communities (Centers for Disease Control and Prevention, 2017). Firearm-related deaths by homicide are highest among Black male youth in urban communities, whereas rates of gun violence in completed suicides are highest among White male youth in rural areas. Parallels exist in deaths by homicide and suicide that have important implications for grief and coping processes among bereaved children and families. Grief may be complicated in deaths by homicide and suicide due to the suddenness of the deaths, lack of recognition (Doka, 1989), social stigma and discrimination (Bordere, 2016, 2019), and mode of death (i.e., non–health-related, preventable). Further, details surrounding deaths by homicide and suicide may be ambiguous or unknown (Boss, 2010) and thus particularly difficult to process and explain to young children.

Grief may also be complicated for children by factors such as nature of relationship to the deceased, prior coping, parental grief (Bugge et al., 2014), poverty and access to social capital, and trauma and loss histories. For example, in a study of predominantly White youth (79%), aged 2 to 12 years with multiple trauma histories (witnessing violence, traumatic grief), Eslinger et al. (2015) found that emotional stress was externally expressed through behavior problems (see also Labar & LeDoux, 2001). Children reared in communities of pervasive violence may be exposed to multiple, cumulative, sudden violence, trauma, and grief across childhood and adolescence (Bordere, 2009). Several researchers have found that traumatic experiences in childhood negatively affect outcomes (PTSD, depression) in adulthood (Briere et al., 2008).

Despite findings on childhood trauma and factors associated with complicated grief in sudden violent loss, a paucity of research addresses outcomes for children bereaved by the deaths of significant persons through homicide and suicide loss. Most research in childhood bereavement focuses on health-related deaths of parents and siblings among largely White youth populations with limited attention to the diverse, co-occurring losses differentially affecting youth of color. An exception is Jenkins et al.'s (2014) study of loss and traumatic grief among Black youth, aged 11 to 15, bereaved both by health-related deaths and violent death losses. Participants reported the death losses of friends, fathers (50%), and siblings related to gun violence as well as health-related death losses of people about whom they cared. Forty-six percent of participants reported the health-related deaths of grandparents or great-grandparents who often function as major sources of support (emotional, social) and socialization of children in Black families. Findings indicated that Black youth experienced trauma around both **types of loss**. For both girls and boys, childhood traumatic grief (CTG) scores were related to lower academic achievement, PTSD, depression, and anxiety. For boys, CTG scores were related to externalizing behaviors.

Summary

Research on loss, grief, and bereavement has bloomed in recent decades. As a result of this upswell in bereavement-related studies, critical inquiry and discussion about theory, clinical practice, and research methods have followed, transforming what we know about the human experience of grief (Neimeyer, 2004). In this chapter, we briefly reviewed the empirical literature on bereavement in families facing losses related to cancer, the death of a child, the death of an older parent, and sudden, violent loss. What we can glean from this collective work is an appreciation for the inimitable experiences of bereaved individuals and families in terms of their response to loss. Although bereavement is certainly one of life's most difficult trials, in time most of us overcome the challenges and heartbreak that we face throughout the grieving process. For some, however, grief can be prolonged, resulting in heightened distress, mental health issues, and increased risk for mortality (Shear, 2012).

CLINICAL APPLICATIONS: CADMONA A. HALL, ALLIE ABRAHAM, DENA DINARDO, MARIANNE CELANO, AND ILEANA UNGUREANU

Clinical Expertise and Interpretation of Evidence: An Overview

In this section of the chapter, we provide an overview of grief and loss with the intention of aiding clinicians in their work with the bereaved. The information, informed by the research evidence and our clinical expertise, provides an understanding of how families experience specific losses as well as clear implications and patterns that are typically present for systemic evaluation and intervention. Clinical vignettes are used to demonstrate the application of empirically evidenced treatment. Although much of what is presented in this chapter applies to many types of losses, we focus on those specific to loss from cancer, the death of a parent, the death of a child, and the sudden, violent death of a family member. Each section includes family dynamics, systemic assessment, and interventions designed to assist the reader with supporting bereaved families.

The discussion of death, although it is a normal and natural part of the life cycle, is often avoided within (North American) societal values. Grief and loss are universal experiences, yet many are unprepared and unaccompanied through the process. At this point in history, many people are removed from a healthy or helpful acknowledgment of the full cycle of life. Most people do not grow their own food or raise livestock, processes that in the past allowed one to witness the life cycle in various ways. In addition, North American value systems have created a death-denying society through advances in science, medicine, and health care, as well as a cultural obsession with youth. Additional values of individualism, strength, and mastery rather than vulnerability continue to create challenges for the bereaved. The practical realities of loss, dying, and death are typically avoided until families are forced to confront them. Even in the midst of shared cultural loss due to increased attention on social injustice such as mass shootings, police brutality and murder, terrorism, and COVID-19, there is an absence of the acknowledgment of grief, loss, and the process of bereavement.

North American cultural values create a climate with a mixed message; death is often sensationalized, even televised, but bereavement and healing are ignored. Knowing and understanding how these values are threaded through the culture aids therapists in understanding the multilayered experiences of clients with whom they are working. Some of these myths include the idea that grief should not be discussed, the bereaved prefer to mourn in private, time heals all wounds, and children are too young to mourn. These myths often leave the bereaved isolated and disconnected at a time when they need the most social connection and support.

Loss is a normal part of experiencing life, and most people learn developmental strategies for how to care for the feelings associated with the loss of what is valued. *Grief* refers to the emotions, thoughts, and behaviors associated with loss. *Mourning* refers to the outward expression of the internal experience, it describes the outward rituals and demonstrations of the grief (i.e., spiritual ceremonies, tattoos, arm bands, wearing of specific colored clothes, or an indicator on the outside of a family home). It is typical for families to grieve both nondeath as well as death related losses. Nondeath losses might be functional or emotional in nature, such as the loss of a job, home, declines in health, as well as losses associated with shattered assumptions such as violations of trust, safety, or fairness and questioning spiritual beliefs. Common emotional, physical, and behavioral responses, as described in the research section require therapist familiarity with grief to name and explore.

Clinical Expertise and Interpretation of Evidence: Grief Framework

Developed by Stroebe and Schut (2015), the dual process model–revised (DPM-R) provides a context for understanding the emotional and functional needs of bereaved families. As reflected in the research section, the DPM-R suggests healthy functioning requires individual and familial adaptations to the loss to move toward healing for bereaved families. According to the DPM-R, **coping** requires tending to two separate but connected elements of healing; the first is those behaviors, thoughts, and emotions directly connected to the loss and the second involves the developmental tasks associated with the new life circumstances. Healthy grief and loss necessitate tending to both elements.

Dimensions of Culture

Grief and loss are universal experiences; however, the **meaning making** of these experiences is influenced by many factors, including family structure, previous history, context, and dimensions of culture. Recognizing the diversity of life experiences due to different positionality of dimensions of culture (e.g., race, gender, sexual orientation, class, age, spirituality, ethnicity, disability, nationality, language) is critical to providing culturally sensitive service to the bereaved. Recognizing the need for social justice in therapy means understanding and assessing how power dynamics, privilege, and marginalization affect the family, and how these dynamics influence the nature of the death and the family's meaning-making and process toward healing (Ungureanu & Hall, 2020). Therapeutic intervention must explore the cultural rituals for dying and commemorating the deceased. Assessment and processing with clients how each dimension of culture informs not only bereavement but the interactional patterns of healthy family functioning is key.

Self of the Therapist

To effectively intervene with clients, it is critical for therapists to address their own experiences of grief and loss. The ability to home in on the needs of clients is directly related to the therapist's ability to recognize their own strengths and growth areas, given that therapists are not immune to the cultural myths associated with grief. Ungureanu and Hall (2020) recommended that therapists explore their thoughts, beliefs, attitudes, and biases about grief and loss and consider exploring the following questions: What are your beliefs about death and dying? What do you believe happens after death? Where do these beliefs come from? What are your beliefs about the right and wrong ways to die, grieve, and heal? How do these beliefs inform your thoughts about different types and causes of death (via suicide, disease, or violence)? How do your dimensions of culture inform your thoughts, beliefs, and expression of grief? It is recommended that therapists evaluate their own knowledge, familiarity, familial history, and experiences of loss. There are several ways to accomplish this such as (a) creating a genogram and exploring the stories and beliefs about death, dying, grief, and loss within their family; (b) journaling or creating a timeline of death and nondeath losses experienced; and (c) using case-consultation and supervision to support the emotional and clinical skills working with the bereaved require. The next sections are designed to aid the therapist in conceptualization and application of the bereavement information presented earlier and in Benson et al.'s research section of this chapter. The authors have selected examples from their clinical work to provide the reader with an overview of common dynamics associated with the type of loss, systemic assessment, and interventions that facilitate healing.

Clinical Expertise and Interpretation of Evidence: Loss Associated With Cancer

For many individuals and families, navigating cancer can be an isolating experience in which each member of the family has their own complex reaction. The importance of normalizing grief reactions in the face of cancer is paramount for treatment success. Families are often charged with making critical decisions at a time in their life when they are the most emotionally flooded (i.e., overwhelmed by the multitude of emotions described in the research section). Naming the importance of receiving emotional support before and after loss is essential for all involved. Additionally, it is typical for there to be an incongruence in grieving style among family members; identifying that grief reactions will vary is a crucial factor in mediating family conflict. As indicated by Walsh and McGoldrick (2004), a major component of the grief process is adapting to the multiple changes and losses on the horizon. It is important to identify the many feelings that will emerge in response to such significant shifts.

Clinical Experience: Observations of Common Interactional Patterns

Although grief is an expected part of bereavement, both the person diagnosed with cancer and their family members are susceptible to both anticipatory and complicated grief. **Anticipatory grief** refers to grief responses that occur before the death, where in addition to grieving the impending death, the griever is also experiencing the nondeath losses that occur (Overton & Cottone, 2016). Families coming to therapy may have limited or no opportunity in which to name and process the impact of anticipatory grief because society has little room to acknowledge loss outside of death. Living with cancer also necessitates learning to live with increasing experiences of loss, such as assumptive losses of what the future will bring and physical loss as health and bodily functioning declines (Hottensen, 2010). Many may experience overt invalidation of their experiences by well-wishers who suggest they should "focus on their loved one while they are still alive." Anticipatory grief may not always occur and may not prevent the experience of grief after a death or shorten the bereavement process.

The experience of grief is both intrapsychic and outwardly expressed through mourning. If one feels that expression of the grief experience is stigmatized on a societal or familial level, patterns of internalization, avoidance, dissociation, or anger are likely to occur. Furthermore, nondeath losses associated with cancer (i.e., multiple surgeries, bodily functioning, job, independence) may be disenfranchised, meaning people receive limited or no social support and their grief goes unacknowledged (Doka, 2002).

Role shifts and losses are inevitable for the person living with cancer and their family, and they are far reaching, having an impact on the relational, emotional, physical, and occupational health of each person in some fashion. When shifts and losses emerge in the system, homeostasis is disrupted. This is a crucial time in the family's functioning. The family's response to this major disruption is a testament to how they have navigated other significant systemic shifts. Stable families with clear communication may grow during stressful periods, whereas unstable families often become more chaotic during stress.

Some family members might function by compensating for other family members who are more avoidant of the changes at hand. This might be observed as a family caregiver overfunctioning or feeling overly protective of their loved one with cancer while another family member takes on a more detached position, proceeding with their normal routine and believing that there is no need for concern. Others might work together and adaptively integrate new roles into their understanding of the system. For adult child caregivers, this role negotiation might lead to feeling burdened or frustrated at having to take on new roles and responsibilities. The experience of observing the shifts and losses for the loved one with cancer can be traumatic.

For the person living with cancer, these shifts will likely be experienced as losses. As they are physically decreasing in functioning, so too is their autonomy. The person living with cancer might view this period of change as an opportunity to become closer to family members and resolve unfinished business, or the opposite can occur, with the patient responding to attempts at connection with rejection, in hopes of protecting themselves and/or their loved ones from the pain of their impending death.

The response to role shifts and losses will often mirror the family's **coping strategies**, overall relational connection, and level of resilience in adapting to major change. The family's preexisting functioning will be important in how successfully they adapt to crises. Important family themes during this time include empathy, compromise, and communication. Families that can empathize with their loved one with cancer, as well as other family members; facilitate compromise in role responsibilities; and openly communicate thoughts and feelings will be most successful. Additional stressors that affect families include different perspectives regarding medical treatment and negotiating caregiving roles. In addition, long-term care has a significant impact on financial status.

Case Context: Characteristics, Culture, and Preferences

Michael, Charmaine, and their adult daughter, Demetria, are an African American family who attended therapy at the recommendation of Charmaine's medical provider after her diagnosis of metastatic breast cancer. The presenting problems include Demetria's frustration and disappointment with what she described as her father's lack of urgency regarding her mother's health. Charmaine's symptoms developed slowly and became so common that both she and her husband avoided them for several years. The diagnosis occurred when Demetria visited and witnessed her mother's symptoms. Since the diagnosis, Demetria has moved back home to take primary responsibility for accompanying her mother to her medical appointments. Subsequently, Michael has taken on the responsibilities of maintaining their home, as Charmaine has become less capable of participating in these activities.

Clinical Decisions: Intervention Implementation

The intake session began by exploring the illness story and discussing relational factors contributing to distress. The therapist was especially mindful of interpersonal interactions and carefully listened for themes of **anticipatory grief** in the dialogue of the family. Covert expressions of anticipatory grief may manifest as anger, blame, denial, or sadness. The therapist's major responsibility was to normalize different grief expressions and disrupt dichotomous beliefs about how one should grieve.

Systemic assessment according to the DPM-R indicated this family struggled with the developmental tasks associated with developing new strategies of emotional expression and connection, accepting the changed needs within the family, and engaging in non–grief-related family interactions. The therapist assessed and reflected patterns of interaction that emerged related to role shifts and losses. Each family member was prompted to express their internal experience navigating such shifts, ultimately helping to increase empathic perspective-taking among the family members. When blame statements were made, such as Michael internalizing blame for Charmaine's illness, the therapist validated the emotions while broadening the experience to the family system:

> Michael, it is not uncommon to look for control in situations that feel uncontrollable, but I suspect you know that this is not your fault. It is nobody's fault. I think underneath the feelings of blame that you all reference in some way, there is a lot of fear. I wonder if we could talk more about that.

A therapeutic challenge was to raise this issue of blame and move it from covert to overt so that it could be appropriately addressed within the system. In addition, this created an opportunity to challenge Demetria and Michael's belief that Charmaine was too fragile to address the blame and shame present in the family. The therapist was curious about the role of blame and its purpose, asking how blame might be contributing in helpful and harmful ways.

Subsequent sessions were designed to address triangulation that occurred— first, between Demetria, Charmaine, and the cancer; and second, between Charmaine, Michael, and the cancer. How might Michael and Demetria be depriving themselves from the empathy and validation they could provide to each other as the only two people in the system tending to the same dynamic. In what ways might Charmaine benefit from the emotional cutoff between her husband and daughter? How might this covert blame distract them from addressing other needs, worries, and concerns that are more frightening? Challenging this unhelpful alliance highlighted for the family that there was another option for the three of them to come together, with cancer being the shared obstacle that all three united to fight against. Following an intervention focused on the shifts, losses, and underlying fear, an inevitable shift in dynamic occurred. The therapist helped the family access a different layer in the dialogue. This created a space where more clinical depth and vulnerability was accessed, ultimately encouraging the family to openly communicate these fears and concerns to facilitate greater connection.

Later sessions focused on strengthening the relationship between Michael and Demetria. These sessions created space for the two to acknowledge their worries and fears and to develop a plan to reach out to extended family for additional support. The therapist also met with Charmaine and Michael separately for several sessions. She helped them explore relationship patterns and new ways to create intimacy. Family sessions resumed to continue to help the family make sense of the anticipated losses collectively and to prepare for upcoming decisions, which included advance directives.

Clinical Expertise and Interpretation of Evidence: Death of a Parent

The healing process for family members after the loss of a parent requires deep, contextual consideration to ensure a functional and effective treatment process. Although literature exists to generally guide clinicians through this process, it often misses the opportunity for the nuanced healing that personalized grief and loss therapy can offer. For these interventions to be successful, therapists must engage in an individualized learning process about the role of the deceased parent, pre- and postmortem communication patterns, unresolved emotional challenges involving the deceased, and divergent aspects of the grief process for the remaining family members (Yamashita et al., 2017).

Clinical Experience: Observations of Common Interactional Patterns
The role of the parent in the family dynamic is a critical point of exploration as the family members move through the healing process. Given that the parent–child relationship is often the longest relationship of the adult child's life, strong bonds are formed around that relationship that significantly influence the identity development of the child. As such, this loss can result in children feeling that they have lost parts of themselves with the loss of their parent, even though such a loss is considered a normative part of the life cycle. It may leave an adult child feeling that they no longer have the support system they once had, the ear they often needed, the perspective they sought, or the person who reminded them about how to take care of themselves and plan for the future.

As a result, adult children may neglect parts of their psychological, physical, or relational health, thereby developing secondary symptoms that could inadvertently serve to distract them from the loss. For example, research shows that adult children often experience increased psychological distress leading to an increase in the use of alcohol (Umberson, 2003). In this example, it may be more tolerable for a son to deal with the backlash at work as a result of showing up late several days in a row from being hungover than it would be to think about or focus on the ways he misses his father. Alternatively, it may be easier for an adult daughter to deal with her husband's disappointment over how much wine she has been drinking since the loss of her mother than it would be for her to focus on the cause of the increase in drinking.

The therapist is also tasked with learning the communication patterns of the family and exploring how they compare with patterns before the loss. Often, communication difficulties are assumed to be "a result of" the trauma surrounding the loss when, in fact, they are most often a mere extension of the communication and emotional processing challenges that existed before the loss. Understanding how the family communicated before the death of the parent thus becomes a critical part in treating the family during the grief process. Once this is discovered, therapists can work to find ways to gently and creatively reveal these aspects of the family back to themselves to correct the false belief that the difficulties are a result of the loss. This type of expanded awareness reduces the feeling of "stuckness" and enables the therapeutic process to loosen the knots that have been further tightened as a result of the loss.

Therapy must attend to the pre- and postmortem alliances that have formed in the family subsystem. The alliance(s) that the deceased parent was a part of can leave the remaining member of that respective subsystem feeling less secure, while the disruption of the alliance may create greater security for other family members. For example, a father may have a close alliance with his oldest daughter, whereas a younger daughter may have a strong alliance with her mother. When the father dies, the oldest daughter may not only be affected by his death, but also by the alienation she may experience as a result of not being a part of the alliance between her mother and her younger sister. These types of structural components in a family can exacerbate feelings of resentment and jealousy between the siblings as they are also **coping** with the grief of the deceased parent.

Depending on each family member's relationship with the deceased parent, a clear and balanced retrospect of the positive and negative attributes of the parent may be unreachable by the grieving family members. Complicating the healing process, this potential imbalance requires intensive time and tenderness when the family feels stuck in recalling who the parent was to each family member. Speaking about the deceased parent in a negative way can be triggering for some who wish to remember or think only of the positive aspects of the parent, whereas a positive appraisal experienced by family members who had a more negative relationship with the deceased could be quite triggering.

An awareness of the unresolved emotional conflicts that existed before the loss of a parent is also an essential component of the overall conceptualization of a family's grief process. It is highly common for family members to feel stuck in that they will never be able to resolve conflicts that existed before the death. They will often perseverate on not having addressed challenges when they thought they should have or when not having said the things that would have resolved a conflict in some way. These thoughts can initiate or exacerbate guilt, which is often a key variable in the stuckness, preventing family members from emotionally moving in a forward direction. As a result, the bereavement process is not only the loss of the parent but the fantasies of events that might have organically resolved the conflicts, such as future weddings, grandchildren, and trips.

Feelings of anger, resentment, and disappointment can often emerge in a family when individuals do not understand or recognize the way their family members are processing their grief. Binary thinking becomes prominent, perpetuating the idea that there is a "right" or "wrong" way to move through the process. As such, it is important to learn about the different ways in which each member of the family is processing the grief because these differences can create significant obstacles in keeping the family dynamics healthy and functional. Resentment may arise toward those who are seemingly moving through the grief "too quickly," resulting in other family members feeling "behind" or "alone" in their process if it is slower or more difficult. Diving deeper into each individual's process may exposes that the "quicker" person may not be healing faster than the slower one but merely avoiding or numbing. Understanding that each person will process grief at their own pace and in their own way is critical for healing the family as a whole.

Understanding variations in processing is especially important for children who witness the living parent "moving on," which may include removing personal items from the home or even exploring new romantic relationships. Children, even adult children, may have a difficult time experiencing how the living parent processes grief, especially if they have never witnessed the living parent suffer such a significant loss. The living parent's **coping mechanisms** derive directly from coping styles that existed during the relationship and even well before. Through the use of a genogram the therapist can help the family identify adaptive strategies for moving forward in treatment. Working with the family and allowing each member to learn more about how each person is processing grief can help to normalize the experience and debunk the myths associated with dichotomous thinking.

Case Context: Characteristics, Culture, and Preferences

Amira, 36, is a South Asian American who entered therapy by herself, sharing that she wished to have some support given her father's (Omar, 62) sudden death 3 months earlier. In addition, she asked for help figuring out how to communicate with her widowed mother, Mariam, 59, and sister, Kayla, 39. She reported that neither her mother nor her sister understood her and that they're "not taking the loss seriously." Last, she shared that mother and sister are "reticent to begin family therapy with her because they do not appreciate her chronic emotional outbursts."

Clinical Decisions: Intervention Implementation

Amira believed she and her mother would never be able to successfully resolve disagreements because the only way they were able to do so in the past was through Omar's facilitation. Thinking systemically, the therapist framed the problem relationally:

> It sounds like it's important to you to bridge this gap in the relationship with your mom and sister. The best way to do this is to have them here and present for the process; it's hard to work on relationships without them. Since you're all grieving have them join us for the healing.

Solidly joining from within the system, the therapist was positioned to temporarily assume the role of the father and support Mariam, Amira, and Kayla through difficult conversations in the present. Although a temporary reliance would be formed with the therapist for this communication to be healthy and effective, the strategy also entailed a communication technique that could ultimately be sustained directly between mother and daughter(s), beyond the course of the family treatment.

The therapist was well positioned to discuss the process of how Omar supported communication between his wife and daughter(s), to increase awareness about his function, how and why it developed, what it achieved, and how new patterns could support a more functional communication structure. For example, Mariam had begun getting rid of her late husband's clothes, tools, and hobby equipment, which left Kayla feeling like her mother was not grieving the loss of her husband. On a deeper level, Amira also felt that her mother was rejecting her, not recognizing that their ability to maintain a close and committed relationship hinged on Omar's presence and ability to "help them" communicate with one another. This represents emotional challenges that existed before the loss but were unrecognized, as is often the case, because family members do not analyze their communication processes unless a need presents or are forced.

The interventions necessary for this particular family focused on the restoration portion of the DPM-R. The family struggled to develop new communication patterns in Omar's absence and the role he played while living. In addition to making Omar's role in the communication patterns overt, the therapist worked to support direct communication between the family members, beginning with having the family members share increasingly emotionally congruent information directly to the therapist. The therapist could then begin to ask questions about the different grief expressions to Miriam: "How has organizing and giving away Omar's belongings affected you?" "How did you decide now was the time to begin the process?" "I'm curious about what felt helpful and what felt hard?" To further expand the conversation, the therapist could then ask, "What's it like describing your emotional experience in front of your daughters?" "What would you like them to understand?" "How do you think they were affected by your decision?" Here the therapist generated curiosity and clarification. Next, the therapist asked Amira how her emotional expression connected to that of her mother. "Are there any ways where you and your mom grieve in similar ways?" "What would it be like to share with your sister and mom what's been going on for you?" "What would you need to believe they could listen and try to understand?" Last, the therapist engaged Kayla by asking, "How does your grief weave through your sister and mother's grieving styles?" "When do you feel safe sharing your own experience?" "What about your sharing this vulnerability with your family, could help you feel more connected to them?" Family members are then encouraged to respond with curiosity and validation. As the family developed greater skill in recognizing each other's pain, the therapists began to transition the family members to converse directly, slowly moving from the center to the outside of the dialogue. Potential questions include the following: "Can the three of you talk together about ways you grieve together and times you grieve alone?" "How has gender informed your expectations of how you're supposed to grieve?" "How have you all shared experiences together that have given you space away from your grief?" "Can you talk about the kind of grief breaks you've taken?" "What has not been shared with each other that would be important for the other members to know?"

Clinical Expertise and Interpretation of Evidence: Death of a Child

The death of a child is a devastating and obscene loss. Lisa Belkin (2010) captured the blasphemy of this loss in her article "Life After a Child Dies" in *The New York Times*: "There is no word in the English language for a parent who loses child. When our parents die, we are orphans. When our spouse dies, we are widowed. When a child dies, we are speechless." A child's death is unique among losses because it is untimely, occurring at the wrong end of the human developmental trajectory, thus yielding prolonged mourning as caregivers grieve during the child's missed developmental milestones (e.g., when the child would have graduated from high school). Support seeking during bereavement is complicated by the fact that a child's death is an almost universally feared experience; friends and even health care providers may have difficulty allowing themselves the empathy needed to be emotionally present for grieving parents. And, as noted in Benson et al.'s research review in this chapter, the death of a child is a shattering experience for the entire family, including siblings.

Clinical Experience: Observations of Common Interactional Patterns
As in other types of losses, there is wide variation among families in the nature, intensity, and timing of grief responses. This variation may be due, in part, to the **age of the child at the time of death, how the child died, the quality of the marital or coparenting relationship, and whether there are other children in the family.** Within families, there are often **individual differences in grieving related to developmental, psychological, and cultural factors**; for example, young children grieve differently from parents. However, the death of a child also affects the family system, changing family roles or ways in which members interact with one another. In addition, preexisting patterns within the family affect the mourning process for its members and for the family as a whole. These two processes can exist simultaneously and recursively; for example, previously adaptive communication patterns may become rigid or exaggerated in the face of loss, contributing to distance or conflict within the family, which in turn can cause family members to withdraw more from one another.

Many families show resilience in mourning the death of a child, reorganizing roles or improving communication patterns to support individual members through the grieving process while strengthening relationship bonds over time. Other families struggle to support one another or even stay together. Although there are many ways in which families can buckle under the pressure of loss, three potentially overlapping systemic formulations are discussed here.

The first formulation occurs when one partner may be paralyzed by grief, while the other partner appears less affected by the loss. This discrepancy may be due to psychological and cultural differences between the caregivers or to relational factors. One parent may withhold, or delay displays of grief to compensate for the more expressive and distressed partner. As a result, parents' grief reactions appear "out of sync," or incongruent, contributing to perceived isolation, misunderstanding, and tension in the couple relationship. Second, one parent copes with grief by relying on maladaptive strategies (e.g., drinking, drug use, overworking, extramarital affairs), which leads to conflict within the relationship when the maladaptive coping is confronted or to distance and tension when it is not. The subsequent partner may assume the maladaptive coping is disconnected from the loss, resulting in fear, confusion, and anger, for example and may create additional relational injuries. Third, the couple attempts to subdue their grief by redirecting anxiety on surviving children. Parents also may distract from their grief by adopting or giving birth to another child, thereby delaying the grieving process or prolonging it. Alternatively, ambivalence about sexual intimacy, childrearing, and family planning may lead to tension in the couple's relationship.

Case Context: Characteristics, Culture, and Preferences
Clara and Juan are a Latinx couple who requested an evaluation of their 9-year-old daughter, Millie, 10 months after the death of their 13-year-old son, Luiz. Presenting problems included social isolation and declining grades in school. Luiz had died in a cycling accident; he had been crossing an intersection when he was hit by a truck, causing fatal injuries. Since the accident, Millie had refused to ride her bike, see friends, or even go outside. During the evaluation, the therapist learned that all family members were having difficulty grieving Luiz's loss. Juan expressed considerable anger about the lack of criminal charges against the truck driver and was actively pursuing a civil suit. Clara had stopped playing tennis and dropped most of her social activities, preferring to spend time with her two remaining children. Robby, age 6, was whining more and had started sleeping in his parents' bed.

As part of Millie's evaluation, the therapist met with the couple. During this meeting Clara expressed her concern that Juan was "obsessed with the lawsuit," drinking regularly in the evenings, and generally not emotionally available to her and the kids. She admitted feeling "depressed and lonely" but said she had difficulty sharing her grief with Juan. Juan expressed anger, disbelief, and guilt about Luiz's death, as he was the one who had taught Luiz to ride a bike and encouraged his independent cycling. He admitted drinking to numb himself from the pain. He cried in a jagged, abrupt manner, accepting physical comfort from his wife, who shed quiet tears as she held him.

Clinical Decisions: Intervention Implementation
In a subsequent session, the therapist shared the systemic formulation stating, "It seems like as a couple you've become 'stuck' in a relationship pattern that makes it difficult for everyone in the family to get the support they needed

to grieve Luiz's death." Both parents had withdrawn from one another, causing them to feel isolated in their grief, particularly in the context of limited social support outside the family. This isolation had led Clara to seek comfort from Robby, Juan to quietly escalate his drinking, and Millie to withdraw from her friends. The couple agreed to therapy to help them change this pattern, improve their communication and connection, and model more adaptive **coping** for Robby and Millie. According to the DPM-R, intervention for this family would tend toward oscillation between loss and restoration, initially focusing on supporting relational expressions of emotion and then developing healthy strategies to address the changed needs as well as the development of new roles.

Early treatment sessions were devoted to helping all four family members express their grief and receive emotional support from one another. The therapist provided some education about grief (e.g., variation in grief responses), normalized family members' emotional reactions, and asked them about Luiz. Questions posed during this time include the following: "Who in the family can tell me a little about Luiz? I'd like to get to know him through your stories." "What was he like as a son and as a brother?" "What happens in the family when someone is feeling sad?" "How do other people respond?" "Are there any rules about how you're allowed to feel and what you're allowed to do when you have thoughts and feelings about Luiz' death?" "What are your culturally significant rituals for grieving?" "How do these rituals feel helpful, and in what ways might they be confining?" "What do you believe about where Luiz is?" "How do you think families heal after the death of a loved one?"

With the therapist's help, the parents were able to encourage the children to resume their normal activities and to help Robby to sleep in his own bed. Clara joined a grief support group for parents and enrolled Robby and Millie in a 1-week summer bereavement camp. Millie's mood improved, and she began to play with friends again.

Later sessions were held primarily with the couple, as Clara and Juan continued to struggle with communication and distancing in their relationship. As Clara received more support outside the family, she began to challenge Juan's drinking. In one session she told Juan, "I feel like I've lost both Luiz and you!" A week later, when she found Juan on the couch passed out from drinking at 6 p.m., she threatened to take both kids and move out if he didn't get help. He subsequently enrolled in outpatient substance abuse treatment and joined AA.

The remaining sessions were devoted to support Juan's sobriety, improving the couple's intimacy and communication, and helping both partners find meaning in their son's death. Questions that began to address the couple dilemmas were as follows: "How has loving Luiz but losing him affected your parenting?" "How has guilt and shame as parents prevented you from turning toward each other for comfort and solace?" "What would it mean to forgive yourself and each other?" "What does intimacy and connection look like for you? What do you want it to look like?" "Is there room for the two of you to grieve differently and yet support each other? Can you describe how you'll know when this is happening?" "Even though Luiz isn't here, he'll always be your son. Are there ways you want to honor him individually and together?" "I wonder if your children might need your help in finding special ways to memorialize Luiz, too?" "How might it be possible to have a good life and look forward to the future while still loving and missing Luiz?" Juan was surprised that the civil suit settlement did not bring him the satisfaction and relief he had hoped for. Clara explained that the accident had challenged her faith because bad things are not supposed to happen to good people who obey the laws, and Luiz had been wearing a helmet. He had also been wearing headphones, listening to music while he rode his bike. Juan and Clara decided to advocate for a new state law prohibiting cyclists' use of listening devices in both ears, and in the following year, "Luiz's Law" was passed by their state legislature.

Clinical Expertise and Interpretation of Evidence: Sudden and Violent Death

A *sudden death* is a death that occurs without warning; it is unexpected and is usually due to accidents, medical situations, or violent deaths through suicide or homicide (i.e., **circumstances**). Usually, sudden deaths are more complicated to grieve, and the bereaved may have symptoms of PTSD through exposure to the unexpected death of a loved one. It complicates the grieving process because it comes without warning that the death is imminent. A violent death, one that happens at the hands of the person (suicide) or by others (homicide), complicates mourning even more by the unnaturalness of the means.

Clinical Experience: Observations of Common Interactional Patterns

Survivors of a violent death may go through a different type of mourning than survivors of a loved one who died after a long battle with an illness. The **anticipatory loss** that families may experience while witnessing a family member dealing with a medical disease is completely absent in a sudden, violent death. There are some specific aspects that are characteristic to grieving a violent death. This type of death shatters a person's **meaning**

making at different levels in a way that is similar to how trauma affects individuals (Janoff-Bulman, 1992).

Family members who experienced a loved one's death by homicide may question assumptions about the world being a benevolent, predictable place. After receiving the news of a violent death, there is a sense of unreality; it may be difficult to make sense of the loss, leading to prolonged experiences of shock and numbness. They may also wonder about what they could have done to prevent the event: "If only I went with him on that trip," "If we wouldn't have had that stupid fight, she would not have stormed out of the house and been run over by that car," leaving the survivors with both a sense of guilt and helplessness. Assumptions about omnipotence and benevolence of God can be shattered as well. Religion and spirituality, important **coping mechanisms** in dealing with violent deaths, can be lost as a resource because of an inability to make meaning of either a perceived impotence of God, or even worst, a nonloving, punishing one. Guilt can also be projected in blame on other people in the family or on institutions: "If they would mark the stop signs more clearly, accidents wouldn't happen," "If his mother would have done a better job teaching him how to be safe in the streets, he wouldn't have ended up shot dead." The emotional experience can be manifested through intense anger and rage that is felt at the perpetrator of death and a desire for justice.

Assessment of the family system dynamics before the loss, especially those directly involving the deceased, is critically important. A more distant or a conflictual relationship between the deceased and other family members can further complicate the bereavement process. A family that has organizational flexibility before death will most likely be able to adjust in a healthier way than a family that had fixed roles and boundaries. For example, when a primary breadwinner is lost to a sudden, violent death, it can create a crisis in the family that can have an impact on both the bereavement and the family sustainability, which will further impede grief. The way the family can use their flexibility to adjust by accessing resources from outside, either extended family or nonfamily related community, becomes significant for the material and emotional health of its members. A similar situation can happen when the person charged with the emotional well-being of the family is lost. Although each loss is significant, the consequences of a loss may be more on the relational level or instrumental.

Another characteristic of violent and sudden death is the "unfinished business" (Worden, 2018) left behind—regrets about all the words left unsaid, or the grudges held that were not resolved. When death is anticipated, there is the potential to resolve unfinished business before the loss.

An aspect that plays a role in delaying bereavement many times in violent deaths is the involvement of judicial processes. Often families hope for justice; however, the judicial system is an adversarial process with no guarantees of fairness. Furthermore, the anger and rage can manifest in violent acts of the survivors, especially when there is a sense of justice not being served. The anger and rage serve to counteract the helplessness at preventing the loss of a loved one as well as reestablishing the assumption that the world is a just place.

Issues of social injustice can be present and complicate grief even more, such as the numerous examples of victims and surviving families of police brutality. In addition, to individual and family aspects of violent death described so far, there is the factor of racialized trauma and inequality that can further add posttraumatic stress disorder symptoms to further complicate the grieving process. Many of these violent deaths go unacknowledged by the public, and families are left with limited recourse and ways to seek justice.

Case Context: Characteristics, Culture, and Preferences
For the Jefferson family, the news of their beloved son Derrell's (age 15) death while coming home from school felt like a bomb exploding in the middle of their living room, with waves that almost destroyed the family. The police officer who rang the bell explained that Derrell had been caught in gang crossfire, an innocent victim. The family comprised grandmother Gladys; her daughter, Seandra; and Derrell's sister, Jamillah (age 12). The family came to therapy at the suggestion of their pastor within days of the funeral services, due to Gladys's concerns about the rest of the family breaking down and Jamillah's running away for several hours, returning shortly before the funeral service. Jamillah's behavior shocked and scared the family.

In their first session, Gladys, the matriarch of the family, explained that she was the one to have to "put herself together and arrange a homegoing for the child, because the other two were beside themselves," referring to Seandra and Jamillah. Honoring the grandmother's position as the matriarch by listening to her point of view first, the therapist learned Gladys's perspective: "Seandra and Jamillah need to come back to reality; life is hard, we grieve and we move on, we don't want to lose someone else, do we?" Next, the therapist was curious about what happened to Jamillah. With her head down and trying to keep the tears back, she explained that she thought her brother wasn't dead, that another kid was killed, probably one that was part of a gang and she knew her brother was a "good kid" and not involved in that mess. Jamillah explained that she tried to tell the family, but when they wouldn't listen, she decided to go look for him.

The therapist validated her feelings and thought process, normalizing that it is "very hard to believe that a young and good kid like Derrell can have something like this happen to him." She then went back to the grandmother and validated her concern about losing someone else in the family and inquired gently about her fear of losing Jamillah, too. The grandmother stayed silent, fighting back tears, while Seandra sobbed. The therapist offered a silent space for crying to happen, then normalized the sadness by saying,

> It is perfectly normal to cry and be sad and be scared and feel confused . . . feel overwhelmed with all sorts of emotions. It is how we honor our love for lost ones, especially when they are taken from us before their time and suddenly.

Clinical Decisions: Intervention Implementation

Assessment based on the DPM-R highlights competing needs in the family for loss and restoration. The timing of the death was recent, and the Jeffersons had limited time to make sense of the loss. However, the nature of the death requires the family to address issues of safety and changed needs within the family. Witnessing the story each family member developed about the loss helped address the sense of unreality of loss, as well as a shared acknowledgment of the occurrence of death (Walsh & McGoldrick, 2004). A key component of treatment is facilitating shared **meaning making** and emotional expression of the loss.

It is important to address the shattered assumptions about life and the world, such as beliefs that the world is a benevolent and just place or people are safe and good. Questions such as "How do you make sense of the fact that Derrell didn't just die, he was killed?" "Is there a way we can talk together about how this affects each of you?" "What do you do to acknowledge the injustice to both Derrell, as well as all of you?" "Is there room to acknowledge the outrage and pain?" The therapist helped the Jeffersons express beliefs about the world that are inclusive of both aspects of their reality. This supported the family in recognizing inequity, as well as fairness, instances of both joy and pain that were true before the loss and subsequent to the death. It is critical for family members to share these thoughts and beliefs among each other and often requires the support from clinicians to do so.

Directly addressing emotions during family therapy and bearing witness to the intensity of the emotional pain (sadness, anger or rage) is instrumental in restoring a sense of togetherness and normalcy for families that find themselves in an almost surreal dimension of suddenly losing someone to violence. Important questions to ask are as follows: "Can we talk together about what Derrell's death means for you as a Black family?" "How have your experiences with racism been affecting how you grieve?" "What parts of this conversation have you had with yourself or at home as a family that have not been named here?" "Where do you go and who do you turn to for comfort?" Cultural aspects related to the family's ethnic and racial identity, specific mourning rituals, and religion play an important role in healthy, uncomplicated bereavement and must be considered in the therapeutic process.

Conclusion

Clinical work with the bereaved is a nuanced and emotionally laden process. Families enter therapy at a vulnerable time in their life cycle and trust that they will be supported in healing. This chapter provided an overarching bereavement framework, applicable across theoretical orientation and family composition. Description of the process of common practice, clinical application, and treatment interventions were used to guide clinicians in their work with the bereaved. Although this chapter focused on specific types of loss (loss due to cancer, death of a parent, death of a child, and sudden and violent loss), many of the strategies are applicable across multiple domains of loss. What this chapter could not convey is the privilege we find in walking with clients in moments of devastation and the gift we experience in watching them move toward healing.

REFERENCES

American Cancer Society. (2019). *Cancer treatment & survivorship facts & figures 2019–2021*. https://www.cancer.org/content/dam/cancer-org/research/cancer-facts-and-statistics/cancer-treatment-and-survivorship-facts-and-figures/cancer-treatment-and-survivorship-facts-and-figures-2019-2021.pdf

Areia, N. P., Fonseca, G., Major, S., & Relvas, A. P. (2019). Psychological morbidity in family caregivers of people living with terminal cancer: Prevalence and predictors. *Palliative & Supportive Care, 17*(3), 286–293. https://doi.org/10.1017/S1478951518000044

Belkin, L. (2010, August 11). Life after a child dies. *New York Times*. https://parenting.blogs.nytimes.com/2010/02/04/when-a-child-dies/?searchResultPosition=1

Benfield, D. G., Leib, S. A., & Reuter, J. (1976). Grief response of parents after referral of the critically ill newborn to a regional center. *The New England Journal of Medicine, 294*(18), 975–978. https://doi.org/10.1056/NEJM197604292941803

Block, S. D. (2001). Perspectives on care at the close of life. Psychological considerations, growth, and transcendence at the end of life: The art of the possible.

Journal of the American Medical Association, 285(22), 2898–2905. https://doi.org/10.1001/jama.285.22.2898

Bluethmann, S. M., Mariotto, A. B., & Rowland, J. H. (2016). Anticipating the "silver tsunami": Prevalence trajectories and comorbidity burden among older cancer survivors in the United States. *Cancer Epidemiology, Biomarkers & Prevention, 25,* 1029–1036. https://doi.org/10.1158/1055-9965.EPI-16-0133

Bonanno, G. A. (2004). Loss, trauma, and human resilience: Have we underestimated the human capacity to thrive after extremely aversive events? *American Psychologist, 59*(1), 20–28. https://doi.org/10.1037/0003-066X.59.1.20

Bordere, T. C. (2009). "To look at death another way": Black teenage males' perspectives on second-lines and regular funerals in New Orleans. *Omega, 58*(3), 213–232. https://doi.org/10.2190/OM.58.3.d

Bordere, T. C. (2016). Social justice conceptualizations in grief and loss. In D. Harris & T. C. Bordere (Eds.), *Handbook of social justice in loss and grief: Exploring diversity, equity, and Inclusion* (pp. 9–20). Routledge.

Bordere, T. C. (2019). Suffocated grief, resilience and survival among African American families. In M. H. Jacobsen & A. Petersen (Eds.), *Exploring grief: Towards a sociology of sorrow* (pp. 188–204). Routledge.

Boss, P. (2004). Ambiguous loss. In F. Wash & M. McGoldrick (Eds.), *Living beyond loss: Death in the family* (2nd ed., pp. 237–246). Norton.

Boss, P. (2010). The trauma and complicated grief of ambiguous loss. *Pastoral Psychology, 59*(2), 137–145. https://doi.org/10.1007/s11089-009-0264-0

Briere, J., Kaltman, S., & Green, B. L. (2008). Accumulated childhood trauma and symptom complexity. *Journal of Traumatic Stress, 21*(2), 223–226. https://doi.org/10.1002/jts.20317

Bugge, K. E., Darbyshire, P., Røkholt, E. G., Haugstvedt, K. T. S., & Helseth, S. (2014). Young children's grief: Parents' understanding and coping. *Death Studies, 38*(1), 36–43. https://doi.org/10.1080/07481187.2012.718037

Burke, L. A., Clark, K. A., Ali, K. S., Gibson, B. W., Smigelsky, M. A., & Neimeyer, R. A. (2015). Risk factors for anticipatory grief in family members of terminally ill veterans receiving palliative care services. *Journal of Social Work in End-of-Life & Palliative Care, 11*(3–4), 244–266. https://doi.org/10.1080/15524256.2015.1110071

Centers for Disease Control and Prevention. (2017). *National Center for Health Statistics, Compressed mortality file, 1999–2016.* CDC Wonder online database. https://wonder.cdc.gov/cmf-icd10.html

Coelho, A., & Barbosa, A. (2017). Family anticipatory grief: An integrative literature review. *The American Journal of Hospice & Palliative Care, 34*(8), 774–785. https://doi.org/10.1177/1049909116647960

Cortese, A. J. (1999). Ethical issues in subculturally diverse society. In T. F. Johnson (Ed.), *Handbook on ethical issues in aging* (pp. 24–58). Greenwood Press.

Davies, B., & Limbo, R. (2010). The grief of siblings. In N. B. Webb (Ed.), *Helping bereaved children: A handbook for practitioners* (3rd ed., pp. 69–90). Guilford Press.

Doka, K. J. (1989). Disenfranchised grief. In K. J. Doka (Ed.), *Disenfranchised grief: Recognizing hidden sorrow* (pp. 3–11). Lexington Books.

Doka, K. J. (2002). *Disenfranchised grief: New directions, challenges, and strategies for practice.* Research Press Publishing.

Eslinger, J. G., Sprang, G., & Otis, M. (2015). Children with multi-trauma histories: Special considerations for care and implications for treatment selection. *Journal of Child and Family Studies, 24*(9), 2757–2768. https://doi.org/10.1007/s10826-014-0079-1

Glick, I. O., Weiss, R. S., & Parkes, C. M. (1974). *The first year of bereavement.* John Wiley and Sons, Inc.

Guldin, M. B., Vedsted, P., Zachariae, R., Olesen, F., & Jensen, A. B. (2012). Complicated grief and need for professional support in family caregivers of cancer patients in palliative care: A longitudinal cohort study. *Supportive Care in Cancer, 20*(8), 1679–1685. https://doi.org/10.1007/s00520-011-1260-3

Harvey, J., & Weber, A. (1998). Why there must be a psychology of loss. In J. Harvey (Ed.), *Perspectives on loss: A sourcebook* (pp. 319–330). Brunner/Mazel.

Hayslip, B., Jr., Pruett, J. H., & Caballero, D. M. (2015). The "how" and "when" of parental loss in adulthood: Effects on grief and adjustment. *Omega: Journal of Death and Dying, 71*(1), 3–18. https://doi.org/10.1177/0030222814568274

Hill, C. D., Thompson, L. W., & Gallagher, D. (1988). The role of anticipatory bereavement in older women's adjustment to widowhood. *The Gerontologist, 28*(6), 792–796. https://doi.org/10.1093/geront/28.6.792

Horsley, H., & Patterson, T. (2006). The effects of a parent guidance intervention on communication among adolescents who have experienced the sudden death of a sibling. *The American Journal of Family Therapy, 34*(2), 119–137. https://doi.org/10.1080/01926180500301519

Hottensen, D. (2010). Anticipatory grief in patients with cancer. *Clinical Journal of Oncology Nursing, 14*(1), 106–107. https://doi.org/10.1188/10.CJON.106-107

Jacobs, S. (1993). *Pathologic grief: Maladaptation to loss.* American Psychiatric Press, Inc.

Janoff-Bulman, R. (1992). *Shattered assumptions: Towards a new psychology of trauma.* Free Press.

Jenkins, E. J., Wang, E., & Turner, L. (2014). Beyond community violence: Loss and traumatic grief in African American elementary school children. *Journal of Child & Adolescent Trauma, 7*(1), 27–36. https://doi.org/10.1007/s40653-014-0001-4

Johansson, A. K., Sundh, V., Wijk, H., & Grimby, A. (2013). Anticipatory grief among close relatives of persons with dementia in comparison with close relatives of patients with cancer. *The American Journal of Hospice & Palliative Care, 30*(1), 29–34. https://doi.org/10.1177/1049909112439744

Johnson, J., Lodhi, M. K., Cheema, U., Stifter, J., Dunn-Lopez, K., Yao, Y., Johnson, A., Keenan, G. M., Ansari, R., Khokhar, A., & Wilkie, D. J. (2017). Outcomes for end-of-life patients with anticipatory grieving: Insights from practice with standardized nursing terminologies within an interoperable internet-based electronic health record. *Journal of Hospice and Palliative Nursing, 19*(3), 223–231. https://doi.org/10.1097/NJH.0000000000000333

Jordan, J. R., & Neimeyer, R. A. (2003). Does grief counseling work? *Death Studies, 27*(9), 765–786. https://doi.org/10.1080/713842360

Labar, K. S., & Ledoux, J. E. (2001). Coping with danger: The neural basis of defensive behavior and fearful feelings. In B. S. McEwan & H. M. Goodman (Eds.), *Handbook of physiology: Section 7. The endocrine system: Vol. 6. Coping with the environment: Neural and endocrine mechanisms* (pp. 139–154). Oxford University Press.

Levy, L. H. (1991). Anticipatory grief: Its measurement and proposed reconceptualization. *The Hospice Journal, 7*(4), 1–28. https://doi.org/10.1080/0742-969X.1991.11882707

Lichtenthal, W. G., & Breitbart, W. (2015). The central role of meaning in adjustment to the loss of a child to cancer: Implications for the development of meaning-centered grief therapy. *Current Opinion in Supportive and Palliative Care, 9*(1), 46–51. https://doi.org/10.1097/SPC.0000000000000117

Lichtenthal, W. G., Currier, J. M., Neimeyer, R. A., & Keesee, N. J. (2010). Sense and significance: A mixed methods examination of meaning making after the loss of one's child. *Journal of Clinical Psychology, 66*(7), 791–812. https://doi.org/10.1002/jclp.20700

Lindemann, E. (1994). The symptomatology and management of acute grief. 1944. *The American Journal of Psychiatry, 151*(Suppl. 6), 155–160. https://doi.org/10.1176/ajp.101.2.141

Malkinson, R. (2001). Cognitive-behavioral therapy of grief: A review and application. *Research on Social Work Practice, 11*(6), 671–698. https://doi.org/10.1177/104973150101100603

Marks, N. F., Jun, H., & Song, J. (2007). Death of parents and adult psychological and physical well-being: A prospective U.S. national study. *Journal of Family Issues, 28*(12), 1611–1638. https://doi.org/10.1177/0192513X07302728

MD Anderson Cancer Center. (2020). *Sexuality and cancer.* https://www.mdanderson.org/patients-family/diagnosis-treatment/emotional-physical-effects/sexuality-cancer.html

Moreno, P. I., & Stanton, A. L. (2013). Personal growth during the experience of advanced cancer: A systematic review. *Cancer Journal, 19*(5), 421–430. https://doi.org/10.1097/PPO.0b013e3182a5bbe7

Morris, A. T., Gabert-Quillen, C., Friebert, S., Carst, N., & Delahanty, D. L. (2016). The indirect effect of positive parenting on the relationship between parent and sibling bereavement outcomes after the death of a child. *Journal of Pain and Symptom Management, 51*(1), 60–70. https://doi.org/10.1016/j.jpainsymman.2015.08.011

Moss, M. S., & Moss, S. Z. (1997). Middle-aged children's bereavement after the death of an elderly parent. In J. Morgan (Ed.), *Readings in thanatology* (pp. 347–355). Baywood.

Mulheron, J., & Inouye, S. K. (2020). Bereavement care in America is broken: A call to action. *National Academy of Medicine.* https://nam.edu/bereavement-care-in-america-is-broken-a-call-to-action/

Nadeau, J. W. (2001). Meaning making in family bereavement: A family systems approach. In M. S. Stroebe, R. O. Hansson, W. Stroebe, & H. Schut (Eds.), *Handbook of bereavement research: Consequences, coping, and care* (pp. 329–347). American Psychological Association. https://doi.org/10.1037/10436-014

National Cancer Institute. (2020). *Side effects of cancer treatment.* https://www.cancer.gov/about-cancer/treatment/side-effects

Neimeyer, R. A. (2004). Research on grief and bereavement: Evolution and revolution. *Death Studies, 28*(6), 489–490. https://doi.org/10.1080/07481180490461179

Neimeyer, R. A., Burke, L. A., Mackay, M. M., & van Dyke Stringer, J. G. (2010). Grief therapy and the reconstruction of meaning: From principles to practice. *Journal of Contemporary Psychotherapy, 40*(2), 73–83. https://doi.org/10.1007/s10879-009-9135-3

Overton, B. L., & Cottone, R. R. (2016). Anticipatory grief: A family systems approach. *The Family Journal, 24*(4), 430–432. https://doi.org/10.1177/1066480716663490

PDQ Supportive and Palliative Care Editorial Board. (2020). Grief, bereavement, and coping with loss (PDQ®): Health professional version. In *PDQ Cancer Information Summaries*. National Cancer Institute. https://www.ncbi.nlm.nih.gov/books/NBK66052/

Reynolds, L., & Botha, D. (2006). Anticipatory grief: Its nature, impact, and reasons for contradictory findings. *Counselling, Psychotherapy, and Health, 2*(2), 15–26. http://www.acrjournal.com.au/resources/assets/journals/Volume-2-Issue-2-2006/V2_I2_Reynolds-et-al_15-26_07_06.pdf

Roach, M. J., & Kitson, G. C. (1989). Impact of forewarning on adjustment to widowhood and divorce. In D. A. Lund (Ed.), *Older bereaved spouses: Research with practical applications* (pp. 185–200). Hemisphere Publishing Corporation.

Robson, P., & Walter, T. (2013). Hierarchies of loss: A critique of disenfranchised grief. *Omega: Journal of Death and Dying, 66*(2), 97–119. https://doi.org/10.2190/OM.66.2.a

Rogers, C. H., Floyd, F. J., Seltzer, M. M., Greenberg, J., & Hong, J. (2008). Long-term effects of the death of a child on parents' adjustment in midlife. *Journal of Family Psychology, 22*(2), 203–211. https://doi.org/10.1037/0893-3200.22.2.203

Rosner, R. (2015). Prolonged grief: Setting the research agenda. *European Journal of Psychotraumatology, 6*(1), 27303. https://doi.org/10.3402/ejpt.v6.27303

Rostila, M., Berg, L., Saarela, J., Kawachi, I., & Hjern, A. (2017). Experience of sibling death in childhood and risk of death in adulthood: A national cohort study from Sweden. *American Journal of Epidemiology, 185*(12), 1247–1254. https://doi.org/10.1093/aje/kww126

Shear, M. K. (2012). Grief and mourning gone awry: Pathway and course of complicated grief. *Dialogues in Clinical Neuroscience, 14*(2), 119–128. https://doi.org/10.31887/DCNS.2012.14.2/mshear

Steffen, E., & Coyle, A. (2017). "I thought they should know . . . that daddy is not completely gone." *Omega: Journal of Death and Dying, 74*(4), 363–385. https://doi.org/10.1177/0030222816686609

Stroebe, M., & Schut, H. (2015). Family matters in bereavement toward an integrative intra-interpersonal coping model. *Perspectives on Psychological Science, 10*(6), 873–879. https://doi.org/10.1177/1745691615598517

Stroebe, M., Schut, H., & Boerner, K. (2017). Cautioning health-care professionals: Bereaved persons are misguided through the stages of grief. *Omega: Journal of Death and Dying, 74*(4), 455–473. https://doi.org/10.1177/0030222817691870

Stroebe, M. S., Hansson, R. O., Schut, H., & Stroebe, W. (Eds.). (2008). *Handbook of bereavement research and practice: Advances in theory and intervention*. American Psychological Association. https://doi.org/10.1037/14498-000

Tomarken, A., Holland, J., Schachter, S., Vanderwerker, L., Zuckerman, E., Nelson, C., Coups, E., Ramirez, P. M., & Prigerson, H. (2008). Factors of complicated grief pre-death in caregivers of cancer patients. *Psycho-Oncology, 17*(2), 105–111. https://doi.org/10.1002/pon.1188

Tsilika, E., Mystakidou, K., Parpa, E., Galanos, A., Sakkas, P., & Vlahos, L. (2009). The influence of cancer impact on patients' preparatory grief. *Psychology and Health, 24*(2), 135–148. https://doi.org/10.1080/08870440701611194

Umberson, D. (1995). Marriage as support or strain? Marital quality following the death of a parent. *Journal of Marriage and the Family, 57*(3), 709–723. https://doi.org/10.2307/353925

Umberson, D. (2003). *Death of a parent: Transition to a new adult identity.* Cambridge University Press. https://doi.org/10.1017/CBO9780511500046

Umberson, D., & Chen, M. D. (1994). Effects of a parent's death on adult children: Relationship salience and reaction to loss. *American Sociological Review, 59*(1), 152–168. https://doi.org/10.2307/2096138

Ungureanu, I., & Hall, C. A. (2020). Grief and loss effects on the couple. In K. S. Wampler (Ed.), *Handbook of systemic family therapy* (Vol. 3, pp. 407–428). John Wiley & Sons Inc.

Valizadeh, L., Zamanzadeh, V., & Rahiminia, E. (2013). Comparison of anticipatory grief reaction between fathers and mothers of premature infants in neonatal intensive care unit. *Scandinavian Journal of Caring Sciences, 27*(4), 921–926. https://doi.org/10.1111/scs.12005

Walsh, F., & McGoldrick, M. (2004). *Living beyond loss: Death in the family.* W. W. Norton & Company.

Weitzman, A., & Smith-Greenaway, E. (2020). The marital implications of bereavement: Child death and intimate partner violence in west and central Africa. *Demography, 57*(1), 347–371. https://doi.org/10.1007/s13524-019-00846-7

Worden, J. W. (2018). *Grief counseling and grief therapy: A handbook for the mental health practitioner.* Springer.

World Health Organization. (2018). *Fact sheets: Cancer.* https://www.who.int/news-room/fact-sheets/detail/cancer

Yamashita, R., Arao, H., Takao, A., Masutani, E., Morita, T., Shima, Y., Kizawa, Y., Tsuneto, S., Aoyama, M., & Miyashita, M. (2017). Unfinished business in families of terminally ill with cancer patients. *Journal of Pain and Symptom Management, 54*(6), 861–869. https://doi.org/10.1016/j.jpainsymman.2017.04.013

Zisook, S. (2000). Understanding and managing bereavement in palliative care. In H. M. Chochinov & B. William (Eds.), *Handbook of psychiatry in palliative medicine* (pp. 321–334). Oxford University Press.

10 EMERGENT AREAS OF CLINICAL PRACTICE IN NEED OF RESEARCH

Medical Changes

SUSAN MCGROARTY, RACHEL HULL, AND CHRISTOPHER ROYER

Unprecedented times are replete with unplanned changes. The COVID-19 pandemic offered a glimpse into the phenomenon of families facing unplanned medical crises who struggled with managing strong emotions such as fear, grief, disappointment, resentment, frustration, and overwhelming confusion amidst ever changing rules and expectations for what life will look like (Moos & Holahan, 2007). Unplanned, unexpected health changes are usually particularly difficult for families. As empathic clinicians, we understand the range of strong emotions families are trying to navigate—each member struggling in their own way and the family struggling as a system. Emerging and extant research can typically provide general guidance at best, since each family is uniquely shaped by factors such as immigration status, gender identity, race, ethnicity, sexual orientation, gender, socioeconomic status, religious/spiritual identities and language. Today's contemporary families often present with a host of diverse intersecting identities within members. To effectively serve these families, we need not only evidence-supported treatments but also clinicians trained in cultural humility and intersectionality with a critical understanding of the long shadow of European hegemony and systemic racism.

https://doi.org/10.1037/0000280-010
Treating Contemporary Families: Toward a More Inclusive Clinical Practice, S. Browning and B. van Eeden-Moorefield (Editors)

This long shadow focuses primarily on the dominance of linear information processing. In a top-down way, experts determine what should be studied, how it should be studied, and how and whether the information should be disseminated. Clinical behavioral health fields, such as psychology, have emulated the Kantian linearity of medicine, as the example. The qualitative methodological paradigms of field and process research are eschewed for lack of random sampling and sophisticated computer analysis. As our society has moved toward a love affair with big data and statistical analyses done on thousands of variables, given the statistical power of big data, research has the sheen of exactitude with no room for uncertainty. However, what does this really tell us, as clinicians, in the trenches walking the path with a family navigating an unplanned transition? The research literature on the phenomenon of unplanned changes and medical concerns is largely absent. Thus, when the family science literature is minimal, clinicians need to rely on expert clinical opinion to guide treatment. In this chapter, we meet two families: one struggling to renavigate communication styles amidst hearing loss and one struggling with vision loss due to diabetic retinopathy. We explore the systemic challenges and discuss their perspectives and interventions to share how research guided their conceptualization and treatment (see Table 10.1).

CLINICAL EXPERTISE AND INTERPRETATION OF EVIDENCE

Deaf/deaf/Hard of Hearing Families

It should be stated at the outset that attempting to address families with a member who is Deaf, deaf, or Hard of Hearing (HoH) in the context of one inclusive work of writing presents an extremely difficult task. An elemental skill in working with this population is clarity on some common terms. A *Deaf* individual (with a capital D) identifies with Deaf culture. "The Deaf community is a subgroup of deaf people whose identity is based on sharing common values, beliefs, and norms and, perhaps more crucially, a common and distinct language" (Munro et al., 2008, p. 307). In the United States, members of Deaf culture communicate using American Sign Language (ASL). The term *deaf* (small d) typically refers to people who possess "the audiological condition of not hearing" (Padden & Humphries, 1988, p. 2). The psychotherapy literature is significantly more robust for clients who identify as Deaf (Boness, 2016). According to Boness (2016), "those who are audiologically deaf but do not identify with the Deaf culture may have their own set of cultural values, separate from ASL proficiency,

TABLE 10.1. Unplanned Medical Changes

Evidence-based area of clinical focus	Type of factor	Appropriateness for use across families	Selected references indicating evidence base
Emotion management/ navigation	General	All[a]	Moos & Holahan, 2007
Clinician's knowledge of Deaf/deaf/Hard of Hearing (HoH) culture	Unique	Deaf/deaf/HoH	Boness, 2016; Munro et al., 2008
Communication between clinician and client	Unique	Deaf/deaf/HoH	Boness, 2016
Feelings of isolation, lack of empathy from others	Unique	Deaf/deaf/HoH	–
Feelings of resentment	Unique	Deaf/deaf/HoH	–
Struggles with multiple losses	Unique	Acquired vision loss	Garcia et al., 2017; Tolman et al., 2005
Relationships with others	Unique	Acquired vision loss	Tolman et al., 2005
Attitudes toward compensation/ relearning to navigate the world/ independence	Unique	Acquired vision loss	Tolman et al., 2005
Role changes	Unique	Acquired vision loss	–

[a]The general factor could work for other family types included in this unit but needs a small adaptation to ensure cultural relevance. Information about potential adaptations are included in the text.

that the psychologists should explore" (p. 566). Another important distinction is differentiating people who are Deaf, deaf, or "hearing," from those who identify as HoH (mild, moderate, severe to profound). Individuals who are HoH often find themselves not identifying with the experience of those who are Deaf, but they also may feel alienated from their hearing peers.

The need to enter the phenomenological world of the Deaf/deaf/HoH individual within the family is probably the most important component of preparing for treatment (Munro et al., 2008). The therapist must prepare to do extra work to facilitate effective and comfortable communication with the patient or family. This preparation can deepen the clinician's empathy in the experience of the "extra work" that the Deaf/deaf/HoH patient is accustomed to doing every day to accommodate to hearing culture. The clinician will likely be working harder to communicate with the patient. It is important to monitor and take care of one's own feelings about doing more work and having to adjust one's systems of clinical interview, etc. Clinicians must address their biases (Boness, 2016).

The issue of ability versus disability may be present in the treatment room to varying degrees. According to Munro et al. (2008), the medical model of deafness must be differentiated from the social model. The medical model defines deafness as an impairment. The social model looks at factors that oppress these individuals (e.g., discrimination, prejudice, stereotypes). It is not the actual reduced hearing that impairs but the discrimination and marginalization society assigns to individuals with this condition. As deafness is an "invisible disability" (Becker, 1981), patients may have minimal to significant relationships with the term "disability," with some embracing and or taking pride in it and some rejecting it. Because of the spectrum of viewpoints, one should avoid assumptions made from bias and ask questions instead. If the clinician is not already aware, it would be helpful to educate oneself on the long history of hard feelings some members of the Deaf community have towards "oralism," and likewise the reverse, with those who advocate inclusion into hearing culture and the subsequent labeling of deafness as disability (Munro et al., 2008; Padden & Humphries, 1988; Retznik et al., 2017). Glickman and Harvey (2008) noted: "Psychotherapy with linguistically competent, employed, deaf persons, who have a range of relationship ties, but who may have marital problems or struggle with nondisabling depression or anxiety, may not be that different than psychotherapy with their hearing counterparts" (p. 130).

Clinical Experience: Observations of Common Interactional Patterns
Family members often devote varying degrees of effort to include the Deaf/deaf/HoH member in conversation. Some family members make great effort to speak slowly and look at the deaf or HoH member when speaking to them if they are lip reading, which is often enhanced through visual cues. Some family members may also learn ASL if that is the Deaf/deaf/HoH member's preferred mode of communication. Others make little effort to accommodate them.

Deaf/deaf/HoH individuals often feel isolated among others who are hearing. In large family gatherings, especially, the Deaf/deaf/HoH member may struggle significantly to follow along in the conversation and eventually just ignore the conversation and retreat to their own internal thoughts. Others may assume the member is not social, avoidant, or disinterested, when in fact they feel left out. This sense of **isolation** may occur in mixed Deaf/deaf/

HoH/hearing relationships. Hearing people seem to struggle to empathize with what it is like to not be able to follow along in conversation and may also experience negative feelings towards the Deaf/deaf/HoH member if they feel like the latter is not interested in what is being said.

In social interactions, the hearing member may be overwhelmed at times with social demands—both interacting as himself or herself in the situation as well as serving as a translator for the Deaf or HoH member in the exchange. Over time, the hearing member may feel resentful. The Deaf/deaf/HoH member may feel resentful if socialization and daily activities are conducted within the backdrop of hearing culture. Depending on how much the hearing member is serving as the gateway to communication, power dynamics may evolve. For example, the hearing member may grow fatigued and selectively translate and/or the Deaf/deaf/HoH member may turn away from connection out of frustration, serving to end the interaction.

Case Context: Characteristics, Culture, and Preferences

Zarah (age 29, White, cisgender, hearing) has been married to Elliot (age 35, White, cisgender, severe-profound HoH) for 2 years. Zarah and Elliot have a 5-year-old daughter, Soraya, who is hearing. Elliot, proficient in sign language after attending a Deaf University, wears high-powered hearing aids and prefers to use speech to communicate. Zarah signs on a proficient level to augment communication. Zarah and Elliot agreed to seek couple therapy because they felt like "two ships in the night." Since the birth of their daughter, Zarah and Elliot agreed that they are more like "roommates." "We work together as parents really well," reported Elliot, "but as soon as I put Soraya to bed, Zarah calls her sister and they talk many nights a week." "Or if I put her to bed, you either work or go on social media," added Zarah.

In their early stages of dating and marriage, Zarah was active in learning how to communicate more easily with Elliot, using such techniques as learning sign to supplement spoken language, making sure to face him when speaking, and using nonverbal gestures if she wanted to gain Elliot's attention. Elliot, too, worked hard in the early days to lip-read, and he wore his hearing aids more frequently throughout the day. As their relationship progressed and both grew more comfortable, Zarah seemed to retreat to hearing-centric communication, making less visible effort. Elliot mirrored her retreat and wore his hearing aids less, at times turning them off during disagreements with Zarah, seemingly to cut off communication. Each resented the other for not making more of an effort, and as the **resentment** grew, Zarah grew more inclined to share with her sister and Elliot more apt to turn to his work or retreat to social media.

Clinical Decisions: Intervention Implementation

The intervention is guided by Munro et al.'s (2008) outline for a constructionist approach to treatment. The authors recommended that "therapists explore ways to work that are culturally and linguistically appropriate rather than rely on empirically supported treatments that have no basis in evidence when used with deaf people" (p. 309). The approach proposes the use of a reflecting team based on Tom Andersen's model, in which processing and discussion is done by the team in front of the client(s). Munro et al. elaborated on the approach:

> Reflecting teams invite an open dialogue in which the team collaborates openly, minimizing the power dynamic between therapist-client. In a sense, the team communicates and openly shares their process, respecting the view of the client and valuing it equally to the views of everyone else. (p. 310)

The first session included Zarah, Elliot, the hearing therapist, and two members of the reflecting team. One member of the reflecting team was hearing (Team Member 1), the other identified as HoH (mild; Team Member 2). The specific inclusion of a HoH member further facilitates conversation towards shared understanding, when possible. In a study by Kersting (1997), it was found easier for deaf students to form relationships with those hearing peers who were familiar with the Deaf/deaf/HoH world and who worked as sign language interpreters or notetakers. Munro et al. (2008) also noted that individuals who are Deaf appreciate efforts made by hearing therapists to use signing.

This five- to seven-session sequence begins with a session clarifying the presenting problem, followed by two to three sessions focused on reducing ambiguity, ending with two to three sessions facilitating a more egalitarian conversation with the goal of constructing a shared understanding of the problem and identifying solutions. In the first session, introductions were made between all parties. Parties sat facing each other in a large circle. This configuration was done strategically so that Elliot could read lips as well as attend to auditory communication or any combination of verbal/symbolic communication.

In the initial session or two, externalizing of the problem was encouraged by asking both members of the couple to use a shared whiteboard in session to clarify the presenting concerns. The addition of the visual aspect of the first session promotes the overarching focus on facilitating an egalitarian atmosphere. In a hearing-centric world, it is easy to privilege the spoken word over the symbolic gesture or visual representation. It was clear that Elliot and Zarah both felt misunderstood by the other. The goal of the first session was to ask detailed, clarifying questions so that both members of the couple would feel understood by the reflecting team, who would then communicate the understanding to Zarah and Elliot at the end of the intake. By the end of Session 1, it became clear that Zarah had some built-up **resentment** towards Elliot for what she perceived as him "not listening" to her when she wanted to talk about things that were bothering her. "It's as if he is so focused on solving the problem, he ignores what I am saying and spends that time while I talk trying to formulate a ready-made solution," reported Zarah. "She couldn't be more wrong," responded Elliot. "I am always listening, but sometimes I feel like it is all about her, she forgets what I go through too."

The goal of Sessions 3 to 4 was to reduce ambiguity in communication between Zarah and Elliot by using the reflecting team as witnesses. "Deaf–hearing relationships are characterized by ambiguity" (Becker, 1981, p. 22). After every few moments of communication (verbal or combination of verbal/sign) from Zarah or Elliot, the therapist and reflecting team members provided clarification of what was being spoken or expressed via symbols. The team identified that Zarah and Elliot were misinterpreting each other's behaviors.

The HoH member of the team (Team Member 2) shared that Zarah seemed to be feeling resentful of the need to slow down when sharing with Elliot due to the need for him to lip-read along with identifying the sounds of her speech. The therapist validated Zarah's frustration with Elliot's use of nonverbal tactics such as turning off his hearing aids and turning away from her.

The hearing member of the team (Team Member 1) proposed that Zarah's turning away from their hearing difference served to increase intimate communication with other members of her family-of-origin (sister). Elliot's turning away from their hearing difference resulted in less demand to accommodate to a hearing-centric world but also brought increased **isolation** and loneliness. The sharing of intimacy without any communication barrier was easier for Zarah, serving then to introduce a contrast when the two reengaged in sharing together. For Elliot, he admitted that social media was an outlet for him, a way to connect with others without so much conflict.

ELLIOT: Zarah's comments are hurtful sometimes. She assumes I am not capable of independent thinking. I am listening to her, and I am also trying to help find solutions for her perhaps. Now, she becomes so upset that I am almost nervous every time we have a discussion because it feels like she has no patience left.

ZARAH: Elliot is right, it does feel sometimes like I am out of patience. I hate to say that, but it feels like I am so alone sometimes.

THERAPIST: I think you are both feeling alone, from the sound of it. What does the team think?

TEAM MEMBER 2:   I think both of you are experiencing isolation, but I think Zarah what your isolation feels like is not really isolation, it is alienation from your spouse. This must be painful, of course, but I think it is important to consider that Elliot's isolation feels more profound. After all, he does not have an alternative person with whom he can share intimacy right now. Social media is definitely not the same, and we know that lots of time spent there can increase negative emotions.

The final sessions held the goal of facilitating an egalitarian conversation using multimodal communication and the reflecting team to support Elliot and Zarah. The reflecting team normalized some of what Zarah called "passive–aggressive" communication on the part of Elliot. The HoH member of the reflecting team offered the feedback to the therapist that defining a non-verbal behavior (turning off his hearing aids) as somehow more "deviant" assumes a hearing perspective, as nonverbal communication and sending nonverbal messages from an HoH individual to a deaf or HoH individual is normal and typical. There was also an important parallel process between addressing and deliberately minimizing the power dynamic in the room and the power dynamics that were promoting discord in the couple relationship.

The team offered suggestions for Zarah and Elliot. Recommendations were discussed openly in the session and were also represented on the whiteboard as a shared exercise. Instead of making two phone calls to Zarah's sister in the next week, Zarah and Elliott would spend that time together sharing. Elliot was to avoid social media during these times together. Zarah and Elliot found the whiteboard surprisingly useful as an aid. She admitted that she talked fast sometimes and said it helped to slow her down. To the extent possible, the team agreed that opening up to extended family about the need for them to spend more time together would be helpful in obtaining support from extended family.

Acquired Vision Loss and Families

Worldwide, over 280 million people have a visual impairment (Bourne et al., 2017; Chan et al., 2018). While some individuals are born with visual loss or blindness, others lose vision gradually or suddenly over the course of their lives (acquired vision loss). Acquired vision loss can be partial or total, and occur over time, such as in cases of macular degeneration or retinitis pigmentosa or abruptly, as in cases of detached retina, stroke, or other traumatic injury. This chapter focuses on acquired vision loss. A core competency when working with this population is the ability to identify and understand some of the common issues and challenges facing patients and family members.

Clinical Experience: Observations of Common Interactional Patterns
Acquired visual impairment can have significant and profound psychological effects. Sleep disruptions, anxiety, and depression are common sequelae, with some people even reporting trauma related symptoms. Visually impaired clients describe struggling with **multiple losses**—from the profound changes associated with job loss, driving ability, personal independence and relational difficulty to the daily hassles and frustrations associated with reduced ability to read, manage finances, run errands, or even to appreciate a change of dress or décor. Given the profound impact of these losses, it is understandable that this population is at high risk for depression (Garcia et al., 2017). Tolman and colleagues (2005) identified three significant factors relating to depression in older adults with macular degeneration: acceptance of the loss, negative impact on relationships, and **attitudes toward compensation**. Depression can also significantly interfere with active coping and motivation to learn adaptive strategies.

Even when depression is not a significant concern, learning new skills such as orientation and mobility can be anxiety provoking for the affected person. Imagine learning to cross a street as a newly blind person. Other activities, such as cooking, taking public transportation, mapping new areas, and gathering information in a world with mostly visual signage all have the potential to cause substantial apprehension. Families may push the affected person to remaster independence skills with reduced awareness of this anxiety, or they may surround and protect, preventing or limiting such skill development.

The **complex emotional reactions of family** members to acquired vision loss may be like family adjustment to other disabilities. Investigating family responses to low vision, Bambara (2009) and her colleagues described "shock-denial, mourning-withdrawal, succumbing-depression, reassessment-reaffirmation, coping-mobilization, and self-acceptance–self-esteem" (p. 138). Other factors that influence family response to vision loss include how quickly the loss is experienced (e.g., trauma vs. slower degeneration), the level of impairment, the level of comorbid medical issues, and the health of the family dynamic prior to the loss.

Common family member reactions of conscious or unconscious anger and **resentment** of the disability and extra caretaking can be expressed directly or indirectly to the affected person. Feelings of being overwhelmed can lead to denying any disability at all (denial of disability). Some family members may experience guilt or blaming if the loss is due to an accident or preventable illness. One partner can shield the affected person from social and community activities due to the extra effort necessary or her or his own embarrassment. Depression in the affected person and/or resentment on the part of the partner or spouse can cause significant conflict or distance in the relationship.

In addition to examining premorbid **family dynamics**, understanding the family's response to the unexpected transition is another important goal. The person who suffers vision loss may hold a key role in emotional, financial, or physical responsibilities within the family, which may cause dramatic changes in one or more of these areas. A power vacuum may arise if the family was centered on the affected member's authority. Responses of nonaffected family members may involve paralysis, an inability to absorb information or solve problems. Problems such as bankruptcy and a sudden change in socioeconomic status are often co-occurring issues. Children can act out in response to the more singular focus on the affected person. There can be a dramatic change in the person's level of independence, and the family may be in danger of fragmenting if the resources and margin are not there to allow for the necessary caretaking.

Since vision loss can profoundly impact personal independence, understanding family values and expectations about independence versus interdependence is another key aspect of treating the family. Depending on a variety of intersecting needs, cultural norms and other factors, families may push for greater or lesser degrees of reacquiring independence following vision loss. Are the affected person and family members in sync with these goals (e.g., learning braille, becoming facile with orientation and mobility strategies, returning to work)? A prudent clinician will try to gauge the level of agreement on these goals early on and work to bring family members to a common space when there is disparity.

Role changes are also an expected consequence of vision loss. Families with visually impaired children often see dramatic role changes in parents (e.g., one parent stops working to care for the child). Adults with vision loss often experience significant role changes (e.g., job, duties around the house, new skills for raising children). Divorce is not uncommon. In addition to varying responses from family members, the time in the family life cycle that the vision loss occurs will also impact family dynamics and coping. Over- or underprotection is one example. For children with vision loss, parental/caregiver response of shielding or overprotection can limit social development. Parents will sometimes confine activities to other visually impaired groups. They may resist reaching out for blindness skills training. At times, families and friends will attribute limitations of blindness to another domain, such as reduced intellect.

Case Context: Characteristics, Culture, and Preferences

Mr. Roland Kim is a 59-year-old, first-generation Korean American man. He came to the United States with his parents at the age of 10 and completed his education in the United States, including a graduate degree in mechanical engineering. He worked for 35 years at the same company, doing design work and inspections. He enjoyed his work, and he reported feeling good about caring for his family financially through the work that he did. He is married to Lin, also a first-generation Korean American, and they have two adult children, Ron and Emily.

Mr. Kim was diagnosed with Type 2 diabetes and hypertension in his 40s. Although compliant with his medications, he struggled with the strict diet for his combined diabetes and high blood pressure. About 8 months ago he began to have pain in both eyes and experienced a progressive loss of vision bilaterally. He was diagnosed with diabetic retinopathy. He is currently able to see large objects and doorways, and he can perform basic activities of daily living (ADLs) with reduced speed, can no longer drive, and has been forced to retire from his job a bit earlier than he had planned. Mr. Kim and his wife were referred for treatment as part of his participation in a multidisciplinary rehabilitation program. His treating therapists felt that he was depressed, unmotivated and not progressing well towards his goals.

Clinical Decisions: Intervention Implementation

During the first family therapy session, Mr. Kim described his life before coming to the United States, stressing the importance that his working-class parents placed on a focused and tenacious pursuit of education and financial independence. As a result, young Mr. Kim was expected to work hard and excel in school, and only excellent grades were permissible. He was able to talk about the little praise he received throughout his primary school years and noted that his parents seemed pleased that he has made a "good career as an engineer." Mrs. Kim also spoke of her husband as a good provider. The family had never gone without, and both children graduated from college. Before the session ended, Mr. Kim stated that his doctors and his family wanted him to apply for social security disability, which he was strongly resisting. He viewed disability income as proof that he was no longer a capable person.

When evaluating treatment options for Mr. Kim and his wife, the therapist considered the brief length of stay in the rehabilitation program (6 weeks), and the presence of cultural factors (e.g., family integrity, conformity, gender). The therapist reflected upon the fierce connection he had with his previous job and earnings under an intergenerational family and cultural lens. There was also concern about Mrs. Kim, and the challenges she may be facing in managing potential **role changes**, such as increased helping around the house, cooperative projects, coping with her own feelings of loss and financial stress, and talking with her husband about his depression.

Observations during the first session were suggestive of a moderate depression. Mr. Kim's main complaints were pain behind the eyes (diabetic retinopathy), fatigue, general aches and pains, and neuropathy, also due to diabetes. Therapists noted that he had not been following through with his homework and that he seemed unmotivated to try new things in the classes he was attending. He was well-liked by the other participants, and the therapists described him as always helpful to those more visually impaired than himself.

The next two sessions explored the family's awareness of his condition and the potential outcomes. An issue that came up early in treatment was Mr. Kim's belief that he might get his sight back. His wife's (accurate and medically confirmed) understanding was that he would be lucky to keep the sight he had. Admitting that he was "angry" at his situation, he became more depressed and less talkative. While this development caused some initial setbacks in Mr. Kim's mood and participation, it was extremely important that he be fully aware of the extent of his vision loss, the unlikely possibility of recovery and the possible paths for his vision loss in the future. Awareness provides a structure to begin therapeutic change in this population. Although education can be more pragmatic and sometimes distressing, the family was now on the same page about Mr. Kim's problems, needs and future options.

The therapist asked Mr. Kim how individuals with disabilities are seen in Korea. He replied that there is generally an agreement that the family will care for the person, "but they don't like doing it." His children were not able to participate in the sessions, as they both lived out of state. However, they both indicated the children seemed to minimize his problems and tried to keep saying positive things to him. Mr. Kim had begun to work harder in therapy when he realized that his condition was not going to improve. The therapist encouraged him to see his efforts as another way to be supportive of his family, as he would be less in need of assistance and care. Mrs. Kim was also convinced that allowing Mr. Kim to do a few things around the house would be good and improve his mood. The therapist encouraged her to participate in some of his rehab therapies to identify areas that he could participate in or take over at home. Lastly, the need for continued medical follow-up around his diabetes and hypertension was addressed. We discussed the tendency of diabetes to cause fatigue and general malaise, and how these can contribute to lack of motivation and poor health habits. Mr. Kim agreed that he would follow up with his doctor, allow his wife to help him monitor his blood sugar (he could not read the numbers on the glucometer) and try to find some ways to exercise and eat a healthy diet.

Mr. Kim ended up meeting many of his goals in his rehabilitation program. He became more motivated and learned some ADL and Orientation and Mobility techniques that would help him maintain greater independence at home and in the community. The therapist also encouraged them to talk to his family doctor about pain management for his eyes, as this was always a hurdle for him. Interestingly, he complained less of pain towards the end of rehab, and therapist and client reviewed how depression can sometimes exacerbate physical symptoms. Mr. Kim reported that he appreciated this perspective as he felt that it gave him another "job" to do, specifically, to identify and talk about his feelings when he could. The therapy was brief and accomplished two major goals: Mr. Kim became a more active participant in his overall rehabilitation, and he was able to use his strengths of a deeply rooted work ethic and the desire to continue supporting his family. These are two cornerstones of adjustment to disability.

CONCLUSION

In this chapter, we set out to deepen the reader's understanding of the experience of providing family therapy to families facing an unexpected medical issue. Perhaps as you read and met our families facing these unplanned life events, you thought about your own personal and/or family experiences. Many therapists enter the field to gain a deeper understanding of their own story. We apply what we learn professionally to our own life experience. These life experiences profoundly shape our views, reactions and biases. Identification, acceptance, and managing our blind spots are core multicultural competencies. In addition to multicultural competencies, understanding our countertransference or personal reactions is another core competency. Furthermore, we again put out the call for researchers in family science to increase the output of information on these family concerns such that clinical intervention will be supported by evidence. Working with families facing unplanned transitions can put us in touch with the fragility of life and how quickly and profoundly life can change. The myths and illusion of control over life can be challenged or shattered. History has shown that for individuals, families, and society, there is opportunity and hope within every crisis, no matter how dark and bleak it may appear. The fictional families in this chapter used their crisis as an opportunity for renewal. As therapists, we are often called upon to carry the backpack of hope for the people we serve, helping them find hope in seemingly hopeless places.

REFERENCES

Bambara, J. K., Owsley, C., Wadley, V., Martin, R., Porter, C., & Dreer, L. E. (2009). Family caregiver social problem-solving abilities and adjustment to caring for a relative with vision loss. *Investigative Ophthalmology & Visual Science, 50*(4), 1585–1592. https://doi.org/10.1167/iovs.08-2744

Becker, G. (1981). Coping with stigma: Lifelong adaptation of deaf people. *Social Science & Medicine. Part B: Medical Anthropology, 15*(1), 21–24. https://doi.org/10.1016/0160-7987(81)90005-3

Boness, C. L. (2016). Treatment of deaf clients: Ethical considerations for professionals in psychology. *Ethics & Behavior, 26*(7), 562–585. https://doi.org/10.1080/10508422.2015.1084929

Bourne, R., Flaxman, S., Braithwaite, T., Cicinelli, M., Das, A., Jones, J., Keeffe, J., Kempen, J. H., Leasher, J., Limburg, H., Naidoo, K., Pesudovs, K., Resnikoff, S., Silvester, A., Stevens, G. A., Tahhan, N., Wong, T. Y., Taylor, H. R., on behalf of the Vision Loss Expert Group. (2017). Magnitude, temporal trends, and projections of the global prevalence of blindness and distance in near vision impairment: A systemic review and meta-analysis. *The Lancet, 5*(9), 888–897. https://doi.org/10.1016/S2214-109X(17)30293-0

Chan, T., Friedman, D. S., Bradley, C., & Massof, R. (2018). Estimates of incidence and prevalence of visual impairment, low vision, and blindness in the United States. *JAMA Ophthalmology, 136*(1), 12–19. https://doi.org/10.1001/jamaophthalmol.2017.4655

Garcia, G. A., Khoshnevis, M., Gale, J., Frousiakis, S. E., Hwang, T. J., Poincenot, L., Karanjia, R., Baron, D., & Sadun, A. A. (2017). Profound vision loss impairs psychological well-being in young and middle-aged individuals. *Clinical Ophthalmology, 2017*(11), 417–427. https://doi.org/10.2147/OPTH.S113414

Glickman, N., & Harvey, M. (2008). Psychotherapy with deaf adults: The development of a clinical specialization. *Journal of the American Deafness and Rehabilitation Association, 41*(3), 129–186.

Kersting, S. (1997). Balancing between deaf and hearing worlds: Reflections of mainstreamed college students on relationships and social interaction. *Journal of Deaf Studies and Deaf Education, 2*(4), 252–263. https://doi.org/10.1093/oxfordjournals.deafed.a014330

Moos, R. F., & Holahan, C. J. (2007). Adaptive tasks and methods of coping with illness and disability. In E. Martz & H. Livneh (Eds.), *Coping with chronic illness and disability: Theoretical, empirical, and clinical aspects* (pp. 107–126). Springer. https://doi.org/10.1007/978-0-387-48670-3_6

Munro, L., Knox, M., & Lowe, R. (2008). Exploring the potential of constructionist therapy: Deaf clients, hearing therapists and a reflecting team. *Journal of Deaf Studies and Deaf Education, 13*(3), 307–323. https://doi.org/10.1093/deafed/enn001

Padden, C., & Humphries, T. (1988). *Deaf in America: Voices from a culture*. Harvard University Press.

Retznik, L., Wienholz, S., Seidel, A., Pantenburg, B., Conrad, I., Michel, M., & Riedel-Heller, S. G. (2017). Relationship status: Single? Young adults with visual, hearing, or physical disability and their experiences with partnership and sexuality. *Sexuality and Disability*, *35*(4), 415–432. https://doi.org/10.1007/s11195-017-9497-5

Tolman, J., Hill, R. D., Kleinschmidt, J. J., & Gregg, C. H. (2005). Psychosocial adaptation to visual impairment and its relationship to depressive affect in older adults with age-related macular degeneration. *The Gerontologist*, *45*(6), 747–753. https://doi.org/10.1093/geront/45.6.747

11 OUTCOME ASSESSMENT IN FAMILY THERAPY

CHARLES FISHMAN, ANGUS CRAIG, SCOTT BROWNING, RACHEL HULL, AND ALLISON ROZOVSKY

This chapter encourages each clinician to become their own local clinical scientist (Stricker & Trierweiler, 1995) by establishing a results-based accountability model that produces evidence-supported practices. Evidence-supported practice is established from the combination of a treatment approach or intervention (with a rationale to explain why clinical change is expected), a grounding in research literature on the presenting problem(s) and population in treatment, and an assessment of the outcome of treatment (how well does the treatment work). Whereas the chapters that follow focus on the treatment intervention and research literature, this chapter addresses outcome assessment. To best demonstrate the assessment process, this chapter describes a method by which therapists can implement outcome assessment, referred to as *results based accountability* (RBA; Friedman, 2005), and introduces a new outcome instrument (the Genogram-Based Interactional Measure [GBIM]), currently being field-tested, that measures interpersonal changes during treatment.

https://doi.org/10.1037/0000280-011
Treating Contemporary Families: Toward a More Inclusive Clinical Practice, S. Browning and B. van Eeden-Moorefield (Editors)

RBA: IS ANYBODY BETTER OFF?

The RBA framework, designed by Mark Friedman (2015), came to prominence in the mid-1990s. RBA was designed initially as a system by which program efficacy could be evaluated and later was applied more specifically to clinical settings (Fishman, 1993). RBA emphasizes the full engagement of all stakeholders during the evaluation or clinical process, especially conceptualization and planning stages, and incorporates systematic measurement of progress (Friedman, 2005, 2015). Engaging in RBA reminds clinicians to stay focused on the key question "Is anybody better off?" (Friedman, 2005). More specifically, any RBA model draws focus to desired goals. The therapist makes use of a table of plans and goals known as the Clinical Scorecard. The scorecard accounts for goals (the informal, agreed-upon outcomes of therapeutic work), plans (the proposed methods of change, particularly the therapeutic model), measures (countable or directly observable outcome data), and targets (outcome scores that stakeholders and therapist agree represent treatment success).

Here, we use a case study to demonstrate RBA. The therapy model used is **intensive structural therapy** (IST; Fishman, 1993). Within this approach, any individual's presentation is not independent of those around them; rather, it is the result of the "demand characteristics of their social context" (Minuchin & Fishman, 1979, p. 79). IST examines family structure and the nature of certain transactional patterns that underlie family dysfunction. Each therapist finds a way to measure clinical change within the theoretical model chosen. This example speaks to therapists utilizing IST. Within IST, an inherent assumption is that families will maintain a homeostasis of certain transactional patterns until there is enough perturbation to the system to reach a threshold for change. One task of the therapist is to identify where it is most effective to intervene, to perturb the system, and hopefully facilitate the development of new transactional patterns that are more functional. The threshold for change in an existing homeostatic structure can be very high, and a family system will often activate to maintain the status quo. Specifically, there is often one agent in the family who activates in service of the existing structure. Within IST, this agent is noted as the **homeostatic maintainer** (HM; Fishman, 1993). Once identified, the HM can be a fruitful target for intervention as, once their maintenance function is mitigated, the wider system may be more readily available to adjust to a new homeostatic position.

CASE STUDY FOR THE RBA

The case of Brad is used to exhibit how the integrated IST-RBA model assesses and formulates a case, before engaging in detailed treatment planning in line with grounded, measurable therapeutic outcomes. Specifically, the scores on the two measures indicate a reduction of family triangulation and improved general family functioning.

Case Background

Brad initially came to the attention of the therapist when he was referred from a previous residential program (in which he'd received 15 months of individual therapy) to a specialist residential program aiming to treat juvenile delinquency and associated psychological disorders. Brad was a 14-year-old young man of New Zealand Maori descent. He was referred to the residential program due to persistent, severe behavioral problems: violence, narcotics abuse, and car thefts. Brad was part of a complex contemporary family. He was one of 11 children, with an age range from 4 to 26 years (with six still residing in the family home). Brad would later give the opinion to the therapist that "every time my parents try to split, I get a new brother or sister which seems to keep them together." The family lived together in the most economically deprived area of the city, in an understandably overcrowded house. Brad's father, Steve, was imprisoned a year before Brad met the therapist. Steve had returned to the family home high on narcotics and sexually assaulted Brad's mother, Mary. Naturally this made joining with this family a complicated task. Mary had received a year's worth of supportive counseling prior to meeting the therapist and was clear with her own desired outcomes: whatever would work best for her son.

Determining Tools to Measure Progress

To encourage a shared sense of support and responsibility in treatment success, the therapist convened all the stakeholders (i.e., the family, social services, educational services) to formally agree on Brad's broad treatment goals (referred to as Targets), before working backwards to elucidate the practical steps (Plans) requisite to the achievement of these goals (Friedman, 2005). The Clinical Scorecard (see Table 11.1) was used to formalize which measures would be used to monitor treatment progress.

TABLE 11.1. Clinical Scorecard

Goal	Plans	Measures	Targets

Well-functioning in all domains	1. Intensive structural therapy will be used to:
	  – Strengthen Mary as a single parent (initially)
	  – Address Steve as the Homeostatic Maintainer
	  – Reduce triangulation of Brad (i.e., strengthen Mary and Steve as a parental system)
	2. Obtain larger accommodation and vehicle
	  – Supports structural distance (i.e., between Mary and her children) in the home
	  – Allows Brad to participate in family activity as a child (i.e., join in on family car rides)
	3. Educational assessment
	  – To rule out cognitive difficulty for Brad
	4. Rugby team
	  – Recontextualize, broaden Brad's system of influence (i.e., away from antisocial peers)
		Family Triangulation Scale (FTS)
		
		Child and Adolescent Functional Assessment Scale (CAFAS)
		
		School attendance rate
			FTS: 10% improvement in 3 months
			
			CAFAS: 20% improvement on all domains in 3 months
			
			Attendance: 20% improvement in 6 months

Goals

The goals for Brad's treatment were broad given the number and complexity of his difficulties. The treatment team agreed that everyone in the system, including Brad himself, wished him to be "well-functioning." The vague nature of this was noted by the therapist but not seen as troublesome given that it would naturally be specified by the other aspects of the model.

Plans

The specific interventions proposed were to initially strengthen Mary in her position as a single parent, then address Steve's role as the HM. Finally, therapy sought to **mitigate triangulation** of Brad between Mary and Steve (a dynamic that persisted even when Steve was incarcerated). A number of wider psychosocial interventions were considered to support therapeutic structural change for Brad's family (discussed further later). Brad was also referred for an **educational assessment** to examine whether there were individual cognitive factors influencing his ability to engage in the scholastic environment.

The therapist initially focused solely on joining with Brad's family and other relevant stakeholders to create a workable therapeutic system. This was a challenging logistical task as the system around Brad was broad: Steve, Mary, her supports, the family's social worker, a police liaison, and his teacher all needed to form a congruent system. Following some negotiation with Steve's correctional facility, he was given permission to attend meetings via phone. Once the Clinical Scorecard was finalized, all stakeholders were invited to attend family therapy sessions. Brad completed a specialized assessment from an educational psychologist, and a program was designed to support him in keeping up with national scholastic standards. It was noted that he possessed no significant educational weaknesses, and any previously noted deficits in his academic performance were secondary to his chronic truancy. The team also facilitated Brad's participation with his local rugby football team (a sport at which he was highly talented). Brad noted later that this team was to become his first nondelinquent peer group in several years. The team noted that this was an effective recontextualization for Brad, whom when surrounded by prosocial influences was able to access prosocial elements of his multitudinous self. That is, when the system around him was as congruently prosocial as possible, he was able to behave in a more positive manner.

In the early phase of family therapy, Steve constantly questioned whether the family required input from any therapist. The early objectives of therapy were, therefore, to reinforce Mary in her position as the sole functioning parent at that time. She engaged with a community support worker who assisted her in reconnecting with culturally-focused social groups. The family's social worker ensured that each child was supported to attend schooling. Mary responded well to this, and armed with more rooms in her house, was able to maintain space for herself.

A few months into treatment, Steve's prison sentence ended. He and Mary participated in a restorative process, and he returned to live within the family home at her request. The therapist then moved the focus of the therapy toward strengthening them as a parental subsystem, facilitating their agreement on how to parent Brad so that he was no longer triangulated between them. Steve persisted in the position of HM. As the system began to provide consequences for misbehavior and add more mature expectations of Brad particularly in his home setting, Steve would often act as a contrarian (e.g., saying that everyone was "overreacting" to Brad's behavior as simply "part of adolescence") activating in support of the status quo. The therapist made use of the IST technique of intensity, perturbing Steve's role, suggesting that he might well be telling everyone else they're overreacting right up until his son acquires a long prison sentence. With Steve and Mary in agreement with the need to unite as a system, their degree of triangulation of Brad steadily declined.

Measures and Targets

The primary measure was a scale of the first author's design, the Family Triangulation Scale (FTS). This scale examines the degree to which the key interactional pattern of triangulation exists within a given family and is based on responses to questions as well as therapist observations. Example items include "To what extent are parents able to come to an agreement on a single point regarding their child?" and "To what extent are parents able to agree on and enforce a specific consequence for their child?" The team also agreed to make use of the Child and Adolescent Functional Assessment Scale (CAFAS; Hodges et al., 1998), which measures behavioral functioning across eight different domains (e.g., school, thinking toward others, mood). Brad's school attendance was included as a final measure. The therapist set the targets using 3-month intervals to assess effectiveness. These targets were set such that Brad's family was their own control group, rather than comparing them to norms implied by clinical cut-off's or thresholds, and were consistent with IST. Outcome measures and goals set this way are about showing that the family, itself, improves through treatment. While Brad was to be the part of the family system most in focus, his changes were to be considered as the result of wider structural change within the family.

Tracking Performance: Turning the Curve

As shown in Figure 11.1, throughout treatment, the therapist tracked scores for the family on the FTS and for Brad on the CAFAS. Each measure was administered once per month of treatment. Conducting family therapy with ongoing assessment allows for precise adjustments to treatment. When the family would drift back into high levels of triangulation, seen via parental over-involvement, the FTS score assisted the therapist with targeted interventions.

Follow-Up

When treatment teams withdraw support, larger systems (e.g., impoverished communities) can exert deleterious influence. Five years after treatment

FIGURE 11.1. Family Triangulation Scale and CAFAS Scores

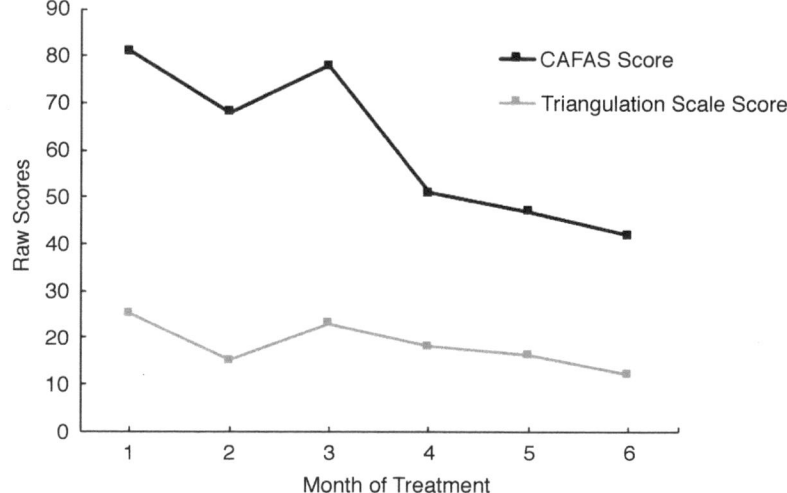

Note. CAFAS = Child and Adolescent Functional Assessment Scale.

concluded, on a chance encounter, Brad hailed his former therapist from across the street. After his cordial greeting, the young man informed the therapist that he had completed his high school education. Upon graduation, he enlisted in the U.S. Navy. No treatment can counteract the effects of large systemic prejudice. It did seem, however, that the restructuring and new congruence of Brad's family created a ballast so he did not revert to his lawbreaking mode of operation.

GENOGRAM-BASED INTERACTIONAL MEASURE

The most common tool in systems therapy is the genogram. The genogram not only creates clarity as to the members of the family and their relationships to one another but also provides a view of all subsystems that might be included in treatment. The GBIM builds on the traditional genogram and articulates how that can be used by practitioners as a quantitative and qualitative assessment measure to assess interactional changes in the family. The quantitative aspects of the instrument are the following: session-by-session feedback, measure of changing systemic dynamics, and a total score of the interactional quality within a family. The qualitative use of the instrument is as an ongoing guide to identify which members (and specific subsystems) require focused intervention. The beginning of this chapter introduced the reader to the benefit of finding a model that allows for each therapist to measure outcomes of treatment. The GBIM is introduced here to add an explicit instrument that is easy to administer and is considered a "practice as usual" methodology. By having two methods of measuring outcomes, clinicians can move toward a seamless evidence support practice integration.

Obtaining an Accurate GBIM

To obtain an accurate GBIM, therapists should first ask family members present to list the family members they consider important to their family system. This step may cause confusion. Members of one's family are important if there are still emotional feelings about the person. For example, a former spouse may no longer seem part of "your family," but due to that person's relationship with your child, there are emotional bonds that remain and should be included in the genogram.

For this step, the primary focus will be the two generations of the family primarily connected to the presenting problem. There are three circumstances in which a third generation (usually the grandparents) will be included in the GBIM: (a) A member of the first generation (grandparent/step-grandparent) attends the initial session, (b) The family reports that there is regular contact with members of the first generation, and (c) The presenting problem involves a member of the first generation explicitly.

Next, the therapist briefly reviews the legend of interactional symbols with family members present. While the process can be done in a full family session, a single family member may be used to create the GBIM. This should take approximately 10 minutes, leaving a few minutes for the family to ask appropriate questions. Afterward, the therapist constructs interaction lines based on information provided by one or more family members about interactional quality.

The therapist presents the baseline GBIM to the family. If the process was done with a single family member, ideally, the therapist and family member agree on the symbols in the GBIM. If multiple family members are present, the therapist/assessor presents the GBIM and looks for agreement. If all members feel a symbol should be changed, the therapist should strongly consider that change. If, however, there are differences of opinion among the family members about the "right" symbol to represent a dyadic relationship, the therapist/assessor's opinion is the recorded response.

The clinician constructs the genogram in direct consultation with members of the family, collecting relational information. Although gathering family history is a component of many models of psychotherapy, application of the GBIM as a dynamic measure of interactional quality requires a clinician who is particularly attentive to capturing potentially nuanced dynamics within the family system. Creating the genogram in this manner is a collaborative intervention in itself, a concept introduced by McGoldrick and colleagues (2008). While the construction of the genogram and assignment of appropriate interactional lines should ideally be a collaborative decision between patient(s) and therapist, the therapist reserves the right to use their clinical judgment to assign the "best-fit" interactional lines. In other words, the process is collegial; the clinician estimates the best score for an interactional dyad. If a family member offers examples that highlight how the relationship is better represented by another score, the clinician is open to alternative perceptions. However, for the sake of reliability of the instrument, the final score is always based on the clinician's perception. The clinician requests information in the following way: "As I complete the GBIM, I would be interested in your opinion on what scores fit best for each relationship."

Scoring

The term "family" is intended to refer to all family configurations, with a particular emphasis on the inclusion of contemporary family types (Browning & Pasley, 2015; Browning & van Eeden-Moorefield, 2017) as well as the traditional "nuclear" family. The specific legend used for this instrument is in Figure 11.2, which incorporates what we consider the most useful and representative interactional symbols. For clinical purposes, a variety of other symbol legends exist (Genopro; DeMaria, Weeks, & Hof, 1999). A numeric value is assigned to each interaction; these scores were established using a Delphi method of weighting expert opinions (Landeta, 2006).

Once each dyadic relationship has been scored, the total number is calculated. This number is then divided by the number of involved dyadic relationships (see Figure 11.3). The higher values represent more positive interactions. Importantly, the score is not meant to establish a norm; rather, this is a score that is designed to be a measure for a specific family. Thus, the family (or some representative of the family) is described fully at intake, and the evolving genogram (see Figure 11.3) is cross-referenced with the family members' consultation. The change in score over time indicates that the overall nature of multiple dyadic relationships is either improving or getting worse. One can visually examine the series of interactions and use that information to determine what specific subsystems are likely to benefit from clinical interventions, or when to capitalize on dyadic strengths to support

FIGURE 11.2. Interactional Legend With Point Values for Assessment

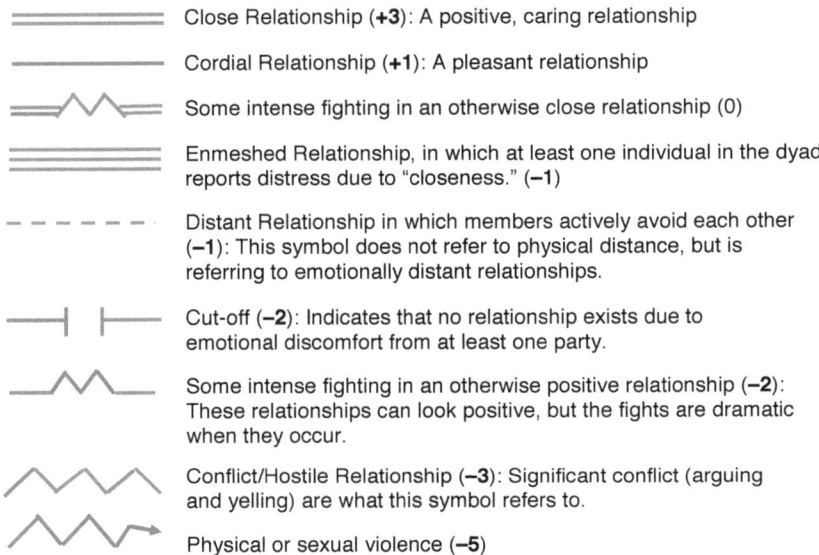

Close Relationship (**+3**): A positive, caring relationship

Cordial Relationship (**+1**): A pleasant relationship

Some intense fighting in an otherwise close relationship (0)

Enmeshed Relationship, in which at least one individual in the dyad reports distress due to "closeness." (**−1**)

Distant Relationship in which members actively avoid each other (**−1**): This symbol does not refer to physical distance, but is referring to emotionally distant relationships.

Cut-off (**−2**): Indicates that no relationship exists due to emotional discomfort from at least one party.

Some intense fighting in an otherwise positive relationship (**−2**): These relationships can look positive, but the fights are dramatic when they occur.

Conflict/Hostile Relationship (**−3**): Significant conflict (arguing and yelling) are what this symbol refers to.

Physical or sexual violence (**−5**)

the family overall. While this numerical analysis is clearly useful, there is substantial gain from qualitative information provided as well. Those using the GBIM will see the general trends from the score going up or down, but it will be in the qualitative examination of the nature of dyadic interactions that will encourage specific clinical interventions.

Validation of the GBIM

The GBIM may be a helpful addition to the field of family therapy as a progress and outcome measure. It is currently being field-tested. There does not appear to be an outcome measure that exists as a single quantitative value. This factor, in itself, makes the GBIM extremely user-friendly. It is simple to calculate, and obtaining the numerical value is not time-consuming. It is recommended that clinicians try to update the GBIM at 8-week intervals; however, clinicians have flexibility in that they may choose to update the number more or less frequently depending on the presenting concerns and the individuals in each case. GBIMs calculated earlier on in the construction process used different versions of the legend than later in the process. Because of this, we intend to report specific data when more research studies are conducted with the final version of the instrument presented here.

FIGURE 11.3. Genogram

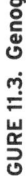

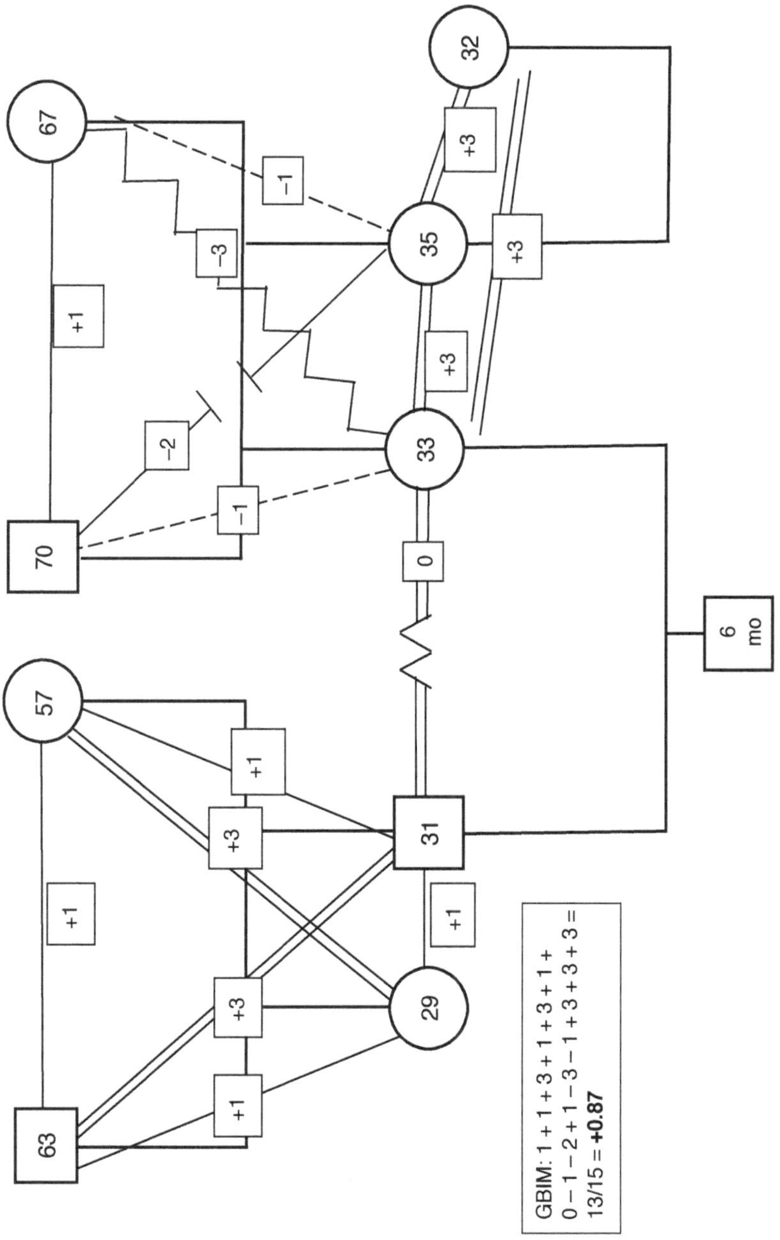

63
57
70
67
31
29
33
35
32
6
mo
+1
+3
+1
+3
+1
+3
+1
0
+1
-2
-1
-3
-1
+3
+3
+3
GBIM: 1 + 1 + 3 + 1 + 3 + 1 +
0 − 1 − 2 + 1 − 3 − 1 + 3 + 3 + 3 =
13/15 = **+0.87**

Note. GBIM = Genogram-Based Interactional Measure.

CASE EXAMPLE FOR THE GBIM

This case is fictional for the purposes of illustrating how the therapist might use the GBIM in clinical work. Figure 11.3 illustrates the accompanying genogram for this case. Throughout the case description, assigned scores for dyadic interactions are included in parenthesis. See Figure 11.3 for further information on assignment of numeric values. Benjamin (age 31) and Norma (age 33) sought treatment to address mistrust and conflict following Benjamin's discovery that Norma was having an "emotional" affair with a work colleague. Benjamin reported feeling distant from Norma throughout her pregnancy and following the discovery that they were pregnant. Norma agreed and said that she felt constantly overwhelmed throughout her pregnancy, admitting that it felt like her colleague was the only one who cared about her. Benjamin admitted that over the months, he found himself dreading going home and would stay later and later in the office working. Since the birth of their son, Malcolm, Norma and Benjamin reported that "the fighting is constant—if we can't find something to disagree on, there's always something else."

In the clinical interview, the therapist discovered through questioning that despite hurtful arguments, Norma and Benjamin enjoy similar activities and have moments when they feel close. The assignment of the "close with conflict" symbol (0) fit with both of their descriptions of their interactions. Although this is the "obvious" choice of dyad within which to conduct treatment, the clinical interview revealed other dyads that could be valuable to approach as a component of treatment. For example, exploration into Norma's family history revealed longstanding and deep family discord. The clinician constructing the genogram would note the conflict between Norma and her mother (−3), as well as distance between she and her father (−1). Despite strained relationships with her parents, Norma and her sister, Jackie, share a deep and powerful bond since childhood (+3). Norma also has a close relationship with Jackie's wife, Megan (+3); however, Norma shared that Jackie and Megan recently moved several states away, making visits less frequent. Benjamin shared somewhat different relational experiences in childhood and the present. He reported a cordial relationship with his mother (+1) and a close relationship with his father (+3), along with a warm and supportive family environment growing up. After creating the initial GBIM, the therapist might note the clusters of positive relationships within Benjamin's family of origin, the cluster of negative or distant relationships in Norma's family of origin, and the exception of the close bonds between the sibling dyad and Jackie's wife.

The family therapist now has a map revealing multiple pathways for intervention. Benjamin and Norma both chose to include their families of origin into the GBIM, as they felt that all of the family members illustrated were significant. The family therapist might also hypothesize that increasing support within additional dyads in the system would help Norma with feeling lonely and overwhelmed. It could also help Benjamin feel less overwhelmed, as he revealed that he felt like he was "never enough" for Norma, which influenced his gradual retreat to the office and into his work. The total score of +0.87 tells the family therapist that the positive dyads outnumber the negative in this family's case, which indicates that support may be available somewhere outside of the presenting dyad. Periodic readministration of the genogram (intervals between 8 weeks would be appropriate, at the clinician's discretion) provides one way to measure progress in family treatment. Tracking the GBIM also gives the clinician a true outcome measure of family functioning, as the score reflects interactional quality within the entire system and not just the presenting client(s).

CONCLUSION

The current psychotherapeutic field is moving toward integration (Wachtel, 2018). With the increase in evidence-supported treatments, perhaps it is more important than ever that each clinician become their own "local clinical scientist" (Stricker & Goldfried, 2019; Stricker & Trierweiler, 1995). The framework outlined in this chapter allows for clinicians to rigorously track outcomes in a way that can be applied with simplicity to whichever psychotherapeutic model they wish to draw upon. While the beginning of the chapter highlighted one particular approach (IST), it was simply used as an example. RBA allows clinicians to become quintessential local clinical scientists, auditing the veracity of whichever model of treatment or integrative approach is chosen. The explicit recommendation of this chapter is that clinicians always determine some method of evaluating the treatment outcome.

REFERENCES

Browning, S., & Pasley, K. (Eds.). (2015). *Contemporary families: Translating research into practice*. Routledge. https://doi.org/10.4324/9781315882369

Browning, S., & van Eeden-Moorefield, B. (Eds.). (2017). *Contemporary families at the nexus of research and practice*. Routledge. https://doi.org/10.4324/9781315668598

DeMaria, R., Weeks, G., & Hof, L. (1999). *Focused genograms: Intergenerational assessment of individuals, couples, and families*. Taylor & Francis.

Fishman, H. C. (1993). *Intensive structural therapy: Treating families in their social context*. Basic Books.

Friedman, M. (2005). *Trying hard is not good enough: How to produce measurable improvements for customers and communities*. Trafford Publishing.

Friedman, M. (2015). *Trying hard is not good enough*. Parse Publishing.

Hodges, K., Wong, M. M., & Latessa, M. (1998). Use of the Child and Adolescent Functional Assessment Scale (CAFAS) as an outcome measure in clinical settings. *The Journal of Behavioral Health Services & Research, 25*(3), 325–336. https://doi.org/10.1007/BF02287471

Landeta, J. (2006). Current validity of the Delphi method in social sciences. *Technological Forecasting and Social Change, 73*(5), 467–482. https://doi.org/10.1016/j.techfore.2005.09.002

McGoldrick, M., Gerson, R., & Petry, S. (2008). *Genograms: Assessment and intervention* (3rd ed.). W. W. Norton & Company.

Minuchin, S., & Fishman, H. C. (1979). The psychosomatic family in child psychiatry. *Journal of the American Academy of Child Psychiatry, 18*(1), 76–90. https://doi.org/10.1016/S0002-7138(09)60479-9

Stricker, G., & Goldfried, M. R. (2019). The gap between science and practice: A conversation. *Psychotherapy, 56*(1), 149–155. https://doi.org/10.1037/pst0000220

Stricker, G., & Trierweiler, S. J. (1995). The local clinical scientist: A bridge between science and practice. *American Psychologist, 50*(12), 995–1002. https://doi.org/10.1037/0003-066X.50.12.995

Wachtel, P. L. (2018). Pathways to progress for integrative psychotherapy: Perspectives on practice and research. *Journal of Psychotherapy Integration, 28*(2), 202–212. https://doi.org/10.1037/int0000089

Index

About the Editors

Scott Browning, PhD, ABPP, is a professor of psychology in the doctoral program at the Center for Professional Psychology at Chestnut Hill College in Philadelphia, Pennsylvania. Dr. Browning has published numerous books, chapters, and articles on topics ranging from stepfamilies, addictions, paradoxical interventions, autism, and empathy. He is the corecipient of the Distinguished Contribution to Family Psychology Award given by Division 43 (the Society for Couple and Family Psychology) of the American Psychological Association. Dr. Browning is a board member of the National Stepfamily Resource Center and on the board of the American Board of Professional Psychology, The Couple and Family Psychology division. He is the recipient of the Lindback Award for Distinguished Teaching. His interest in intersectionality comes, in part, from his deep interest in training psychotherapists to increase empathic perspective.

Brad van Eeden-Moorefield, MSW, PhD, CFLE, is a professor and associate department chair for social justice initiatives in the Department of Family Science and Human Development at Montclair State University. Dr. van Eeden-Moorefield's research uses social justice tools to merge research and practice in support of strengthening historically minoritized families. His most recent scholarship addresses stepfamilies headed by queer couples. Broadly, his research focuses on identifying how factors in the social world (e.g., stigma, stereotypes, policy) influence everyday family life and how both impact various indicators of individual (e.g., depression, happiness) and family well-being (stability). He has authored multiple works in journals such as the *Journal of Family Psychology*, *Family Relations*, the *Journal of Family Issues*, and *Sex Roles*. Dr. van Eeden-Moorefield also guest edited special issues on "Intersectional Variations in the Experiences of Queer Families" and "Transformative Family Scholarship: Theory, Practice, and Research at the Intersection of Families, Race, and Social Justice." He has served on several editorial boards and is a former journal editor. Dr. van Eeden-Moorefield was the 2020 National Council on Family Relations (NCFR) program chair and served on the NCFR Board of Directors and the NCFR Diversity and Inclusion Committee.